Drug Hypersensitivity

Editor

ELIZABETH J. PHILLIPS

IMMUNOLOGY AND ALLERGY CLINICS OF NORTH AMERICA

https://www.immunology.theclinics.com/

May 2022 • Volume 42 • Number 2

ELSEVIER

1600 John F. Kennedy Boulevard • Suite 1800 • Philadelphia, Pennsylvania, 19103-2899

http://www.theclinics.com

IMMUNOLOGY AND ALLERGY CLINICS OF NORTH AMERICA Volume 42, Number 2

May 2022 ISSN 0889-8561, ISBN-13: 978-0-323-98737-0

Editor: Katerina Heidhausen

Developmental Editor: Jessica Cañaberal

Immunology and Allergy Clinics of North America (ISSN 0889–8561) is published quarterly by Elsevier Inc., 360 Park Avenue South, New York, NY 10010-1710. Months of issue are February, May, August, and November. Periodicals postage paid at New York, NY and additional mailing offices. Subscription prices are $354.00 per year for US individuals, $844.00 per year for US institutions, $100.00 per year for US students and residents, $432.00 per year for Canadian individuals, $100.00 per year for Canadian students, $861.00 per year for Canadian institutions, $456.00 per year for international individuals, $861.00 per year for international institutions, $220.00 per year for international students. To receive student/resident rate, orders must be accompanied by name of affiliated institution, date of term, and the *signature* of program/residency coordinator on institution letterhead. Orders will be billed at individual rate until proof of status is received. Foreign air speed delivery is included in all *Clinics* subscription prices. All prices are subject to change without notice. **POSTMASTER:** Send address changes to *Immunology and Allergy Clinics of North America,* Elsevier Health Sciences Division, Subscription Customer Service, 3251 Riverport Lane, Maryland Heights, MO 63043. **Customer Service: 1-800-654-2452 (U.S. and Canada); 314-447-8871 (outside U.S. and Canada). Fax: 314-447-8029. E-mail: journalscustomerservice-usa@elsevier.com (for print support); journalsonlinesupport-usa@elsevier.com (for online support).**

Reprints. For copies of 100 or more, of articles in this publication, please contact the Commercial Reprints Department, Elsevier Inc., 360 Park Avenue South, New York, New York 10010-1710. Tel. 212-633-3874, Fax: 212-633-3820, E-mail: reprints@elsevier.com.

Immunology and Allergy Clinics of North America is covered in MEDLINE/PubMed (Index Medicus), Current Contents/Life Sciences, Science Citation Index, ISI/BIOMED, Chemical Abstracts, and EMBASE/Excerpta Medica.

Contributors

EDITOR

ELIZABETH J. PHILLIPS, MD, FIDSA, FAAAAI
John A. Oates Chair in Clinical Research, Professor of Medicine, Pharmacology, Pathology, Immunology, and Microbiology, Director, Center for Drug Safety and Immunology and Personalized Immunology, Vanderbilt University Medical Center, Nashville, Tennessee, USA

AUTHORS

HYDAR ALI, PhD
Professor, Department of Basic and Translational Sciences, University of Pennsylvania, School of Dental Medicine, Philadelphia, Pennsylvania, USA

ANNICK BARBAUD, MD, PhD
Département de dermatologie et allergologie, Sorbonne Université, INSERM, Institut Pierre Louis d'Epidémiologie et de Santé Publique, AP-HP.Sorbonne Université, Hôpital Tenon, Paris, France

FATIMA BASSIRA, MPH
Division of General Internal Medicine and Primary Care, Department of Medicine, Brigham and Women's Hospital, Somerville, Massachusetts, USA

MOSHE BEN-SHOSHAN, MD, MSc
Division of Allergy, Immunology and Dermatology, Montreal Children's Hospital, Montreal, Québec, Canada

KNUT BROCKOW, MD
Department of Dermatology and Allergy Biederstein, School of Medicine, Technical University of Munich, Munich, Germany

MARIA A. BRUUSGAARD-MOURITSEN, MD
Department of Dermatology and Allergy, Allergy Clinic, Copenhagen University Hospital - Herlev and Gentofte, Copenhagen, Denmark

KATHERINE N. CAHILL, MD
Assistant Professor of Medicine, Division of Allergy, Pulmonary, and Critical Care Medicine, Department of Medicine, Vanderbilt University Medical Center, Nashville, Tennessee, USA

MARIANA C. CASTELLS, MD, PhD
Director of Drug Hypersensitivity and Desensitization Center, Professor of Medicine, Division of Allergy and Clinical Immunology, Department of Medicine, Harvard Medical School, Brigham and Women's Hospital, Boston, Massachusetts, USA

YEN PO CHIN, MD, MBI
Division of General Internal Medicine and Primary Care, Department of Medicine, Brigham and Women's Hospital, Harvard Medical School, Massachusetts, USA

CHALATIP CHOMPUNUD NA AYUDHYA, DDS, DScD
Instructor, Department of Oral Diagnosis, Faculty of Dentistry, Naresuan University, Phitsanulok, Thailand

WEN-HUNG CHUNG, MD, PhD
Cancer Vaccine and Immune Cell Therapy Core Lab, Department of Medical Research, Chang Gung Memorial Hospital, Linkou, Taiwan; Department of Dermatology, Drug Hypersensitivity Clinical and Research Center, Chang Gung Memorial Hospital, Linkou, Taipei and Keelung, Taiwan; Department of Dermatology, Xiamen Chang Gung Hospital, Xiamen, China; Department of Dermatology, Drug Hypersensitivity Clinical and Research Center, Chang Gung Memorial Hospital, Linkou Branch, College of Medicine, Chang Gung University, Taoyuan, Taiwan; Whole-Genome Research Core Laboratory of Human Diseases, Chang Gung Memorial Hospital, Keelung, Taiwan

ANA M. COPAESCU, MD, PhD(c)
Department of Medicine, Division of Allergy and Clinical Immunology, McGill University Health Centre (MUHC), McGill University, Montreal, Québec, Canada

KRISTEN B. COREY, MD
Division of Allergy, Pulmonary, and Critical Care Medicine, Department of Medicine, Vanderbilt University Medical Center, Nashville, Tennessee, USA

KATHERINE L. DENIRO, MD
Allergy/Immunology Clinical Fellow, Assistant Professor, Division of Dermatology, University of Washington, Seattle, Washington, USA

ANNA K. DEWAN, MD
Department of Dermatology, Vanderbilt University Medical Center, Nashville, Tennessee, USA

SHERRIE JILL DIVITO, MD, PhD
Department of Dermatology, Brigham and Women's Hospital, Harvard Medical School, Boston, Massachusetts, USA

SOFIANNE GABRIELLI, MD(c), MSc
Division of Allergy, Immunology and Dermatology, Montreal Children's Hospital, Montreal, Québec, Canada

LENE H. GARVEY, MD, PhD
Department of Dermatology and Allergy, Allergy Clinic, Copenhagen University Hospital - Herlev and Gentofte, Department of Clinical Medicine, University of Copenhagen, Copenhagen, Denmark

SHUEN-IU HUNG, PhD
Cancer Vaccine and Immune Cell Therapy Core Lab, Department of Medical Research, Chang Gung Memorial Hospital, Linkou, Taiwan; Department of Dermatology, Drug Hypersensitivity Clinical and Research Center, Chang Gung Memorial Hospital, Linkou, Taipei and Keelung, Taiwan; Department and Institute of Pharmacology, National Yang-Ming University, Taipei, Taiwan; Department of Medical Research, Cancer Vaccine and Immune Cell Therapy Core Lab, Chang Gung Memorial Hospital, Linkou Branch, Taoyuan, Taiwan

DOUGLAS B. JOHNSON, MD
Department of Medicine, Vanderbilt University Medical Center, Nashville, Tennessee, USA

MATTHEW S. KRANTZ, MD
Division of Allergy, Pulmonary and Critical Care Medicine, Department of Medicine, Vanderbilt University Medical Center, Nashville, Tennessee, USA

REBECCA KURUVILLA, MB ChB, MRCP
Academic Clinical Fellow, Department of Pharmacology and Therapeutics, Wolfson Centre for Personalised Medicine, The University of Liverpool, Liverpool, United Kingdom

RANNAKOE J. LEHLOENYA, MD, FCDerm (SA)
Division of Dermatology, Department of Medicine, Groote Schuur Hospital, University of Cape Town, Combined Drug Allergy Clinic, Groote Schuur Hospital, Cape Town, South Africa

PASQUALE MULE, MSc(c), BSc
Division of Allergy, Immunology and Dermatology, Montreal Children's Hospital, Montreal, Québec, Canada

SHUAIB NASSER, MD, MBBS, FRCP
Department of Allergy, Cambridge University Hospitals NHS Foundation Trust, Cambridge, United Kingdom

BENJAMIN C. PARK, BS
School of Medicine, Vanderbilt University, Nashville, Tennessee, USA

HELENA B. PASIEKA, MD, MS
Departments of Dermatology and Medicine, Uniformed Serviced University, Bethesda, Maryland, USA; Department of Dermatology, MedStar Washington Hospital Center/ Georgetown University Hospital, The Burn Center, MedStar Washington Hospital Center, Washington DC, USA

JONNY PETER, MD, PhD
Combined Drug Allergy Clinic, Division of Allergy and Clinical Immunology, Department of Medicine, Groote Schuur Hospital, University of Cape Town, Cape Town, South Africa; Allergy and Immunology Unit, University of Cape Town Lung Institute, Cape Town, South Africa

ELIZABETH J. PHILLIPS, MD, FIDSA, FAAAAI
John A. Oates Chair in Clinical Research, Professor of Medicine, Pharmacology, Pathology, Immunology, and Microbiology, Director, Center for Drug Safety and Immunology and Personalized Immunology, Vanderbilt University Medical Center, Nashville, Tennessee, USA

SIR MUNIR PIRMOHAMED, PhD, FRCP, FMEDSCI
David Weatherall Chair of Medicine, Department of Pharmacology and Therapeutics, Wolfson Centre for Personalised Medicine, The University of Liverpool, Liverpool, United Kingdom

CONNOR PROSTY, MD(c), BSc
Faculty of Medicine, McGill University, Montréal, Québec, Canada

ALLISON RAMSEY, MD
Division of Allergy/Immunology, Rochester Regional Health, Clinical Assistant Professor of Medicine, University of Rochester, Rochester, New York, USA

ANTONINO ROMANO, MD, PhD
Oasi Research Institute-IRCCS, Troina, Italy

KATHRYN SCOTT, PhD
Project Manager, Department of Pharmacology and Therapeutics, Wolfson Centre for Personalised Medicine, The University of Liverpool, Liverpool, United Kingdom

COSBY A. STONE, Jr., MD, MPH
Division of Allergy, Pulmonary and Critical Care Medicine, Department of Medicine, Vanderbilt University Medical Center, Nashville, Tennessee, USA

JASON A. TRUBIANO, BBiomedSci, MBBS, PhD
Associate Professor, Department of Infectious Diseases, Centre for Antibiotic Allergy and Research, Department of Medicine, Austin Health, University of Melbourne, Heidelberg, Victoria, Australia

SHERIL VARGHESE, B.A
Division of General Internal Medicine and Primary Care, Department of Medicine, Brigham and Women's Hospital, Boston, Massachusetts, USA

CHUANG-WEI WANG, PhD
Cancer Vaccine and Immune Cell Therapy Core Lab, Department of Medical Research, Chang Gung Memorial Hospital, Linkou, Taiwan; Department of Dermatology, Drug Hypersensitivity Clinical and Research Center, Chang Gung Memorial Hospital, Linkou, Taipei and Keelung, Taiwan; Department of Dermatology, Xiamen Chang Gung Hospital, Xiamen, China

LIQIN WANG, PhD
Division of General Internal Medicine and Primary Care, Department of Medicine, Brigham and Women's Hospital, Harvard Medical School, Boston, Massachusetts, USA

DEVA WELLS, MD
Dermatology Resident Physician, Division of Dermatology, University of Washington, Seattle, Washington, USA

BARBARA C. YANG, MD
Clinical Research Fellow in Allergy and Immunology, Division of Allergy and Clinical Immunology, Department of Medicine, Harvard Medical School, Brigham and Women's Hospital, Boston, Massachusetts, USA

LI ZHOU, MD, PhD
Division of General Internal Medicine and Primary Care, Department of Medicine, Brigham and Women's Hospital, Harvard Medical School, Boston, Massachusetts, USA

Contents

Preface: Drug Hypersensitivity: A Glass Half Full xiii

Elizabeth J. Phillips

Recognizing Drug Hypersensitivity in Pigmented Skin 219

Rannakoe J. Lehloenya, Elizabeth J. Phillips, Helena B. Pasieka, and Jonny Peter

The imagery of pigmented skin is underrepresented in teaching materials such as textbooks, journals, and online references, and this has resulted in poorer diagnostic and management outcomes of skin pathology, including delayed cutaneous drug hypersensitivity reactions. In this review, we use clinical images to highlight factors that impact clinical presentations and sequelae of drug hypersensitivity reactions in pigmented skin compared with nonpigmented skin. We describe clinical features in some anatomic sites that aid diagnosis or are associated with more severe sequelae. Finally, we discuss strategies that may aid the diagnosis and management of these reactions in pigmented skin.

Anaphylaxis to Excipients in Current Clinical Practice: Evaluation and Management 239

Maria A. Bruusgaard-Mouritsen, Shuaib Nasser, Lene H. Garvey, Matthew S. Krantz, and Cosby A. Stone Jr.

Excipients are the inactive ingredients in a drug or product that help to stabilize, preserve, or enhance the pharmacokinetics and bioavailability of the active ingredients. Excipient allergy is rare and hence often missed or misdiagnosed due to lack of awareness of the need to carefully review all drug ingredients. For the patient, excipient allergy can be frightening and potentially disruptive to health care delivery. This narrative review provides a clinically oriented, international, collaborative perspective on excipient allergy testing, management of future health care safety, limitations in our testing modalities, and barriers to optimal care.

Mas-Related G Protein–Coupled Receptor-X2 and Its Role in Non-immunoglobulin E–Mediated Drug Hypersensitivity 269

Chalatip Chompunud Na Ayudhya and Hydar Ali

A diverse group of Food and Drug Administration–approved cationic drugs including antibiotics, neuromuscular blocking drugs, opioids, antidepressants, and radiocontrast media activate mast cells and cause hypersensitivity reactions by both an immunoglobulin E IgE-dependent and independent manner. The recent discovery that these drugs activate mast cells via the G protein–coupled receptor known as Mas-related GPCR-X2 (MRGPRX2) has represented a paradigm shift of how drug hypersensitivity reactions are viewed. This article provides an overview of the current status of the role of MRGPRX2 on non-IgE-mediated drug hypersensitivity. Potential risk factors and evaluation for suspected MRGPRX2-mediated drug reactions are also discussed.

Hypersensitivity Reactions and Immune-Related Adverse Events to Immune Checkpoint Inhibitors: Approaches, Mechanisms, and Models   285

Benjamin C. Park, Cosby A. Stone Jr, Anna K. Dewan, and Douglas B. Johnson

Immune checkpoint inhibitors (ICI) are a major class of cancer therapeutics that may cause durable responses in a growing proportion of patients with metastatic cancer. These monoclonal antibodies remove negative regulators on T cells and may cause autoimmunelike toxicities that affect all organ systems, but are less commonly associated with traditional hypersensitivity reactions. Herein, we discuss the pathophysiology, clinical presentation, and management of toxicities of ICI and discuss their broader context within drug hypersensitivity.

Skin Testing Approaches for Immediate and Delayed Hypersensitivity Reactions   307

Annick Barbaud and Antonino Romano

In evaluating adverse drug reactions (ADRs), patch tests (PTs), skin prick tests (SPTs), and intradermal tests (IDTs) are useful tools for identifying responsible drugs and finding safe alternatives. Their diagnostic value depends on the clinical features of the ADR and on the drug tested. PTs have a good sensitivity in assessing acute generalized exanthematous pustulosis and drug rash with eosinophilia and systemic symptoms. SPTs done with all drugs except opiates are used for immediate hypersensitivity reactions. IDTs seem sensitive for immediate hypersensitivity reactions to beta-lactam antibiotics, iodinated contrast media, heparins, general anesthetics, and platinum salts.

Telemedicine in Drug Hypersensitivity   323

Deva Wells, Katherine L. DeNiro, and Allison Ramsey

This review focuses on the current applications of telemedicine for drug hypersensitivity reactions. Telemedicine holds promise as a tool to risk-stratify patients with drug hypersensitivity, for both evaluation of penicillin allergies and severe cutaneous adverse reactions. Although telemedicine may not fully replace in-person assessment owing to the need for testing, challenges, and in-person physical examination or skin biopsy, it may allow for risk stratification whereby some in-person visits may not be necessary. Electronic consults have also emerged along with telemedicine as a tool for drug allergy evaluations.

Pharmacogenomics of Drug Hypersensitivity: Technology and Translation   335

Rebecca Kuruvilla, Kathryn Scott, and Sir Munir Pirmohamed

Hypersensitivity reactions are caused by many structurally unrelated drugs used for many different diseases. These reactions vary in severity and can be fatal. Only a minority of patients are affected by drug hypersensitivity reactions. Predisposition seems to be mediated by genetic factors, particularly within the HLA system. Apart from HLA-B*57:01 testing, which is routine to prevent abacavir hypersensitivity, uptake of HLA testing into clinical practice has been slow and challenging. As genomic medicine becomes mainstream, it will be important for genetic testing in this area to move from the current reactive strategy to a more pre-emptive approach.

Advances in the Pathomechanisms of Delayed Drug Hypersensitivity   357

Chuang-Wei Wang, Sherrie Jill Divito, Wen-Hung Chung, and Shuen-Iu Hung

Delayed drug hypersensitivity continues to contribute to major clinical problems worldwide. The clinical presentations of delayed drug hypersensitivity are diverse, ranging from mild skin rashes to life-threatening systemic reactions. The pathomechanism of delayed drug hypersensitivity involves human leukocyte antigens (HLA) presentation of drugs/metabolites to T cell receptors (TCR), resulting in T-cell activation. The pathogenesis of delayed drug hypersensitivity also has reactivation of the virus, and activation of many immune mediators. In this review, we discuss the immune pathogenesis, molecular interactions of HLA/drugs/TCR, and downstream signaling of cytotoxic proteins/cytokines/chemokines, as well as disease prevention and management for delayed drug hypersensitivity.

A Risk-Based Approach to Penicillin Allergy   375

Jason A. Trubiano

Penicillin allergy can be risk stratified in the hospital or outpatient setting to identify low-, moderate-, and high-risk phenotypes. Following ascertainment of risk, dedicated penicillin allergy testing strategies can be deployed successfully for each risk type—direct oral challenge (low risk), skin testing and oral challenge (moderate risk), and specialist review and/or skin testing (high risk).

Allergy to Radiocontrast Dye   391

Knut Brockow

Radiocontrast media (RCM) are common elicitors of immediate and non-immediate hypersensitivity reactions, manifesting predominantly as urticaria/anaphylaxis or exanthems, respectively. In the minority of patients with immediate hypersensitivity reactions to RCM allergy is demonstrated by positive skin tests. However, data show that assessment by an allergist/immunologist is beneficial for managing patients with previous immediate and nonimmediate hypersensitivity reactions. For future RCM-enhanced examinations in patients with previous reactions, structurally different, skin test–negative preparations should be applied. The efficacy of this strategy is confirmed by drug provocation tests or exposures confirming or excluding RCM hypersensitivity and demonstrating tolerability of alternative RCM.

The Who, What, Where, When, Why, and How of Drug Desensitization   403

Barbara C. Yang and Mariana C. Castells

Hypersensitivity reactions to drugs have increased in the past 25 years due to increased exposures and availability of efficient, targeted, and personalized medications. Rapid drug desensitization is a clinical procedure that allows for the safe administration of a drug in patients with a history of such hypersensitivity reactions. Desensitization allows the continued use of first-line therapies, leading to higher efficacy of treatment, fewer side effects, cost-effectiveness, and increased quality of life and life expectancy of patients when compared with the use of second-line therapy. In this review, we discuss the who, what, where, when, why, and how of drug desensitization.

Aspirin-Exacerbated Respiratory Disease: A Unique Case of Drug Hypersensitivity   421

Kristen B. Corey and Katherine N. Cahill

This review of aspirin-exacerbated respiratory disease (AERD) describes the clinical characteristics and pathophysiology of the acute and chronic disease process, highlighting its similarities and unique differences in comparison to classic IgE mediated hypersensitivity. There is a specific focus on the comparison of mediator production over time and the method and mechanisms of desensitization in each diagnosis that serves to aid the clinician in differentiating and managing aspirin reactions in AERD from those related to true immediate hypersensitivity.

Pediatric Drug Allergy   433

Connor Prosty, Ana M. Copaescu, Sofianne Gabrielli, Pasquale Mule, and Moshe Ben-Shoshan

Drug allergies are reported in approximately 10% of children and carry significant health and economic impacts. However, only a minority of these reported drug allergies are established on diagnostic workup. Classically, drug allergies were diagnosed by skin prick and/or intradermal tests. However, recent data reveal that a direct ingestion challenge is often an appropriate diagnostic strategy in cases of reported nonsevere reactions to penicillin derivatives in children. This article will review the prevalence, diagnosis, and management of the main culprits of pediatric drug allergies: antibiotics and nonsteroidal anti-inflammatory drugs (NSAIDs). We will also review severe cutaneous adverse reactions to drugs in children.

The Use of Electronic Health Records to Study Drug-Induced Hypersensitivity Reactions from 2000 to 2021: A Systematic Review   453

Fatima Bassir, Sheril Varghese, Liqin Wang, Yen Po Chin, and Li Zhou

Electronic health records (EHRs) have revolutionized the field of drug hypersensitivity reaction (DHR) research. In this systematic review, we assessed 140 articles from 2000-2021, classifying them under six themes: observational studies (n=61), clinical documentation (n=27), case management (n=22), clinical decision support (CDS) (n=18), case identification (n=9), and genetic studies (n=3). EHRs provide convenient access to millions of medical records, facilitating epidemiological studies of DHRs. Though the goal of CDS is to promote safe drug prescribing, allergy alerts must be designed and used in a way that supports this effort. Ultimately, accurate allergy documentation is essential for DHR prevention.

IMMUNOLOGY AND ALLERGY CLINICS OF NORTH AMERICA

FORTHCOMING ISSUES

August 2022
Asthma and COPD Overlap: An Update
Louis-Philippe Boulet and Nicola Hanania,
Editors

November 2022
Pregnancy and Allergy
Edward S. Schulman, *Editor*

February 2023
Environmental Issues and Allergy
Jill A. Poole, *Editor*

RECENT ISSUES

February 2022
Allergic and Non-Allergic Systemic Reactions including Anaphylaxis
Panida Sriaroon, Dennis K. Ledford, and
Richard F. Lockey, *Editors*

November 2021
Pediatric Immunology and Allergy
Elizabeth Secord, *Editor*

August 2021
Skin Allergy
Susan Nedorost, *Editor*

SERIES OF RELATED INTEREST

Medical Clinics
https://www.medical.theclinics.com/

THE CLINICS ARE AVAILABLE ONLINE!
Access your subscription at:
www.theclinics.com

Preface

Drug Hypersensitivity: A Glass Half Full

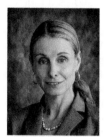

Elizabeth J. Phillips, MD, FIDSA, FAAAAI
Editor

Drug hypersensitivity is a specialty that intersects with multiple fields and underpins the safe and effective use of drugs in every discipline in medicine. Drug hypersensitivity has been both a driver and a beneficiary of the stunning advances that have graced all of science. After more than a century of accelerated drug development, we benefit from an enhanced understanding of the prevention, classification, mechanisms, diagnosis, and management of immediate and delayed hypersensitivity reactions, which led to safer drugs and better patient outcomes across multiple disciplines. We have seen improved knowledge and implementation of skin testing strategies for both immediate and delayed reactions. For hypersensitivity to penicillin and other drugs associated with a label of an immediate hypersensitivity reaction, the allergy is either temporary and wanes over time, or may never have been. Removal of the drug allergy label ("delabeling") has become the norm in the twenty-first century and is a powerful antibiotic stewardship tool. Risk stratification, taking into account the time since the reaction, type of reaction, and use of ancillary therapy such as epinephrine, is a key tool to determine the most efficient delabeling strategy. This has been particularly relevant to the field of pediatric drug allergy where many antibiotic allergy labels are the result of viral infections. Indeed, 75% of children with antibiotic allergy labels have acquired these allergy labels by the age of three, although most of these unverified reactions, including serum sickness-like reactions, can be eventually delabeled. Increased understanding of the mechanisms and occurrence of non-IgE-mediated mast cell activation is fueled by the discovery that many drugs, such as injectable cationic peptides, neuromuscular blocking agents, vancomycin, opioids, radiocontrast dyes, and fluoroquinolones, are small molecule ligands for the mas-related G-protein-coupled receptor (MRGPRX2). This has contributed to our understanding and management of immediate reactions in the perioperative setting and allergy to radiocontrast dyes. With regards to other non-IgE-mediated reactions, such as aspirin and nonsteroidal

Immunol Allergy Clin N Am 42 (2022) xiii–xiv
https://doi.org/10.1016/j.iac.2022.01.007
0889-8561/22/© 2022 Published by Elsevier Inc.

exacerbated respiratory disease, we have seen significant advances in pathomechanisms and treatment. Desensitization is a targeted tool that has evolved to become more efficient, smarter, and faster. The almost universal use of electronic health records has created new and scalable opportunities to study drug hypersensitivity that promise both reproductions across health care systems and a new tool to understand the epidemiology and ecological and biological risk factors. New patient communication strategies have been facilitated by advances in the electronic health record. The provision of telehealth promises to be repurposed as a tool to enable a wide array of drug hypersensitivity services from delabeling of penicillin allergy in the outpatient setting to institutional triage of severe cutaneous adverse drug reactions. This has come to the forefront in the current COVID-19 pandemic to improve access to drug and vaccine allergy services, such as risk stratification and advice for potential COVID-19 vaccine hypersensitivity reactions. Knowledge of genetic risk and immunopathogenesis of drug hypersensitivity has increased exponentially over the last two decades, and we now benefit from the use of pharmacogenetics and HLA typing to enable pre-prescription screening, risk stratification, and diagnosis. Knowledge of immunopathogenesis also promises to enable earlier diagnosis and targeted treatments. The discovery and use of promising immunotherapies for cancer unveiled new phenotypes of immune-related adverse events and have helped us understand mechanisms and approaches. Drug hypersensitivity affects diverse populations across different ages, sexes, and skin pigmentation. In particular, our understanding and recognition of these differences among different skin pigmentation types with regards to drug reaction phenotypes and immediate and delayed skin and patch testing modalities are fundamental to competency in the practice of Allergy and Immunology and related disciplines.

I am confident that this issue of the *Immunology and Allergy Clinics of North America* will be of great interest and use to clinicians, researchers, and patients. I am extremely grateful to all the authors who contributed their invaluable expertise and time to produce such a high-quality product. I would like to thank Dr Lanny Rosenwasser, who created the opportunity to publish this issue on "Drug Hypersensitivity," and Jessica Canaberal, for her outstanding editorial support.

Elizabeth J. Phillips, MD, FIDSA, FAAAAI
Center for Drug Safety and Immunology
Vanderbilt University Medical Center
1161 21St Avenue South
Medical Center North, A-2200
Nashville, TN 37232, USA

E-mail address:
Elizabeth.j.phillips@vanderbilt.edu

Recognizing Drug Hypersensitivity in Pigmented Skin

Rannakoe J. Lehloenya, MD, FCDerm (SA)[a,b,*],
Elizabeth J. Phillips, MD[c,d], Helena B. Pasieka, MD, MS[e,f,g,h],
Jonny Peter, MD, PhD[b,i,j]

KEYWORDS

- Drug hypersensitivity reactions • Pigmented skin • Clinical presentation • Sequelae

KEY POINTS

- Deeply pigmented skin tones are underrepresented in clinical learning materials around the world, resulting in deficiencies by clinicians to recognize and manage many skin disorders in patients with pigmented skin.
- Competence in identifying disorders in pigmented skin depends on repeated visual exposure to pathology in deeply pigmented skin.
- Factors that make skin pathology in pigmented skin to present differently from nonpigmented skin include the subtlety of erythema, quantity and quality of melanin and melanocytes, predilection to scarring and dyspigmentation, as well as propensity to dryness and itching.

Continued

Funding: R.J. Lehloenya is supported by South African Medical Research Council and nonrated researcher support from the South African National Research Foundation.
[a] Division of Dermatology, Department of Medicine, Groote Schuur Hospital, University of Cape Town, Dermatology ward G23, New Groote Schuur Hospital, Observatory, Cape Town 7925, South Africa; [b] Combined Drug Allergy Clinic, Groote Schuur Hospital, Dermatology ward G23, New Groote Schuur Hospital, Observatory, Cape Town 7925, South Africa; [c] Center for Drug Safety & Immunology, Vanderbilt University Medical Center, Nashville, TN; [d] Institute for Immunology & Infectious Diseases, Murdoch University, Murdoch, Western Australia, Australia; [e] Department of Dermatology, Uniformed Serviced University, Bethesda, MD, USA; [f] Department of Medicine, Uniformed Serviced University, Bethesda, MD, USA; [g] Department of Dermatology, MedStar Washington Hospital Center/Georgetown University Hospital, Washington, DC, USA; [h] The Burn Center, MedStar Washington Hospital Center, Washington, DC, USA; [i] Division of Allergy and Clinical Immunology, Department of Medicine, Groote Schuur Hospital, University of Cape Town Lung institute, George Street, Mowbray, 7925, Cape Town, South Africa; [j] Allergy and Immunology Unit, University of Cape Town Lung Institute, Old Main Building, Groote Schuur Hospital, Anzio Road, 7925, Cape Town, South Africa
* Corresponding author. Dermatology ward G23, New Groote Schuur Hospital, Observatory, Cape Town 7925.
E-mail address: rannakoe.lehloenya@uct.ac.za

Immunol Allergy Clin N Am 42 (2022) 219–238
https://doi.org/10.1016/j.iac.2022.01.005
0889-8561/22/© 2022 Elsevier Inc. All rights reserved.
immunology.theclinics.com

Continued

- Although not fully characterized for cutaneous drug reactions dermoscopy and Wood lamp are potential adjuvant tools to aid diagnosis.
- Optimization and modification of skin (immediate and delayed prick and intradermal drug allergy testing) and drug patch testing protocols may improve diagnostic sensitivity for inconclusive cases.

BACKGROUND

There is an increasing awareness of the underrepresentation of pigmented skin in both undergraduate and postgraduate teaching, textbooks, journal articles, online resources, and even the materials used to do online searches.[1–5] The clinical presentation of cutaneous disorders often varies in different skin types. The variations range from subclinical, subtle, to distinctive. Defining, understanding, and recognizing these differences ultimately helps improve diagnostic and management outcomes. Knowledge about the normal variations in the color, texture, and responses of the skin and its appendages is also necessary to understand abnormalities. The underexposure of clinicians to darker skin types, can lead to a delayed diagnosis and worse quality of care for patients with pigmented skin.[2] Dermatology practice to a large extent depends on repeated exposure and familiarity with the clinical presentation of skin findings either during direct contact with the patient or viewing live or stored images. In this review, we describe factors that impact clinical presentations of delayed drug hypersensitivity reactions in pigmented skin aided by clinical pictures and anatomic sites that warrant special consideration in addition to strategies that may aid the diagnosis.

DEFINING PIGMENTED SKIN

The terminology and all criteria used to classify human skin and appendices (including hair, nails and mucosae) have limitations. These limitations are usually based on color, geographic origin, or social groups like race and ethnicity, all of which are not clear-cut and may not be readily apparent. The Skin of Color Society defines people of color as "individuals of Asian, Hispanic/Latino, African, Native American, Pacific Island descent, and mixtures thereof."[6]

Fitzpatrick skin type (FST) was originally developed to assess the susceptibility of the skin to burn during phototherapy.[7] Despite its limitations, FST is the most widely used classification system of skin color because there is no other widely adopted system for describing skin color that can be applied to all skin types.[8] For the purpose of this review, pigmented skin refers to FST IV (light brown skin, burns minimally, tans easily), V (brown skin that rarely burns and tans darkly easily), and VI (dark brown or black skin that never burns and always tans darkly).[7]

CLINICAL SPECTRUM OF CUTANEOUS DRUG HYPERSENSITIVITY REACTIONS
Immediate Hypersensitivity Reactions

Flushing, urticaria, and angioedema
Cutaneous manifestations of immediate IgE- and non-IgE-mediated drug hypersensitivity include flushing, pruritis (localized or generalized), urticaria, and angioedema. Urticaria and angioedema are characterized by intermittent, localized swelling in the superficial and deep layers of the skin, caused by a temporary increase in vascular

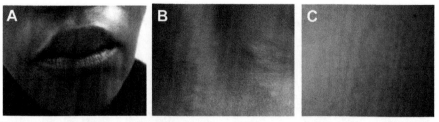

Fig. 1. (A) Lip angioedema, (B) urticaria, (C) morbilliform eruption.

permeability.[9] Urticaria and angioedema develop secondary to mast cell mediators, bradykinin, or other vasoactive mediators, for example, leukotrienes in nonsteroidal anti-inflammatory drug-associated urticaria and angioedema; angiotensin-converting enzyme inhibitor angioedema is overrepresented in black Africans.[10] Urticarial "wheals" can range in size from a few millimeters to large coalescing lesions of greater than 20 cm; all anatomic areas of the skin can develop urticaria. Similarly, angioedema swellings secondary to drugs can involve different anatomic areas but most commonly lips, face, eyes, limbs, intestine, and genitalia[10] (**Fig. 1**A, B).

Delayed Hypersensitivity Reactions

1. *Maculopapular exanthem/morbilliform eruption:*
   The commonest cutaneous manifestations to drugs involve a benign, self-limiting morbilliform drug eruption (also called maculopapular or exanthematous). The most common primary lesion is a pink to red flat macule or papule. The rash is bilateral and symmetric and usually starts on the trunk and then spreads to the limbs and neck. Systemic features are limited to itch and transient peripheral blood eosinophilia without organ involvement.[11] Fever is uncommon, and when present, it is low grade (**Fig. 1**C).
2. *Drug reaction with eosinophilia and systemic symptoms (DRESS)*/drug-induced hypersensitivity syndrome (DiHS) is most typically characterized by a constellation of fever, eosinophilia, atypical lymphocytosis, internal organ involvement, and a widespread rash of varying severity and morphology. The rash of DRESS/DiHS is widely polymorphic and ranges from morbilliform, eczematous, lichenoid, purpuric plaques, vesicles, pustules, targetoid lesions, cheilitis, erythroderma, to exfoliative dermatitis. However, indurated erythematous papules and plaques are most typical. Facial swelling, particularly of the central face, with nasolabial fold effacement is common. Systemic features include fever, lymphadenopathy, leukocytosis, eosinophilia, atypical lymphocytosis, hepatitis, nephritis, pancreatitis, pneumonitis, and myocarditis with varying frequency.[12] The rash has a long duration, usually lasting more than 14 days, and it can also relapse as a single finding. The spectrum of skin lesions in DRESS is shown in **Fig. 2**A–D.
3. *Stevens-Johnson syndrome (SJS) and toxic epidermal necrolysis (TEN)* form a spectrum defined by the affected body surface area (BSA), where SJS affects less than 10% BSA, SJS/TEN overlap 10% to 30%, and TEN affects more than 30%.[13,14] Features of SJS/TEN include a prodrome of malaise, low-grade fever, sore throat, and oral pain that is followed in subsequent days by the development of a rash. The morphology of the rash is most commonly atypical targetoid lesions with dusky purple center that go on to blister and detach. Progression and coalescence of these lesions leads to skin detachment and deiptheliazation in sheets. A notable association is the development of mucositis of at least 2 surfaces, including

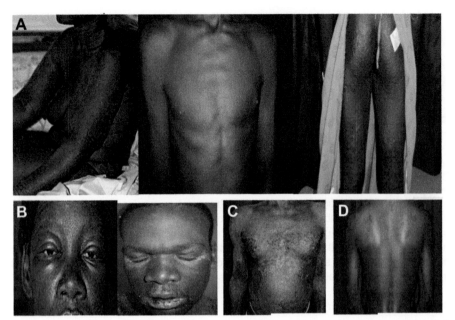

Fig. 2. DRESS. (*A*) Indurated purpuric erythema in DRESS. (*B*) Periorbital and central facial edema and scale in DRESS. (*C*) Extensive scale in a patient with resolving DRESS. (*D*) Lichenoid repair on the back post-DRESS.

of the eyes, oropharynx, nares, or genitourinary or perianal mucosae.[15] This deep-itheliazation can range from a small percentage of BSA to nearly complete skin loss. Secondary internal organ involvement, including hepatitis and nephritis, may accompany the eruption, but is not as common as in DRESS/DiHS.[16,17] **Fig. 3**A–G shows the cutaneous and mucosal lesions of SJS/TEN in pigmented skin.

4. *Fixed drug eruption (FDE)* typically presents as very well-circumscribed, circular erythematous macules or dusky indurated plaques on the skin or mucosal surfaces as shown in **Fig. 4**A–G; they can be pruritic or tender. Occasionally the central portion will be bullous. If severe and extensive, the lesions can vesiculate and become confluent and bullous resembling SJS/TEN, but typically without mucositis as defined for SJS/TEN. The latter is referred to as bullous FDE (BFDE) or generalized BFDE (GBFDE). **Fig. 4**J–L shows BFDE and GBFDE. On reexposure to the drug, FDE recurs on the same sites within a few hours, sometimes with new lesions at other sites as shown in **Fig. 4**N. Persistent hyperpigmentation is a major feature of FDE, although hypopigmentation does occur (**Fig. 4**I).[18] However, this is not so marked with BFDE (**Fig. 4**M, N).

5. *Lichenoid drug eruption (LDE)* refers to a poorly characterized group of delayed hypersensitivity reactions affecting the skin, hair, and mucosa that resemble lichen planus hence the synonym drug-induced lichen planus. LDE presents as pruritic, violaceus, symmetric papules or plaques that mainly affect the trunk and extremities and sometimes the mucosa (**Fig. 5**). On the skin, the lesions are often photo-distributed or photoaccentuated.[19,20] Prolonged exposure to the offending drug can result in postinflammatory hyperpigmentation and hypopigmentation, both of which are reversible[21,22] (**Fig. 5**).

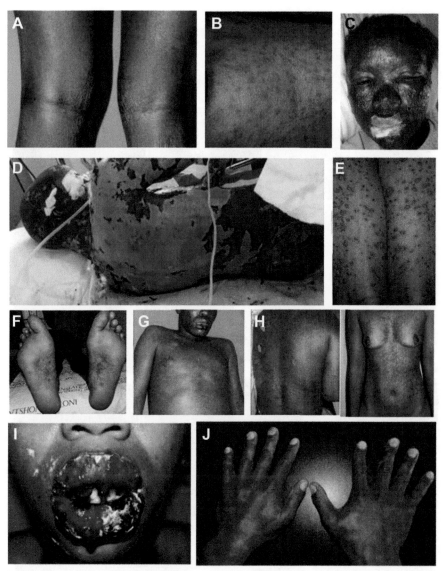

Fig. 3. Spectrum of lesions seen on the skin in SJS/TEN (*A*) Dusky erythema in a patient with early SJS/TEN. (*B*) Dusky purpuric erythema in a patient with early SJS/TEN. (*C*) Early blisters and edema in SJS/TEN before the lesions turn purpuric and dusky. (*D*) Extensive skin detachment in TEN. (*E*) Purpuric targetoid lesions with blisters, some becoming confluent, in SJS/TEN. (*F*) Epidermal necrosis on the feet in patient with SJS/TEN with Fitzpatrick skin type VI highlighting discernible erythema. (*G*) Duskier, more superficial epidermal necrosis and hemorrhagic cheilitis in a darker patient with SJS/TEN. (*H*) SJS/TEN lesions in different stages of evolution highlighting early indurated erythematous lesions, more advanced larger duskier lesions, progression to confluent blisters, and finally epidermal detachment and positive Nikolsky sign. (*I*) Severe hemorrhagic cheilitis. (*J*) Postinflammatory hyperpigmentation and nail dystrophy in resolved TEN.

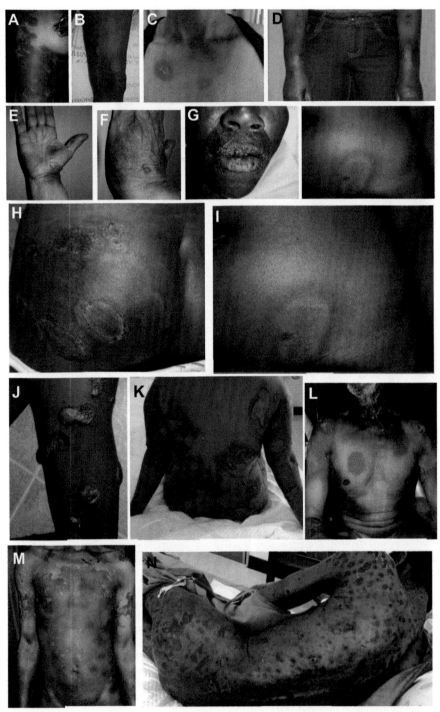

Fig. 4. Variations in clinical presentation of FDE and bullous fixed drug eruption (BFDE) and generalized BFDE in pigmented skin (*A*). Round hyperpigmented lesions of FDE. (*B*) Round hyperpigmented lesions of FDE with blister formation. (*C*) Erythematous round lesions of

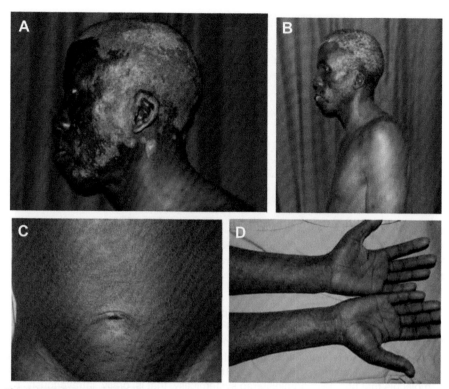

Fig. 5. LDE with depigmentation. The lesions initially developed during the first prolonged exposure to the offending drug, resulting in areas of depigmentation and hyperpigmentation. (*A*) Recurrence with violaceous patches within the depigmented areas from the first episode. (*B*) Three months after completion of prolonged treatment showing repigmentation. (*C, D*) Violaceous flat-topped papules and plaques in 2 patients with LDE.

6. *Acute generalized exanthematous pustulosis (AGEP)* is characterized by an eruption of nonfollicular, sterile pustules on a background of indurated erythema. Although the pustules can be generalized, there is a predilection for the flexures and intertriginous areas. In 20% to 25% of cases, a mucosal surface is affected, whereas palmoplantar involvement is uncommon. Systemically, fever, neutrophilia, leukocytosis, eosinophilia, and hypocalcemia are more common findings compared with nephritis, hepatitis, and respiratory distress. Assuming the

---

FDE with blistering and scale. (*D*) Indurated erythematous round lesions of FDE. (*E*) Palmar erythema in FDE. (*F*) Indurated, hyperpigmented round lesion of FDE with peripheral erythema suggesting ongoing disease process. (*G*) Resolving FDE on the lips. (*H*) Recurrent FDE showing lesional hyperpigmentation with peripheral hypopigmentation of old lesions, hyperpigmentation, erosions, and scale in recent lesions and peripheral edema in ongoing active lesions. (*I*) Postinflammatory hypopigmentation in a healed lesion of FDE. Variants of BFDE. (*J*) Round intact blister of GBFDE (*L*) Loss of epidermis in GBFDE. (*M*) Postinflammatory hyperpigmentation in GBFDE. (*N*) Severe postinflammatory hyperpigmentation following recurrent GBFDE.

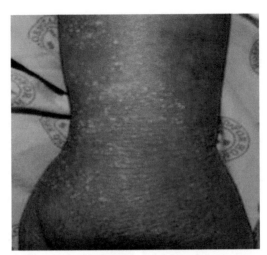

Fig. 6. AGEP showing pustules on the background of indurated erythema, which extends beyond the area affected by pustules. Note the brighter erythema in the nonindurated area.

offending agent has been withdrawn, spontaneous resolution within 14 days with very superficial desquamation is typical[23,24] (**Fig. 6**).

7. *Symmetric drug-related intertriginous and flexural exanthema (SDRIFE)*, previously known as baboon syndrome, is a form of systemic contact dermatitis that occurs in contact-sensitized individuals on exposure to the same allergen or a cross-reacting molecule that has been administered systemically, that is, orally, intravenously, by inhalation, per rectum, intravesically, or transcutaneously. Criteria for diagnosis have been published, and clinical features include erythema of the perianal area and/or inguinal area, involvement of at least one other flexure, symmetry of affected areas, and absence of systemic symptoms and signs. The lesions can be papular, pustular, or vesicles, and rarely bullous[25,26] (**Fig. 7**).

8. *Drug-induced lupus erythematosus (DILE)* is a lupuslike syndrome with a temporal relationship to ongoing exposure to a specific drug. The reaction resolves on

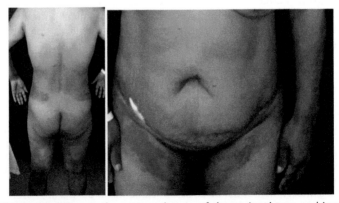

Fig. 7. SDRIFE highlighting erythematous plaques of the perianal area and inguinal areas and symmetric involvement of the waist, axillae, and popliteal fossae.

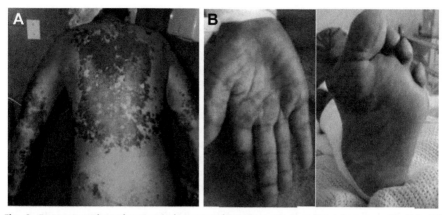

Fig. 8. Drug-exarcebated systemic lupus erythematosus in a patient known with SLE. (*A*) Extensive epidermal necrosis of the trunk and arms. (*B*) Tender erythema and skin necrosis of the hands and feet.

cessation of the offending drug. DILE is categorized into systemic, subacute cutaneous, and chronic cutaneous variants. Skin signs of the systemic variant are infrequent and include photosensitivity, purpura, panniculitis, and urticarial or small vessel vasculitis. SJS/TEN-like variants have been reported[27] (**Fig. 8**). The subacute form presents as annular or scaly photodistributed or photoaccentuated lesions. The edges of the lesions may blister. The discoid presentation is the most infrequent and delayed, often months after initiating the offending drug. The lesions are similar to those in the classic form of discoid cutaneous lupus erythematosus, mainly affecting the scalp, face, ears, upper trunk, and arms.[28,29]

FACTORS THAT INFLUENCE CLINICAL PRESENTATION AND SEQUELAE OF CUTANEOUS DRUG HYPERSENSITIVITY IN PIGMENTED SKIN

1. Erythema

    Erythema is the superficial, blanchable redness of the skin as a result of dilated blood vessels. The quantity of blood flowing through the skin, blood pooling, its oxygen saturation, the photoreflective properties of the dermis, and the overlying epidermis all determine the characteristics of the erythema. Erythema, occurring in the context of immediate or delayed drug hypersensitivity, is potentially more challenging to detect in pigmented skin, and inflammation that typically manifests as pink or red lesions in lighter skin may appear hyperpigmented in darker skin and has a progressively duskier, violaceous hue[30–32] (**Fig. 8**). The same principles apply to flushing, which occurs in the absence of an inflammatory response.

2. Purpura

    Purpura refers to bleeding under the skin. In contrast to erythema, purpura is not blanchable. Early lesions of epidermal necrosis as seen in SJS/TEN and BFDE present as purpuric lesions (**Fig. 3**A,B). One of the differentiating factors between viral exanthems and DRESS/DiHS is indurated erythema with purpuric areas (**Fig. 2**A). The purpuric areas represent areas characterized by scattered necrotic keratinocytes histologically. Purpura enhances visibility of a rash in darker skin.

3. Edema

Central facial edema is a feature characteristic of DRESS/DiHS, and its detection does not depend on skin color (**Fig. 2**B). In DRESS/DiHS, erythema in the presence of edema is more visible. Edema, characterized by spongiosis histologically, is another differentiating factor between viral exanthems and DRESS/DiHS. In DRESS/DiHS the edematous areas present with indurated erythema; this can also be seen in FDE (**Figs. 2**A and **4**).

4. Dyspigmentation

The way that melanocytes react to cutaneous inflammation or trauma can result in unchanged, increased, or decreased melanin production. Melanocytes that are highly susceptible to damage are more likely to result in hypopigmentation, whereas those that are more resilient tend to result in hyperpigmentation. This theory is referred to as the chromatic tendency theory, and it seems to be genetically determined and inherited in an autosomal dominant pattern.[33]

a Postinflammatory hyperpigmentation (PIHP) is broadly classified as epidermal or dermal. In epidermal PIHP there is increased epidermal pigmentation and increased melanogenic activity by melanocytes. In dermal PIHP there is increased dermal pigmentation, decreased epidermal pigmentation, as well as increased melanogenic activity. In both types, the number of melanocytes is the same; this suggests that increased melanogenic activity is a common denominator in PIHP. Dermal pigmentation seems to be associated with vacuolar degeneration of the basement membrane, weakening or loosening of the basement membrane, perivascular lymphocytic infiltrate, as well as higher numbers of mast cells and macrophages in lesional skin.[34] Historically, it was believed that the skin had an incredible capacity to degrade melanin; this is characterized by the near absence of melanin granules in the stratum granulosum and stratum corneum, even in hyperproliferative conditions like psoriasis. Basal keratinocytes contain up to 10 times the number of melanosomes found in the granular and corneal layers.[35] It has previously been reported that an autophagy-based pathway is responsible for melanophage degradation and this pathway is impaired in darker skin types.[36,37] However, recent studies suggest that melanin granules are redistributed to keratinocytes that are retained in the basal layers when undergoing mitosis as opposed to those migrating vertically. Thus, melanin was distributed preferentially to the daughter keratinocyte retained within the basal layer, whereas the second daughter cell destined to leave the basal layer for differentiation through upward stratification lacked significant amounts of melanin.[35] This suggests that rather than degrade melanin, the human skin actually recycles it in the lower layers of the skin. However, under inflammatory conditions that stimulate increase in mitotic activity of keratinocytes, both daughter cells inherited similar melanin granule loading. Thus, in stressful times the uneven distribution of melanin to keratinocyte daughter cells during mitosis is lost, driving more pigment into the upper layers of the skin[35] (**Fig. 9**). Pooling of blood and other pigments like hemosiderin also contribute.[30,38]

b Postinflammatory hypopigmentation is an acquired partial loss of skin pigmentation occurring following inflammation of the skin. The severity of this condition is related to the extent and degree of the inflammation; it can occur in all skin types but is more common and prominent in darker skin, possibly because of the color contrast with the normal skin. The pathogenesis is not clear, but theories include inhibition of melanogenesis rather

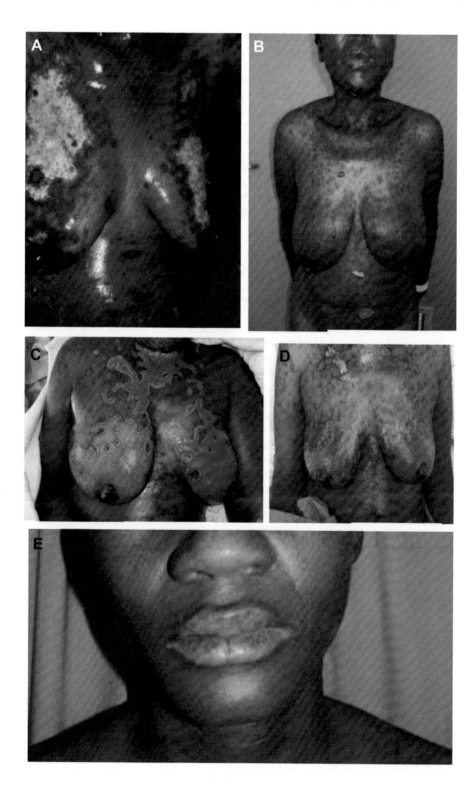

than destruction of melanocytes and chromatic tendency theory described earlier.[33,39] With severe persistent inflammation, however, there may be loss of melanocytes and permanent hypopigmentation. Hypopigmentation can become a sequela of any of the cutaneous drug hypersensitivity reactions detailed earlier (**Fig. 9**).

c Universal depigmentation has rarely been reported as sequelae in SJS/TEN.[40] Localized depigmentation occurs more commonly in areas that are scarred (**Fig. 9**). The lower lip is more prone to depigmentation after SJS/TEN, and this seems to be more common in those with prolonged time to resolution (author's observation). LDE is associated with reversible depigmentation in cases of prolonged exposure to the offending drug as seen in the treatment of tuberculosis[22] (**Fig. 5**); this is likely a result of melanocyte damage at the dermoepidermal junction by the infiltrating lymphocytes as mentioned earlier.

5. Borders

Detection of the border of any lesion provides important information for accurate differentiation between the pathologic and normal skin because the border of a lesion is an important and informative feature to properly define the morphology of a lesion allowing one to generate a differential diagnosis.

6. Contrast

Similarly, contrast enhances border detection. Better contrast may be beneficial for diagnosis of erythema in a lighter skin with DRESS/DiHS but have a detrimental cosmetic outlook for postinflammatory hypopigmentation in a darker skin as sequalae for the same disorder.

7. Keloids and hypertrophic scarring

Although keloids and hypertrophic scarring have been described in all skin types, they are more common in individuals of African, Asian, Hispanic, and Mediterranean descent in that order. Keloid formation is estimated to be up to 15 times more prevalent in dark-skinned individuals.[38,41,42] SJS/TEN primarily affects the epidermis, thus hypertrophic scarring and keloid formation are rarely reported,[43–48] suggesting that in some instances there is significant dermal involvement resulting in cicatricial changes in the absence of infection or other cicatricializing factors[49] (**Fig. 9**).

8. Scale

Visualization and characterization of scale is an important diagnostic clue in many skin conditions. Pigmented skin is associated with higher transepidermal water loss and more prone to scale and xerosis.[38] As part of the normal process of cornification, the melanin pigment that is deposited in keratinocytes in the deeper layers of the epidermis is degraded and recycled.[50] As a result, the scale in pigmented skin is devoid of melanin and becomes more visible on the background of contrasting darker skin[50]; this is seen in DRESS/DiHS, resolving AGEP, and SDRIFE among others (**Fig. 3**).

9. Xerosis

Fig. 9. A) Areas of hyperpigmentation and depigmentation on the chest after resolution of SJS/TEN. The depigmented areas showed scarring with absence of hair follicles. Evolution of delayed healing and scarring in TEN. (*B*) Day 3 after onset of symptoms, (*C*) day 38, (*D*) day 120. (*E*) Lichenoid repair on healing lips post-SJS/TEN.

Xerosis is more common in pigmented skin, particularly FST V and VI.[38] Xerosis has also been reported as a common sequalae beyond the acute stage of SJS and DRESS.[51] It is not clear if xerosis postcutaneous drug hypersensitivity reactions is more common in pigmented skin.

10. Pruritus

Itch is a common feature of many cutaneous drug reactions during the acute stages, with some classes of drugs like immune checkpoint inhibitors associated with higher incidences.[52] Chronic pruritus has been reported in up to 53% of patients with SJS/TEN.[51] Darker skin is generally more prone to pruritus, and this has been attributed to higher transepidermal water loss, lower ceramide levels, lower pH in the stratum corneum, and larger mast cells.[38,53,54] Considering the debilitating effects of pruritus on the quality of life, a better understanding of the epidemiology of chronic pruritus across skin types will improve care.

11. Lichenoid repair

Lchenoid repair refers to a violaceous color seen during healing of pigmented skin, mainly following a blistering disorder like SJS/TEN as well as severe DRESS, and is often followed by PIHP (**Fig,** 2D and **Fig. 9E**).

ANATOMIC SITES THAT WARRANT SPECIAL CONSIDERATION
Eyes

There are data emerging to suggest that phototypes V and VI are more likely to develop late ocular complication of SJS/TEN, namely, visual loss and severe cicatrizing conjunctivitis.[49]

Lips

In SJS/TEN the lips tend to be last to form new epithelium, with the lower lip healing after the upper lip. Patients with fuller lips tend to take the longest to achieve full epithelialization. People of African descent genetically tend to have greater lip volume even into old age, the latter due to the increased melanin protection against solar elastosis.[55–57] Lip volume can impact that perception of angioedema of the lips, and it is important to enquire from patients or review other pictures to detect more subtle swelling. We postulate that lip volume correlates with the delayed lip healing in SJS/TEN. Depigmentation of the lips post-LDE and post-SJS/TEN is not uncommon (**Figs. 1A, 5**, and **9E**). Involvement of the lips in isolation or as part of wider skin involvement in FDE is frequent.

Palms and soles

In individuals with dark skin, the palms and soles are generally much less pigmented. Consequently erythema and epidermal necrosis as seen in SJS/TEN and FDE, for example, are detectable much earlier and more easily (**Figs. 3F and 4E**). A hallmark of SJS/TEN is tenderness of the palms and soles.

Nails

Melanonychia or brown-black discoloration of the nail plate in people of African descent ranges from 2.5% before age 3 years to 96% in those older than 50 years, and it is more common in those of skin of color. On the other hand, melanonychia in FST I and II is rare.[58] Development of diffuse melanonychia seems to be accelerated after severe drug hypersensitivity reactions in pigmented skin. Drug-induced melanonychia is typically associated with pigmentation of the skin and other mucosa. Common implicated drugs include chemotherapeutic agents (cyclophosphamide, doxorubicin, daunorubicin, busulfan, taxanes, capecitabine, cisplatin, bleomycin, 5-fluorouracil, methotrexate, and dacarbazine). Antiretrovirals implicated include zidovudine. Cases that are reversible, as well as those that persist for months, have been described.

STRATEGIES THAT MAY AID THE DIAGNOSIS AND MANAGEMENT OF CUTANEOUS DRUG HYPERSENSITIVITY IN PIGMENTED SKIN

Dermoscopy

Dermoscopy is a common technique used in dermatology practice to examine pigmented skin lesions. The skin surface is evaluated using a dermatoscope. Based on current literature, dermoscopic findings in inflammatory disorders are mainly similar between darker and lighter skin types. The major differences relate to frequencies of vascular features, predominant background colors, and pigmentary changes.[59] It has been suggested that multispectral dermatoscopes with yellow and red light are better suited for darker skin types. These longer wavelengths penetrate deeper into the dermis, and yellow corresponds to the absorption peaks of melanin and close to that of hemoglobin making it suitable for visualization of dermal vasculature and pigmentation with better contrast.[60] The dermoscopic features of severe cutaneous adverse drug reactions have recently been described.[61] However, the field is in its infancy and there is a paucity of data reporting dermoscopy of SCAR in different skin types.

Wood Lamp

Examination under Wood lamp accentuates dyspigmentation and helps distinguish between hypopigmented and depigmented lesions much earlier than would be clinically apparent. In addition, it can be used to evaluate hyperpigmentation to determine if the pigment is epidermal or dermal. Epidermal hyperpigmentation enhances with Wood lamp, whereas it remains muted when dermal.

Prick and Intradermal Testing

Prick and intradermal testing are typically used for the diagnosis of immediate hypersensitivity reactions with criteria for positivity described as (1) wheal of at least 5 mm with flare greater than wheal or (2) wheal greater than 3 mm from baseline with a flare at least 5 mm greater than baseline. The positive histamine control and the flare of positive skin tests both prick and intradermal may be more subtle in pigmented skin (Fig. 10A–C). A recent study highlighted an association with HLA-DRB1*10:01 with immediate reactions to penicillins. HLA-DRB1*10:01 is carried twice as frequently in those of African origin; however, no data exist specifically about risk of immediate hypersensitivity reactions to penicillins in those of African race. Delayed intradermal testing is used as an in vivo tool to aid in the diagnosis of a delayed hypersensitivity reaction. A delayed intradermal positive test is defined as any wheal occurring greater than 6 hours following application that is persistent greater than 24 to 72 hours; this may be more difficult to appreciate in darkly pigmented skin. Postinflammatory hyperpigmentation can occur in particular at the site of a positive patch test or delayed intradermal test.

Patch Testing

Patch testing is often used to identify the offending drug cutaneous hypersensitivity reactions. In pigmented skin patch testing requires additional skills and experience because color changes are more subtle and erythema not as prominent (Fig. 10D). Papular or perifollicular eruption is often an early presentation of a positive test rather

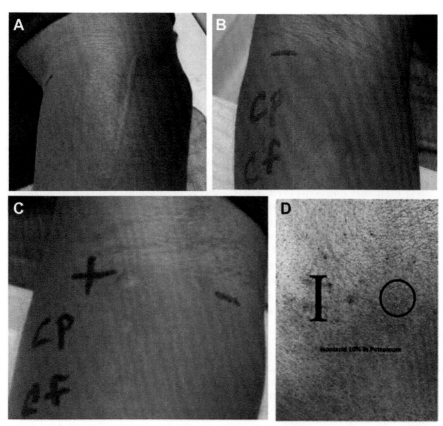

Fig. 10. Prick, intradermal, and patch testing in pigmented skin. (*A*) Negative prick testing with positive histamine control to cefazolin (Cp) and ceftriaxone (Cf) and (*B*) positive intradermal test to Cf 2.5 mg/mL and negative to Cp 1 mg/mL in a man with ceftriaxone anaphylaxis 2 months prior. (*C*) Dermatographism. (*D*) Positive patch test to isoniazid at 10% in petrolatum.

than erythema.[62–64] Numerous strategies can be applied to improve detection of positive reactions including adequate lighting, angled views, palpation, and rereading the test 24 to 48 hours later. To enhance sensitivity in suspected false-negative results, tape stripping of the skin with moderately adhesive tape like 3M Blenderm surgical tape (3M Medica, 3M Deutschland GmbH, Neuss, Germany; width, 25 mm) before application of the patch test and "repeated open application test" (ROAT) have also been used.[64–66] ROAT was initially developed for allergic contact dermatitis and has not been standardized for delayed systemic drug hypersensitivity. We have successfully used a repeat application method by reapplying the drug allergen and controls in a Finn chamber over the same area 48 hours after the initial application in indeterminate cases to enhance sensitivity.[65] The test is read 24 and 48 hours after the second application. The timing and reading of the second test still need validation.

SUMMARY

Diagnosis of immediate and delayed drug hypersensitivity reactions is challenging at the best of times, but the underrepresentation of pigmented skin imagery in general makes it even more challenging in this population. We have used clinical images to describe these reactions and testing responses in pigmented skin, highlight factors that make it more challenging, as well as describe clinical features that can aid diagnosis, management, and awareness of sequelae. Ultimately the best solution to the problem is a proportional representation of pigmented skin in all dermatology learning and reading material and to have a spectrum of skin pigmentation types represented side by side for accurate context and comparison.

The IMARI-Africa project is part of the EDCTP2 program supported by the European Union (Grant number TMA2017SF-1981). The IMARI-SA Registry and Biorepository is supported by the National Institute Of Allergy And Infectious Diseases of the National Institutes of Health under Award Number R01AI152183. J.P. is supported by the South African Medical Research Council, the National Research Foundation and receives funding from NIH K43TW011178. E.J.P. reports grants from National Institutes of Health (P50GM115305, R01HG010863, R01AI152183, R21AI139021, U01AI154659) and from the National Health and Medical Research Council of Australia. She receives Royalties from Uptodate and consulting fees from Janssen, Vertex, Biocryst, and Regeneron. She is codirector of IIID Pty Ltd that holds a patent for HLA-B*57:01 testing for abacavir hypersensitivity and has a patent pending for Detection of Human Leukocyte Antigen-A*32:01 in connection with Diagnosing Drug Reaction with Eosinophilia and Systemic Symptoms without any financial remuneration and not directly related to the submitted work. Funders played no role in any aspect of this review.

CLINICS CARE POINTS

- Underexposure of clinicians to clinical learning material showing deeply pigmented skin tones negatively impacts management of cutaneous disorders in patients with pigmented skin. This can be improved by increasing training exposure to disorders in pigmented.

- Factors that make skin pathology in pigmented skin to present differently from non-pigmented skin include the subtlety of erythema; quantity and quality of melanin and melanocytes; predilection to scarring and dyspigmentation; as well as propensity to dryness and itching.

- Although not fully characterized for cutaneous drug reactions dermoscopy and Wood's lamp are potential adjuvant tool to aid diagnosis.

- Optimization and modification of skin (immediate and delayed prick and intradermal drug allergy testing) and drug patch testing protocols may improve diagnostic sensitivity for inconclusive cases.

CONFLICT OF INTEREST

The authors have no conflict of interest to declare. Required disclaimers: (1) The opinions and assertions expressed herein are those of the author [H.B.P.] and do not reflect the official policy or position of the Uniformed Services University of the Health Sciences or the Department of Defense. (2) This work was prepared by a military or civilian employee of the US Government as part of the individual's official duties and therefore is in the public domain and does not possess copyright protection (public domain information may be freely distributed and copied; however, as a courtesy it is requested that the Uniformed Services University and the author be given an appropriate acknowledgment).

REFERENCES

1. Kurtti A, Austin E, Jagdeo J. Representation of skin color in dermatology-related Google image searches. J Am Acad Dermatol 2021;S0190-9622(21)00582-X. https://doi.org/10.1016/j.jaad.2021.03.036. Epub ahead of print.
2. Fathy R, Lipoff JB. Lack of skin of color in Google image searches may reflect under-representation in all educational resources. J Am Acad Dermatol 2021; S0190-9622(21)00981-6. https://doi.org/10.1016/j.jaad.2021.04.097. Online ahead of print.
3. Mhlaba JM, Pontes DS, Patterson SS, et al. Evaluation of a skin of color curriculum for dermatology residents. J Drugs Dermatol 2021;20(7):786–9.
4. Reilley-Luther J, Cline A, Zimmerly A, et al. Representation of Fitzpatrick skin type in dermatology textbooks compared with national percentiles. Dermatol Online J 2020;26(12).
5. Chang MJ, Lipner SR. Analysis of Skin Color on the American Academy of Dermatology Public Education Website. J Drugs Dermatol 2020;19(12):1236–7.
6. Skin of Color Society Professional Dermatology Organization | Skin Of Color Society. 2020 [Available at: https://skinofcolorsociety.org/about-socs/our-mission/.
7. Fitzpatrick TB. The validity and practicality of sun-reactive skin types I through VI. Arch Dermatol 1988;124(6):869–71.
8. Ware OR, Dawson JE, Shinohara MM, et al. Racial limitations of fitzpatrick skin type. Cutis 2020;105(2):77–80.
9. Peter J, Krause K, Staubach P, et al. Chronic urticaria and recurrent angioedema: clues to the mimics. J Allergy Clin Immunol Pract 2021;9(6):2220–8.
10. Stone C Jr, Brown NJ. Angiotensin-converting Enzyme Inhibitor and Other Drug-associated Angioedema. Immunol Allergy Clin North Am 2017;37(3):483–95.
11. Blumenthal KG, Peter JG, Trubiano JA, et al. Antibiotic allergy. Lancet 2019; 393(10167):183–98.
12. Kardaun SH, Sekula P, Valeyrie-Allanore L, et al. Drug reaction with eosinophilia and systemic symptoms (DRESS): an original multisystem adverse drug reaction. Results from the prospective RegiSCAR study. Br J Dermatol 2013;169(5): 1071–80.
13. Bastuji-Garin S, Rzany B, Stern RS, et al. Clinical classification of cases of toxic epidermal necrolysis, Stevens-Johnson syndrome, and erythema multiforme. Arch Dermatol 1993;129(1):92–6.
14. Roujeau JC. Stevens-Johnson syndrome and toxic epidermal necrolysis are severity variants of the same disease which differs from erythema multiforme. J Dermatol 1997;24(11):726–9.
15. Roujeau JC. The spectrum of Stevens-Johnson syndrome and toxic epidermal necrolysis: a clinical classification. J Invest Dermatol 1994;102(6):28S–30S.
16. Nalitye Haitembu BN, Porter MN, Basera W, et al. Pattern and impact of drug-induced liver injury in South African patients with Stevens-Johnson syndrome/ toxic epidermal necrolysis and a high burden of HIV. J Allergy Clin Immunol Pract 2021;9(12):4483–5.e1.
17. Saeed H, Mantagos IS, Chodosh J. Complications of Stevens-Johnson syndrome beyond the eye and skin. Burns 2016;42(1):20–7.
18. Peter JG, Lehloenya R, Dlamini S, et al. Severe delayed cutaneous and systemic reactions to drugs: a global perspective on the science and art of current practice. J Allergy Clin Immunol Pract 2017;5(3):547–63.
19. Halevy S, Shai A. Lichenoid drug eruptions. J Am Acad Dermatol 1993;29(2 Pt 1): 249–55.

20. Cheraghlou S, Levy LL. Fixed drug eruptions, bullous drug eruptions, and lichenoid drug eruptions. Clin Dermatol 2020;38(6):679–92.

21. Lehloenya RJ, Kgokolo M. Clinical presentations of severe cutaneous drug reactions in HIV-infected Africans. Dermatol Clin 2014;32(2):227–35.

22. Lehloenya RJ, Todd G, Mogotlane L, et al. Lichenoid drug reaction to antituberculosis drugs treated through with topical steroids and phototherapy. J Antimicrob Chemother 2012;67(10):2535–7.

23. Hotz C, Valeyrie-Allanore L, Haddad C, et al. Systemic involvement of acute generalized exanthematous pustulosis: a retrospective study on 58 patients. Br J Dermatol 2013;169(6):1223–32.

24. Roujeau JC, Bioulac-Sage P, Bourseau C, et al. Acute generalized exanthematous pustulosis. Analysis of 63 cases. Arch Dermatol 1991;127(9):1333–8.

25. Aquino M, Rosner G. Systemic contact dermatitis. Clin Rev Allergy Immunol 2019;56(1):9–18.

26. Winnicki M, Shear NH. A systematic approach to systemic contact dermatitis and symmetric drug-related intertriginous and flexural exanthema (SDRIFE): a closer look at these conditions and an approach to intertriginous eruptions. Am J Clin Dermatol 2011;12(3):171–80.

27. Bojinca VC, Bojinca M, Gheorghe M, et al. Stevens-Johnsons syndrome or drug-induced lupus - a clinical dilemma: a case report and review of the literature. Biomed Rep 2018;9(1):37–41.

28. Bataille P, Chasset F, Monfort JB, et al. Cutaneous drug-induced lupus erythematosus: clinical and immunological characteristics and update on new associated drugs. Ann Dermatol Venereol 2021;148(4):211–20. https://doi.org/10.1016/j.annder.2021.02.006.

29. Dalle Vedove C, Simon JC, Girolomoni G. Drug-induced lupus erythematosus with emphasis on skin manifestations and the role of anti-TNFalpha agents. J Dtsch Dermatol Ges 2012;10(12):889–97.

30. Stamatas GN, Kollias N. Blood stasis contributions to the perception of skin pigmentation. J Biomed Opt 2004;9(2):315–22.

31. Rawlings AV. Ethnic skin types: are there differences in skin structure and function? Int J Cosmet Sci 2006;28(2):79–93.

32. Alexis AF, Blackcloud P. Psoriasis in skin of color: epidemiology, genetics, clinical presentation, and treatment nuances. J Clin Aesthet Dermatol 2014;7(11):16–24.

33. Ruiz-Maldonado R, Orozco-Covarrubias ML. Postinflammatory hypopigmentation and hyperpigmentation. Semin Cutan Med Surg 1997;16(1):36–43.

34. Park JY, Park JH, Kim SJ, et al. Two histopathological patterns of postinflammatory hyperpigmentation: epidermal and dermal. J Cutan Pathol 2017;44(2):118–24.

35. Joly-Tonetti N, Wibawa JID, Bell M, et al. An explanation for the mysterious distribution of melanin in human skin: a rare example of asymmetric (melanin) organelle distribution during mitosis of basal layer progenitor keratinocytes. Br J Dermatol 2018;179(5):1115–26.

36. Ebanks JP, Koshoffer A, Wickett RR, et al. Epidermal keratinocytes from light vs. dark skin exhibit differential degradation of melanosomes. J Invest Dermatol 2011;131(6):1226–33.

37. Murase D, Hachiya A, Fullenkamp R, et al. Variation in Hsp70-1A expression contributes to skin color diversity. J Invest Dermatol 2016;136(8):1681–91.

38. Wesley NO, Maibach HI. Racial (ethnic) differences in skin properties: the objective data. Am J Clin Dermatol 2003;4(12):843–60.

39. Grimes PE, Bhawan J, Kim J, et al. Laser resurfacing-induced hypopigmentation: histologic alterations and repigmentation with topical photochemotherapy. Dermatol Surg 2001;27(6):515–20.
40. Smith DA, Burgdorf WH. Universal cutaneous depigmentation following phenytoin-induced toxic epidermal necrolysis. J Am Acad Dermatol 1984; 10(1):106–9.
41. Chike-Obi CJ, Cole PD, Brissett AE. Keloids: pathogenesis, clinical features, and management. Semin Plast Surg 2009;23(3):178–84.
42. Ud-Din S, Wilgus TA, Bayat A. Mast cells in skin scarring: a review of animal and human research. Front Immunol 2020;11:552205.
43. Hofs W. [Multiple keloids following "toxic epidermal necrolysis" (Lyell)]. Dermatol Wochenschr 1966;152(6):121–8.
44. Paquet P, Jacob E, Quatresooz P, et al. Delayed reepithelialization and scarring deregulation following drug-induced toxic epidermal necrolysis. Burns 2007; 33(1):100–4.
45. Lang PG Jr. Severe hypersensitivity reactions to allopurinol. South Med J 1979; 72(11):1361–8.
46. Habre M, Ortonne N, Colin A, et al. Facial scars following toxic epidermal necrolysis: role of adnexal involvement? Dermatology 2016;232(2):220–3.
47. Kavanagh GM, Page P, Hanna MM. Silicone gel treatment of extensive hypertrophic scarring following toxic epidermal necrolysis. Br J Dermatol 1994;130(4): 540–1.
48. Neiner J, Whittemore D, Hivnor C. Buried alive: functional eccrine coils buried under scar tissue? J Am Acad Dermatol 2011;65(3):661–3.
49. Thorel D, Delcampe A, Ingen-Housz-Oro S, et al. Dark skin phototype is associated with more severe ocular complications of Stevens-Johnson syndrome and toxic epidermal necrolysis. Br J Dermatol 2019;181(1):212–3.
50. Benito-Martinez S, Salavessa L, Raposo G, et al. Melanin transfer and fate within keratinocytes in human skin pigmentation. Integr Comp Biol 2021;61(4):1546–55.
51. Olteanu C, Shear NH, Chew HF, et al. Severe physical complications among survivors of stevens-johnson syndrome and toxic epidermal necrolysis. Drug Saf 2018;41(3):277–84.
52. Geisler AN, Phillips GS, Barrios DM, et al. Immune checkpoint inhibitor-related dermatologic adverse events. J Am Acad Dermatol 2020;83(5):1255–68.
53. Sutaria N, Parthasarathy V, Roh YS, et al. Itch in skin of colour: a multicentre cross-sectional study. Br J Dermatol 2021;185(3):652–4.
54. McColl M, Boozalis E, Aguh C, et al. Pruritus in black skin: unique molecular characteristics and clinical features. J Natl Med Assoc 2021;113(1):30–8.
55. Connor AM, Moshiri F. Orthognathic surgery norms for American black patients. Am J Orthod 1985;87(2):119–34.
56. Kar M, Muluk NB, Bafaqeeh SA, et al. Is it possible to define the ideal lips? Acta Otorhinolaryngol Ital 2018;38(1):67–72.
57. Isiekwe GI dO, Isiekwe MC. Lip dimensions of an adult nigerian population with normal occlusion. J Contemp Dent Pract 2012;13(2):188–93.
58. Leyden JJ, Spott DA, Goldschmidt H. Diffuse and banded melanin pigmentation in nails. Arch Dermatol 1972;105(4):548–50.
59. Nwako-Mohamadi MK, Masenga JE, Mavura D, et al. Dermoscopic Features of Psoriasis, Lichen Planus, and Pityriasis Rosea in Patients With Skin Type IV and Darker Attending the Regional Dermatology Training Centre in Northern Tanzania. Dermatol Pract Concept 2019;9(1):44–51.

60. Nirmal B. Yellow light in dermatoscopy and its utility in dermatological disorders. Indian Dermatol Online J 2017;8(5):384–5.
61. Errichetti E, Stinco G. Dermatoscopy in life-threatening and severe acute rashes. Clin Dermatol 2020;38(1):113–21.
62. Otrofanowei E, Ayanlowo OO, Akinkugbe A, et al. Clinico-etiologic profile of hand dermatitis and patch response of patients at a tertiary hospital in Lagos, Nigeria: results of a prospective observational study. Int J Dermatol 2018;57(2):149–55.
63. Yu SH, Khanna U, Taylor JS, et al. Patch testing in the African American Population: a 10-year experience. Dermatitis 2019;30(4):277–8.
64. Scott I, Atwater AR, Reeder M. Update on contact dermatitis and patch testing in patients with skin of color. Cutis 2021;108(1):10–2.
65. Hannuksela M, Salo H. The repeated open application test (ROAT). Contact Dermatitis 1986;14(4):221–7.
66. Dickel H, Bruckner TM, Erdmann SM, et al. The "strip" patch test: results of a multicentre study towards a standardization. Arch Dermatol Res 2004;296(5):212–9.

Anaphylaxis to Excipients in Current Clinical Practice

Evaluation and Management

Maria A. Bruusgaard-Mouritsen, MD[a],
Shuaib Nasser, MD, MBBS, FRCP[b], Lene H. Garvey, MD, PhD[a,c],
Matthew S. Krantz, MD[d], Cosby A. Stone Jr, MD, MPH[d,*]

KEYWORDS

- Excipient • Allergy • Polyethylene glycol • Polysorbate • Carboxymethylcellulose
- Mannitol • Povidone • Protamine

KEY POINTS

- Excipient allergy is uncommon and often missed or misdiagnosed due to lack of awareness of the need to carefully review the drug ingredients; this is particularly important when clear reactions have occurred to structurally unrelated drugs.
- The primary challenge in excipient allergy evaluation is to access drug product information and to identify ingredients most likely to be the culprits in a given reaction. It is important to consider the pretest probability, along with the limitations of the testing modality being used.
- Skin testing protocols/panels that are validated, harmonized across health care systems, and readily available are needed. In the meantime, it is recommended that future publications to the literature also provide at least some data on skin testing results from healthy controls.
- Given how uncommon these reactions are, there is a clear need for international collaborations between the allergists and immunologists who see the patients, excipient allergy researchers, and the laboratory testing industry to meet a need for confirmatory tests.

Funding Sources: Dr C.A. Stone receives funding from AHRQ/PCORI 1K12HS026395-01 and the American Academy of Allergy, Asthma and Immunology Foundation.
^a Department of Dermatology and Allergy, Allergy Clinic, Copenhagen University Hospital - Herlev and Gentofte, Hospitalsvej 8, 1st Floor, 2900 Hellerup, Copenhagen, Denmark;
^b Department of Allergy, Cambridge University Hospitals NHS Foundation Trust, Box 40, CB2 0QQ, Cambridge, UK; ^c Department of Clinical Medicine, University of Copenhagen, Denmark;
^d Division of Allergy, Pulmonary and Critical Care Medicine, Department of Medicine, Vanderbilt University Medical Center, Nashville, TN, USA
* Corresponding author. Division of Allergy, Pulmonary and Critical Care Medicine, Vanderbilt University, 1161 21st Avenue South T-1218, MCN, Nashville, TN 37232-2650.
E-mail address: cosby.a.stone@vumc.org

Immunol Allergy Clin N Am 42 (2022) 239–267
https://doi.org/10.1016/j.iac.2021.12.008
0889-8561/22/© 2021 Elsevier Inc. All rights reserved.
immunology.theclinics.com

INTRODUCTION

Excipients are inactive ingredients of drugs that are not under the same regulation as the parent drug and are used to stabilize, preserve, or enhance the pharmacokinetics, bioavailability of the active ingredients, and palatability of the preparation. In the event of a reaction to a particular drug, it is typically assumed that the reaction is due to the active ingredient, and for many drugs and drug classes that assumption is correct. However, many excipients are also potential allergens and should not be overlooked in patients with a compatible medical history (**Table 1**).

Excipient allergy is overall rare and hence often missed or misdiagnosed due to lack of awareness of the need to carefully review the drug ingredients. In addition, some excipients also have an unearned reputation for being "inert" that may cause them to be dismissed from a suspect line-up. For these reasons, excipient allergy can often be overlooked by everyone involved, despite a history of life-threatening reactions. For example, patients often have repeated anaphylaxis to bowel preparations using polyethylene glycol (PEG) before they are referred for evaluation. Further, anaphylaxis to injectable corticosteroids is typically attributed to the active ingredient but is actually more commonly caused by the excipients.

For the patient, excipient allergy can be frightening and potentially disruptive to health care delivery. It may present as multiple reactions to structurally unrelated drugs, as reactions to only some formulations or doses of a specific drug, or as reactions to drugs not usually associated with allergy such as laxatives and injectable corticosteroids. Because of variations in drug formulation that have arisen across different national health care systems and pharmacopoeias, the same allergy may also present with reactions to different drugs, in different geographic settings.

Although the underlying mechanism of anaphylaxis is not apparent in all cases of immediate excipient hypersensitivity, immunoglobulin E (IgE)–mediated anaphylaxis does seem to be the most likely and has been reported for the allergens selected in this review, which are PEGs, polysorbates, carboxymethylcellulose, mannitol, povidone, protamine, gelatin, and galactose-alpha, 1,3, galactose (alpha-gal) (**Fig. 1**, **Table 2**). The authors have also included other (PEG) derivatives such as poloxamers, due to multicenter observations from the investigators that these compounds may have cross-reactivity with PEGs. Although the authors focus on excipients to which anaphylaxis has been demonstrated repeatedly or to their potentially cross-reactive substances, this review does not exclude the possibility that other excipients with rare allergic potential (such as tromethamine[1] or hypromellose[2]) could emerge over time. As our knowledge grows, evidence for the allergenicity of an excipient should ideally pass through a sequence of initial reports, validation, and confirmation of the mechanism.

POLYETHYLENE-CONTAINING EXCIPIENTS

These excipients share the common structural feature of repeating ethylene oxide units and include PEGs, polysorbates, and poloxamers (**Fig. 2**).

Polyethylene Glycols (Macrogols)

PEGs also called macrogols, are polymers of repeating ethylene oxide units, in which the number of ethylene repeats, each weighing 44 g/mol, determines the molecular weight of the compound. The term macrogol was initially chosen to refer to the PEG used as an excipient in drugs and devices to differentiate from PEG used as an excipient in cosmetic products. The nomenclature of PEGs is based on either the number of repeating units (eg, PEG 76, as typically used in topical products) or the molecular weight 76 x 44 g/mol = PEG 3350 typically used in pharmaceutical products.[3]

Table 1	
Clinical history where excipient allergy should be considered	
Excipient	**History/Presentation**
Any excipient in general	• Repeated, severe reactions to structurally distinct drugs/products • Severe allergic reactions where allergy to the active ingredient has been excluded • Severe allergic reaction to some formulations or doses of drug, but not others • Severe, unexplained allergic reactions in relation to surgery or invasive procedures
PEG (macrogol)	• Anaphylaxis to PEG-containing bowel preparations, laxatives • Anaphylaxis to injectable corticosteroids (methylprednisolone acetate most common) • Anaphylaxis to other injectable products containing PEG • Anaphylaxis to implantable devices containing PEG • Anaphylaxis to oral tablets or effervescing tablets • Anaphylaxis to PEGylated liposomal echocardiogram contrast or other PEGylated drugs • Anaphylaxis to medroxyprogesterone acetate injections • Anaphylaxis to ultrasound gels • Allergic reactions to polysorbates or poloxamers
Polysorbate 80	• Anaphylaxis to monoclonal antibodies • Anaphylaxis to disinfectant solutions • Anaphylaxis to intraarticular depot steroids such as methylprednisolone acetate and triamcinolone acetonide • Dexamethasone-lidocaine preparations for intramuscular and intraarticular injection • Subcutaneously injected erythropoietin • Rarely, anaphylaxis to vaccines (only one confirmed case reported) • Allergic reactions to PEGs or poloxamers
Poloxamers	• Anaphylaxis to radiopharmaceuticals, bone cements • Anaphylaxis to injectable drugs containing poloxamers. • Allergic reactions to PEGs or polysorbates
Carboxymethylcellulose (Carmellose, croscarmellose, E466)	• Anaphylaxis to injectable medications (corticosteroids) • Anaphylaxis to CMC-containing barium sulfate for imaging • Anaphylaxis to other injectable products (eg, benzathine penicillin, leuprolide depot) containing CMC • Rarely, anaphylaxis to foods containing CMC • Possibly, anaphylaxis to other drugs containing CMC
Mannitol	• Anaphylaxis to 20% mannitol • Anaphylaxis to intravenous paracetamol • Less commonly, anaphylaxis to foods containing mannitol

(continued on next page)

Table 1 (*continued*)	
Excipient	**History/Presentation**
Povidone-iodine	• Anaphylaxis to intraarticular corticosteroid (paramethasone) • Anaphylaxis to oral tablets • Anaphylaxis to facial creams • Anaphylaxis to eyedrops • Anaphylaxis to topical povidone-iodine for wound antisepsis
Gelatin	• Anaphylaxis to gelatin-containing foods (marshmallows, wine gums/gummy bears, foods molded with gelatin) • Anaphylaxis to gelatin-containing vaccinations • Anaphylaxis to intraoperative colloid plasma expanders, hemostatics (gelfoams, sponges)
Alpha-gal	• Delayed onset anaphylaxis to mammal-derived meat, dairy, or gelatin • Anaphylaxis to cetuximab, infliximab, other partially humanized mAbs • Anaphylaxis to porcine-derived pancrelipase • Anaphylaxis to heparin • Anaphylaxis to gelatin-containing vaccines (MMR vaccine, varicella vaccine, varicella zoster vaccine) • Anaphylaxis to bovine collagen • Anaphylaxis to gelatin capsules and gelatin-based colloid plasma expanders

Abbreviation: mAb, monoclonal antibody.

Understanding this structural concept is crucial, because a wide variety of excipients in current use also contain chains of repeating ethylene of various lengths, such as PEG sorbitans (polysorbates), poloxamers, PEG castor oils (cremophor), and others. Cross-reactivity among polyethylene compounds is currently the most important unknown for PEG allergy, affecting our ability to advise patients on what truly needs to be avoided.

PEGs have many properties and are found in a wide variety of products. They are used as surface coating and pill binders in tablets, as the active ingredient in laxatives, and can be conjugated directly to an active ingredient to prolong or potentiate the active ingredient's mechanism of action (PEGylation). On a publicly available database of Food and Drug Administration–regulated products,[4] a focused search for PEG 3350 content (on August 17th, 2021) finds 1434 products available in the United States, of which laxatives, bowel preparations, film coated tablets, topical gels, and parenteral steroids are typical representatives. Although not strictly speaking an excipient, PEG-lipid compounds are used in messenger RNA (mRNA) technologies to construct the lipid nanoparticle carrier system. The intent is to stabilize the construct and protect those lipid microspheres from complement activation. The mRNA vaccines against COVID-19 are the first widely used vaccines using this technology.

Poloxamers

Poloxamers, as other PEG derivatives, are commonly used in pharmaceutical and cosmetic products as surfactants, stabilizers, and solubilizers.[5] Poloxamers are co-polymers arranged in a triblock structure formed by a hydrophobic central chain of

The Usual Suspects?
Allergenic Excipients Implicated in Rare Cases of Anaphylaxis

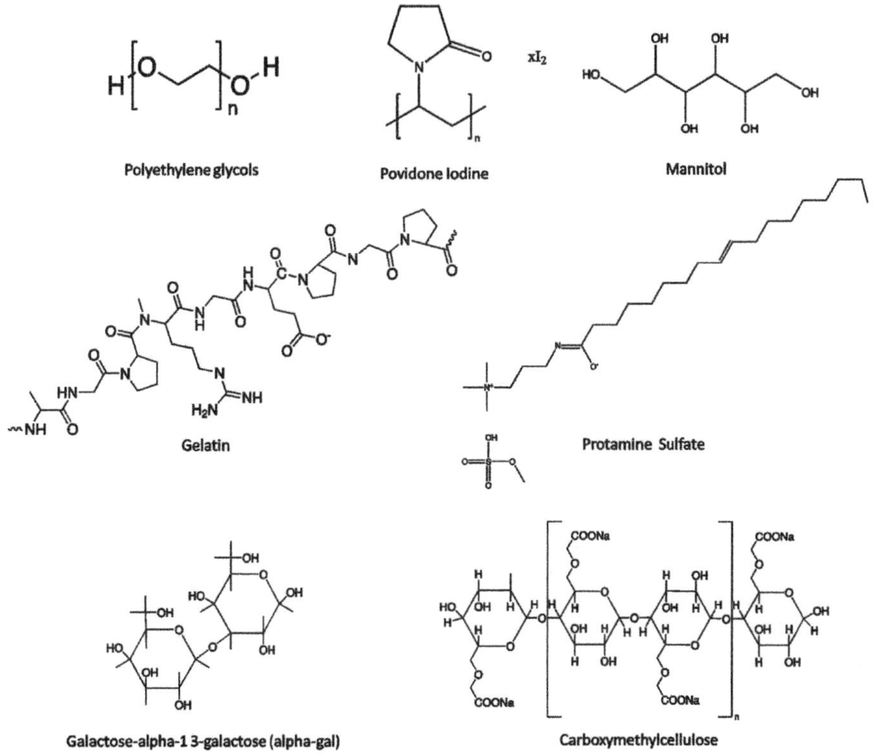

Fig. 1. Key allergenic excipients covered in this review.

polypropylene glycol surrounded by 2 hydrophilic chains of PEG[5] (see **Fig. 2**). Although there are more than 50 poloxamers with a similar chemical structure, they differ in their molecular weight (MW) due to the variable number of polypropylene glycol and PEG units. Therefore, each type of poloxamer has a different hydrophilic-lipophilic balance. Poloxamer 188 and poloxamer 407 are the most prevalent due to their great solubility in water.[6] MW vary from 1100 to 14,000 g/mol. The generic term "poloxamer" is commonly followed by a numerical value of 3 digits: the first 2 digits, multiplied $\times$ 100, indicates the MW of the hydrophobic core of propylene glycol, and the last digit, multiplied $\times$ 10, gives the percentage of the hydrophilic PEG content. Poloxamer 188 contains roughly 80% ethylene oxide repeats by weight, with two 75-repeat polyethylene chains ($\sim$6600 g/mol out of an average 8400 g/mol), and poloxamer 407 contains around 70% ethylene oxide repeats by weight, with two 98-repeat polyethylene chains ($\sim$8624 g/mol out of an average 12,600 g/mol).[7]

Polysorbates

Polysorbates are surfactants commonly used as emulsifiers, solubilizers, and stabilizers in cosmetic and pharmaceutical products as well as food agents.[8] Polysorbate

Table 2
Overview of allergy to key excipients

Excipient	Presentation	Knowns/Unknowns	Management of Proven Allergy
Polyethylene Glycol–Derived Compounds			
Polyethylene glycols (macrogols)	The most common presentations of PEG allergy are with immediate type reactions, including anaphylaxis to PEG-containing bowel preparations or laxatives,[3,37–41] or after injecting corticosteroids containing PEG as an excipient.[42–48] Patients may also present with PEG allergy after multiple drug reactions to oral tablets[41,48] or effervescing oral products containing high-molecular-weight PEGs, such as PEG 4000–20,000 range.[30] Some rarer presentations include anaphylaxis to intravenous PEGylated liposomal echocardiogram contrast,[49] medroxyprogesterone acetate injections (excipient PEG 3350),[41,50] and ultrasound gels in contact with mucous membranes (PEG 8000).[51] PEGs contained in implantable devices are potentially of concern.	• One key feature of PEG allergy is that reactivity both on skin testing and oral consumption increases with increasing length of the polyethylene chain and thereby higher molecular weight.[47,52] • A key unknown is whether a lower limit of reactivity exists, that is, if there is a point of PEG molecular weight that is universally safe for all patients with immediate hypersensitivity. Patient-specific IgG antibody binding studies previously demonstrated increase in binding as PEG molecular weight increased beyond 2000g/mol in a couple of patients.[47] • A study of skin test reactivity to PEG over time showed that the threshold for skin test reactivity increased over time on lack of exposure but that it also decreased in a few patients, possibly due to inadvertent reexposure to PEG.[52]	• Management of patients with confirmed polyethylene glycol allergy requires considerable and continued input from the treating allergist. • The patient and their provider will need to learn new skills of label reading and hunting down ingredient lists from reputable sources, such as package inserts or databases. • It is recommended that medical alert bracelets or warning cards be provided, as they can be helpful in the event of a patient's altered mental status during a time when acute treatment is needed. • Because PEGs can be encountered frequently in medical settings and with over-the-counter products, resulting in severe and life-threatening allergic reactions, it is recommended that patients be provided with epinephrine autoinjectors and trained in their use.[48]

- The length of the polyethylene chain that a patient is capable of reacting to may also determine clinical cross-reactivity with polysorbate 80 (which typically has 20 ethylene repeats and a polyethylene MW of ~880 g/mol.)
- The mechanism for PEG anaphylaxis is thought to be IgE mediated[44,53] and due to the severity of clinical reactions to PEG and risk of systemic reactions (even on SPT). A reliable in vitro test would safely differentiate patients with true PEG allergy from those with multiple drug allergies.

Poloxamers

Anaphylaxis to poloxamer has been described in the literature in 2 cases with anaphylaxis to poloxamer 238 in radiopharmaceuticals (1 case confirmed with skin testing).[54,55] Among 17 patients diagnosed with allergy to PEG (skin prick test positive to PEG 3000 and/or PEG 6000 and a clinical history of an allergic reaction to a PEG-containing product) at the Allergy Clinic at Gentofte Hospital, Denmark, 15/17 patients were positive to

- Poloxamers are likely to be skin test positive in PEG-allergic patients. The clinical relevance of this sensitization in patients who have only reacted to PEG is not clear, but poloxamer skin test reactivity seems to be related to PEG MW.
- Further, in 3 patients initially testing negative to low-MW PEGs or positive-only to high-MW PEGs (2 patients), poloxamer 407 was positive. Therefore, poloxamer 407 may be a predictor for PEG allergy, as

- Avoidance of poloxamer. Additional testing with analogue structures (PEGs and polysorbates) and management as per PEG allergy if cross-reactivity is detected.

(continued on next page)

Table 2
(continued)

Excipient	Presentation	Knowns/Unknowns	Management of Proven Allergy
	poloxamer 407 (PEG MW 4444 g/mol) at time of diagnosis. Of these, 3/15 patients have had anaphylaxis to a poloxamer-containing pharmaceutical before diagnosis, in one case presenting as a perioperative cardiac arrest after insertion of poloxamer 407–containing bone cement during hand surgery.[48] Similarly, all 4 PEG-allergic patients (PEG 3350, PEG 8000) tested to poloxamer 407 by SPT at Vanderbilt University Medical Center have tested positive (unpublished observations).	the 3 patients were positive to low-MW PEGs at retesting (**Fig. 3**) (unpublished observation).	
Polysorbates	Rarely, immediate hypersensitivity to polysorbates has been described in the literature in monoclonal antibodies, disinfectant solutions, intraarticular depot steroids such as methylprednisolone acetate and triamcinolone acetonide, dexamethasone–lidocaine preparations for intramuscular and intraarticular injection and subcutaneously injected erythropoietin.[56–58]	• Polysorbate 80 may be skin prick test positive (see **Fig. 3**) or IDT positive when sterile triamcinolone acetonide is used in PEG-allergic patients. However, the clinical relevance of this sensitization is not clear. • Although skin test reactivity may be related to MW to some extent, there seem to be other factors involved, as both polysorbate 20 and polysorbate 80 contain similar amounts of PEG (between 20–24 PEG; MW: 880 g/mol–1056 g/mol), but patients and controls test negative to polysorbate 20.	• Avoidance of relevant polysorbates until clinical reactivity can be evaluated further. Additional testing with analogue structures (PEGs and poloxamers).

- It is possible that the conformation of the molecule or perhaps the binding site between the PEG chain and the lipophilic group may be important for the allergenicity of the molecule and that the length of the PEG chain may affect reactogenicity in settings outside of the skin.

Non–polyethylene-derived compounds

| Carboxymethylcellulose (CMC) | Skin test–proven anaphylactic reactions have most commonly been associated with parenteral drugs and oral suspensions containing several CMC, for example, to injectable corticosteroids or to oral barium sulfate contrast suspensions.[30,59,60] Most of the reported cases have shown oral tolerance for CMC despite anaphylaxis on parenteral exposure. Rare cases of anaphylaxis to ice creams[61] and popsicles/ice lollies[62] due to CMC has also been reported. | • Validated skin testing protocols are needed, but patients are rare.
• Further validation of IgE testing is another area for potential improvement.
• It is unknown whether sensitized patients react to low-dose CMC–containing foods and CMC film–coated tablets or whether reactions only occur on parenteral or high-dose mucosal/enteral exposure. Most tolerate all oral exposures.
• Cross-reactivity to other methylcelluloses is not well described. One patient with anaphylaxis to hypromellose (hydroxypropylmethylcellulose) tested negative to CMC.[2] | • Because CMC is a common additive to foods and medications, it is recommended that the rare patients who react at lower doses via the oral route should be provided with an epinephrine autoinjector and counseled on strict avoidance.
• Individuals with parenteral sensitivity to CMC such as the patient in Fig. 4 who have demonstrated tolerance to small amounts of oral CMC and other celluloses such as hypromellose can be advised to read labels and avoid injectable medications and high-dose mucosal/enteral drugs containing CMC. |

(continued on next page)

Table 2
(continued)

Excipient	Presentation	Knowns/Unknowns	Management of Proven Allergy
Mannitol	Most case reports of anaphylaxis to mannitol describe reactions to intravenous infusion of 20% mannitol as treatment of raised intracranial pressure and cerebral edema.[63] However, only a few cases have been confirmed on allergy testing, so the level of certainty is low. A more recent report describes 2 patients who presented with anaphylaxis to intravenous paracetamol containing mannitol as an excipient,[64] whereas another report described a patient with anaphylaxis after oral consumption of effervescing paracetamol tablets containing mannitol and to a mannitol-based artificial sweetener.[12] This highlights that patients may react to mannitol as a "hidden" excipient. The natural occurrence of mannitol in many plants increases the risk of anaphylaxis on ingestion of certain foods in sensitized individuals; cases of anaphylaxis to pomegranate and cultivated mushrooms have been described.[63]	• Mannitol is a hidden excipient in many products and foodstuffs and natural foods. • It is likely that the allergy is simultaneously rare but also underdiagnosed. • The diagnosis should be considered in patients with intermittent episodes of urticaria, unexplained anaphylaxis, or confirmed allergic reactions to seemingly unrelated products. • Two of the well-investigated cases of mannitol allergy describes reactions to both tablet and natural foods/food supplements[12,63] and 2 cases with anaphylaxis to intravenous administration of mannitol both reported intolerance to mushrooms.[64]	• Avoidance of mannitol in both food and medications.

Povidone	Povidone anaphylaxis has been described after intraarticular injections of corticosteroids[65] oral tablets,[66] facial creams,[66] eyedrops[67] and topical povidone-iodine swabs for wound antiseptics.[68]	• Patients allergic to povidone may be cross-reactive to crospovidone (called E1202 when used in food according to the European Directive on food additives). Therefore, SPT with crospovidone should be performed.[66] • Although iodine-containing, povidone is not cross-reactive with radiocontrast materials.	• Patients should be instructed in avoidance of povidone by label-checking products and should receive an allergy warning card with povidone (and crospovidone) and relevant synonyms listed and an adrenaline autoinjector.[66]
Protamine	Anaphylaxis to protamine typically presents at reversal of heparin-anticoagulation during open-heart surgery or with insulin injections.[69] In one case series of 3 patients who developed anaphylaxis during cardiac surgery, all 3 patients were taking long-acting insulins containing protamine as an excipient, which was the likely source of allergic sensitisation.[70] Previous investigators had also suggested that sensitization to protamine occurs through insulin injections.[71,72] The incidence of allergic or anaphylactic reactions to protamine in patients on protamine-containing insulins is reported to be 0.6% to 2%.[73,74]	• It was previously thought that protamine allergy might be associated with fish allergy or with vasectomy, but this now seems to be untrue.	• In those who are allergic to protamine, avoidance of protamine during cardiac surgery anticoagulation reversal and the use of non–protamine-containing insulins are the mainstays of management. • Desensitization to NPH insulin has been reported, in the event that alternative insulins are not available. • However, it is unclear whether this also results in desensitization to protamine.[75]

(continued on next page)

Table 2
(continued)

Excipient	Presentation	Knowns/Unknowns	Management of Proven Allergy
Gelatin	A typical gelatin-allergic patient will present with reactions that are rapid in onset and overtly related to gelatin such as gelatin-containing foods (marshmallows, wine gums/gummy bears, foods molded within gelatin) or medications (vaccinations, capsules, intraoperative hemostatics, or gelatin-based colloids).[35] The pattern of sensitization and time to reaction is thought to be more like a typical food allergy and unrelated to tick bites, unless alpha-gal allergy is an underlying reason/contributing factor for the gelatin allergy.	• It is not currently clear how often gelatin allergy exists independently of alpha-gal allergy, as they are frequently found together.[76] • It is also unclear whether individual patients might be sensitized to one type of mammalian gelatin but tolerate others.	• Avoidance of gelatin, test for alpha-gal allergy. • Because gelatin can be found in unexpected places, it is recommended that patients read labels and carry an epinephrine autoinjector. • Fish-based gelatins can be used as an alternative in those with mammalian gelatin allergy.

| Alpha-gal | A typical alpha-gal patient presents with delayed-onset of what is normally associated with immediate IgE type hypersensitivity reactions (urticaria, angioedema, diarrhea, shortness of breath, anaphylaxis) in relation to oral intake of red meat, dairy, or gelatin.[23] Parenteral exposure, however, results in rapid onset symptoms.[23,25,29,36] Most alpha-gal patients do not react to dairy, and even fewer will react to gelatin.[23] Cofactors for reactions include exercise, alcohol, and nonsteroidal anti-inflammatory medications.[23] Prior to more recent widespread awareness of alpha-gal allergy in endemic areas,[77] many patients carried a diagnosis for years as idiopathic anaphylaxis or intermittent urticaria/angioedema.[78] Because of the delayed onset of symptoms, one hallmark for which alpha-gal should be considered is allergic reactions that awaken patients from sleep (due to consumption of meat with the evening meal prior to going to bed.) | • Active drugs and excipients that contain alpha-gal due to processes that use mammalian ingredients are slowly becoming clearer from translational studies using patient serum or monoclonal IgE specific for alpha-gal.[79]
• Concern for alpha-gal contamination of other mammalian-derived excipients beyond gelatin needs to be proved and would be very rare to precipitate reactions at a minimum.
• Further, the degree to which any one alpha-gal–containing drug can precipitate a reaction in an individual patient is less clear.
• Content of alpha-gal does not always guarantee a reaction in a patient, and cofactors such as alcohol may be necessary to elicit reactions in some cases.
• Beyond this, patient-specific factors for these contextually driven responses remain unknown.
• Other red meat allergies, such as those mediated by specific IgE to mammalian albumin, may not have the same drug cross-reactivity patterns observed in alpha-gal. | • Most alpha-gal patients do not react to the small amounts of alpha-gal contained in gelatin-containing products or dairy products, which means they do not have to avoid these ingredients orally.
• The risk increases, however, when drugs are delivered parenterally or have a higher alpha-gal content or with cofactors.
• When there is no treatment alternative, skin testing with observed drug challenge before drug use has been used as a strategy,[27] along with drug desensitization.[80] |

Abbreviation: NPH, neutral protamine Hagedorn; SPT, skin prick test.

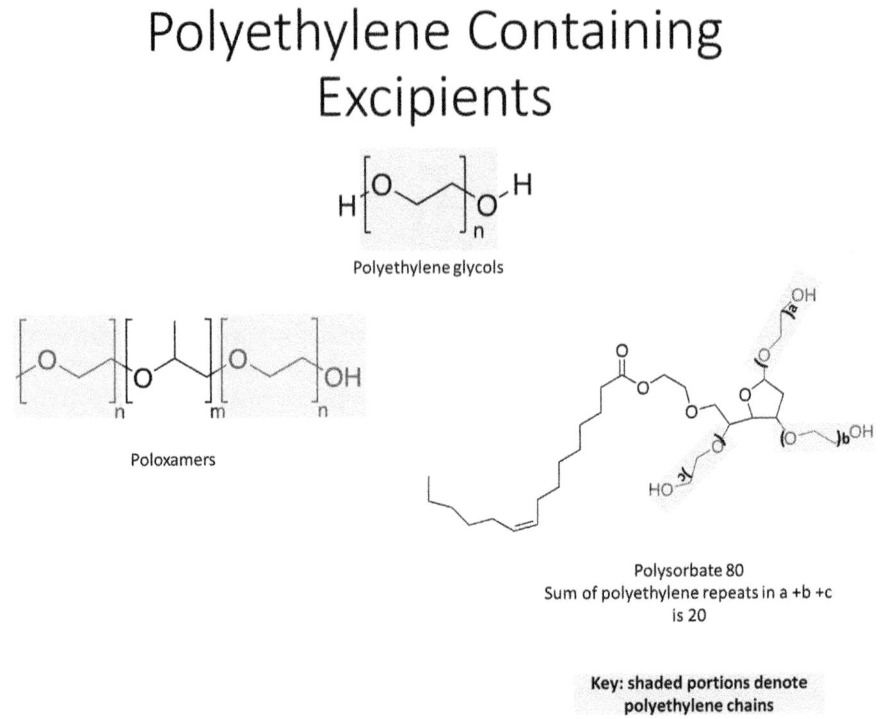

Polyethylene Containing Excipients

Polyethylene glycols

Poloxamers

Polysorbate 80
Sum of polyethylene repeats in a +b +c
is 20

Key: shaded portions denote
polyethylene chains

Fig. 2. Key polyethylene containing excipients: the polyethylene glycols, poloxamers, and polysorbates.

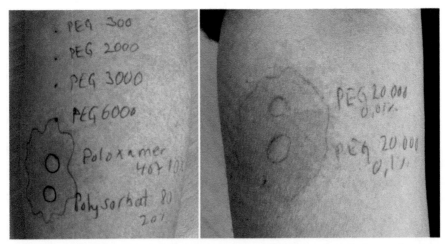

Fig. 3. Skin prick test results in patient diagnosed 2 weeks after anaphylaxis to a depot steroid injection containing PEG 3350. Note that SPT is negative to PEG 6000 and lower MW, but positive to polysorbate 80, poloxamer 407 and PEG 20.000 at 0.01% and 0.1% solution. Patient consent obtained. SPT, skin prick test.

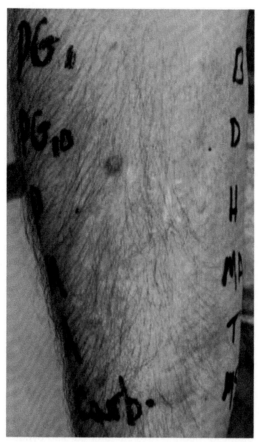

Fig. 4. Positive intradermal skin testing to carboxymethylcellulose (Carb), in a patient with anaphylaxis to triamcinolone injection containing carboxymethylcellulose (T), with otherwise negative corticosteroid testing. Patient consent obtained.

80 has been used in vaccines and biological pharmaceutical drugs for years, although only one case of anaphylaxis linked with polysorbate 80 in a vaccine had ever been reported before this becoming a concern during the COVID pandemic,[9,10] suggesting it is a rare allergen. Polysorbates are derived from pegylated sorbitan esterified with a lipophilic group of fatty acids, for example, lauric acid in the case of polysorbate 20 or in the case of polysorbate 80, oleic acid[8] (see **Fig. 2**). The generic term "polysorbate" is followed by a number, for example, 20, 40, 60, or 80. This number represents not the number of repeating ethylene oxide units but qualitatively the lipophilic group associated with the pegylated sorbitan portion. Polysorbates such as polysorbate 80 have 20 to 24 PEG units linked to the lipophilic group of fatty acids with a PEG MW between 880 g/mol and 1056 g/mol.

NONPOLYETHYLENE-DERIVED EXCIPIENTS
Carboxymethylcellulose (E466—Europe, Carmellose/Croscarmellose—Australia and Asia, Cellulose Gum—Many Countries)

Carboxymethylcellulose (CMC) is an organic polysaccharide compound derived from cellulose via an alkali-catalyzed reaction with chloroacetic acid.[11] CMC is found as an ingredient in film-coated tablets, ophthalmic drops, oral suspensions, foods, and as a stabilizer for some injectable, parenteral drugs. It is confusing for patients and physicians alike that different regions have different names for CMC.

Mannitol

Mannitol is a sugar occurring naturally in many plants, fruits, vegetables, and fungi. Medical uses include inducing osmotic diuresis, reducing raised intracranial or intraocular pressure and as an inhalational irritant used in bronchial inhalational challenge to assess airway hyperreactivity. It is used as a food additive labeled E421 according to the European Directive on food additives[12] and as a low calorie sweetener due to poor intestinal absorption.[13] Mannitol is also used as an inactive ingredient in a wide variety of tablets where it functions as a sweetener, diluent, tonicity agent, and a bulking agent. In addition, it is used in anticoagulant blood bags as part of the red cell preservative.[4]

Povidone

Povidone is also known as polyvinylpyrrolidone or when used in food, E1201 according to the European Directive on food additives. It is a hydrophilic polymer originally developed as a plasma expander. Povidone is currently used in medications as a synthetic vehicle for suspension and dispersal of drugs, in other tablets as a binder and disintegrator, as povidone-iodine in skin disinfectants used before surgery and wound antiseptic solutions, as a lubricant in ophthalmic solutions (including eye drops and contact lenses) and in cosmetic products, and as a food additive.[4] A common myth of patients and health care providers is cross-reactivity between povidone and radiocontrast dyes. There is no relationship.

Protamine

Protamine is a highly cationic peptide historically derived from salmon spermatozoa but now produced primarily through recombinant technologies. Protamine is administered as an active agent for heparin reversal after cardiac bypass surgery. It is also used in various preparations of intermediate duration insulins (such as neutral protamine Hagedorn insulin) as an excipient that slows insulin absorption, but not in newer fast or long-acting insulins.[4,14] Protamine is not used as an excipient outside of insulin preparations.[4]

Gelatin

Gelatin is an animal-derived product made by denaturing collagen from mammal/fish skins and bones using heat and dilute acids or bases. As an excipient, its intended role is to stabilize the active ingredients or to comprise the bulk of an oral drug–containing tablet, capsule, or chewable candy/wine gum formulations. As an active ingredient, gelatin has use in topically and intraoperatively applied hemostatic drugs.[15] Gelatin is found in topical gelatin-based hemostatic products containing porcine[16–19] or bovine[18–21] gelatin. It is also found in gelatin-containing vaccines.[9]

Alpha-Gal

Galactose-alpha-1,3 galactose (alpha-gal) is a disaccharide added by alpha 1,3 galactosyl transferase to the surface of nonprimate mammalian cell membranes and cellular synthesized peptides. Because many drugs contain mammalian derived active or inactive ingredients, alpha-gal can be considered an unintended excipient allergen.

Alpha-gal allergy is found in many countries all over the world and is related to the bite of endemic ticks that produce sensitization due to the presence of alpha-gal in their salivary glands and gut.[22,23] Patients may (but will not always) recall an inflamed tick bite in the weeks or months preceding the onset of their alpha-gal symptoms and can also occasionally experience recall urticaria at the site of the bite during a subsequent reaction to alpha-gal.[24] In terms of drugs, alpha-gal allergen is found in products with mammal-derived ingredients or manufacturing processes using mammalian cell lines, such as cetuximab,[25] infliximab,[26] porcine-derived pancrelipase,[27] heparin,[28] MMR vaccine,[29] varicella vaccine,[30] bovine collagen,[31,32] gelatin capsules,[33,34] and gelatin-based colloid plasma expanders.[35] Varicella zoster vaccine was previously found to contain alpha-gal,[36] in a version that is no longer commercially available in the United States. Because of the use of mammalian ingredients and mammalian cell lines in pharmaceutical manufacturing processes, and a large number of affected patients in endemic areas, there is currently an unmet need to evaluate drugs more widely for this allergen in both the preapproval and postmarketing phases.

OVERALL MANAGEMENT OF EXCIPIENT ALLERGY

In general, patients with a proven excipient allergy need to be adequately educated on the name of their allergen, its potential cross-reactivities, how to read medication and food labels including the presence of different nomenclature used in different countries (eg, CMC), how to risk assess and identify their target allergen within a product, and how to engage their families and health care providers in keeping them safe. Epinephrine autoinjectors are recommended for excipients that are difficult to avoid and when the index reaction is severe. Wallet cards or medical alert bracelets can protect patients from unintentional medical exposures in the event of altered mental status. Key times at which a patient is at highest risk of exposure include health care encounters with new providers or interactions in which new medications will be given (the operating theater, provider from a new specialty becoming involved in the patient's care, during hospital admissions). Consultation with the allergist in these situations can reduce patient's and nonallergy provider's anxiety, while improving safety.

Recently, 2 cases of anaphylaxis to mRNA COVID vaccines (which use a PEG 2000 lipid nanoparticle) have been reported in patients with subsequently confirmed PEG 2000 lipid emulsion. Routine PEG skin testing for all reactors seems to be low yield and may delay subsequent doses, as most cases of immediate hypersensitivity seem to be non-IgE mediated. However, select higher risk patients whose history suggests a preexisting PEG allergy, those with severe immediate mRNA vaccine reactions, or those who refuse immunization without skin testing may still benefit from testing to PEG.

LIMITATIONS AND BARRIERS TO OPTIMAL EXCIPIENT ALLERGY MANAGEMENT

When considering the need to test for an excipient allergy, there are some key elements and limitations that currently need to be accounted for.

First, the differences across health care systems are myriad. The primary challenge in even evaluating *the possibility* of an excipient allergy is knowing how to access the necessary information in the drug product information and to identify ingredients most likely to be allergenic. Once the ingredient list has been located, it is then important to remember that requirements to declare the inactive ingredients of the drug, the amounts, and molecular weights (especially with PEGs) may vary geographically. Another barrier at this stage is that there can be many synonyms and cross-reactive compounds (eg, PEG is often called macrogol when it is used in medicines due to a naming convention, and the poloxamers and polysorbates also contain PEGs of varying lengths). Therefore, it is important to determine all possible names by which an

Table 3
Quantity/concentrations of excipients used in the literature and by investigators for allergy testing

Excipient	Notes on Testing	Skin Prick Test (SPT)	Intradermal	Blood Testing Modalities	Oral Challenge in Skin Test Negative Patients
Polyethylene-Derived Compounds					
Polyethylene glycols of various molecular weights (300–20,000)	• Testing strategies to assess the possibility of PEG allergy (see **Fig. 3**) are under active study, with investigators recently reporting the utility of using PEGs of the highest molecular weight possible as a key feature for improving clinical sensitivity when SPT to lower MW are negative.[52] • Cross-reactivity to polysorbate 80 and poloxamers, which share long chains of repeating ethylenes can possibly be determined by skin testing. • Translation of skin test cross-reactivity into clinical cross-reactivity on drug challenge remains to be determined. • Titrated SPT must be performed stepwise and with caution, as systemic reactions can be induced. • When PEG allergy is suspected, the patient should ideally be skin prick tested with the suspected culprit product, low-MW PEGs (PEG 300, PEG 2000) and with higher MW (PEG 3000 and PEG 6000), and the PEG derivatives poloxamer 407 and polysorbate 80 due to possible cross-sensitization. If SPT is positive, the diagnosis is confirmed. • If SPT with low-MW PEGs is negative but clinical suspicion is strong, SPT with high-MW PEGs (PEG 20,000 0.1–200 mg/mL in stepwise, increasing concentrations) is recommended. If SPT is positive, the diagnosis is confirmed (see **Fig. 3**). • Once SPT is positive, further testing with higher MW PEGs is not necessary, as this may induce systemic reactions due to the increasing allergenicity in increasing MW PEGs.	• See Bruusgaard et al. as primary reference.[52] Initial test with PEG 300 (1000 mg/mL), 2000 (500 mg/mL), 3000 (500 mg/mL), and 6000 (500 mg/mL) increasing to PEG 20,000 in 10-fold step increases from 0.1 up to 200 mg/mL. Testing is stopped on reaching a positive test • Gentofte Allergy Clinic, Denmark (unpublished data) > 600 negative controls on PEG 300, 3000, and 6000, > 200 negative controls on PEG 2000 and > 30 negative controls on PEG 20,000 in aforementioned concentrations	• Not routinely performed, sterile-grade reagents not available. • Anaphylaxis has been reported.	• Under research[47,49,53]	
Polyethylene glycol 3350 (using commercially available OTC products)		• 1.7–170 mg/mL when starting from 17 gm packet mixed with 100 cc sterile water	• Not routinely performed, unless sterile-grade reagents are available. • Anaphylaxis has been reported.		Challenges using Gaviscon (alginic acid) double action tablets (20,000)[41] Open titrated challenges using PEG 3350[45] 850 mg oral challenge, using 5 mL of 170 mg/mL concentration has been used by investigators

Excipient	Notes on Testing	Skin Prick Test (SPT)	Intradermal
			(Krantz, Stone) after 1st dose mRNA vaccine anaphylaxis, before 2nd dose vaccine attempt.[81] Note: common side effect of sticky mouth sensation.
Methylprednisolone acetate (PEG 3350 containing)	• 0.4 mg/mL, 4mg/mL of methylprednisolone acetate can be used[47] but not enough evidence on irritant doses.	• 0.4 mg/mL, 4 mg/mL	• If SPT is continuously negative, IDT or graded challenges can be considered.[52] • The use of intradermal corticosteroid preparations containing PEG 3350 and polysorbate 80 has been reported in some cases[47] but may come with a risk of irritant responses when the steroids are used in the range of 1–10 mg/mL.
Poloxamer 407	• Not routinely performed, sterile-grade reagents not available	• 100 mg/mL[21] • Gentofte Allergy Clinic, Denmark > 600 negative controls	
Poloxamer 188	• Not routinely performed, sterile-grade reagents not available	• 100 mg/mL • Gentofte Allergy Clinic, Denmark > 10 negative controls	
Polysorbate 80	• Not routinely performed, sterile-grade reagents not available	• 200 mg/mL[21] • Gentofte Allergy Clinic, Denmark > 600 negative controls	
Triamcinolone acetonide (contains polysorbate 80)	• 0.1 mg/mL, 1mg/mL of triamcinolone acetonide can be used[47] but not enough evidence on irritant doses.	• 0.1 mg/mL, 1 mg/mL	

(continued on next page)

Table 3
(continued)

Excipient	Notes on Testing	Skin Prick Test (SPT)	Intradermal	Blood Testing Modalities	Oral Challenge in Skin Test Negative Patients
Non–polyethylene-derived compounds					
Carboxymethylcellulose	• Skin testing concentrations have not been validated, but skin prick testing can be performed using CMC powder dissolved in saline. • Certain medications, such as eye drops containing CMC as the only ingredient, along with injectable corticosteroids containing CMC, have been useful in the investigators' experience (**Fig. 4**). • Specific IgE testing has been used in a research capacity and seems to have potential utility.[60]	• Skin prick tests using technique with CMC powder dissolved in saline • Skin prick tests with undiluted CMC single-ingredient eye drops • Gentofte Allergy Clinic, Denmark > 600 negative controls with eyedrops 10 mg/mL	• No published protocols. • Use sterile products containing CMC. (**Fig. 5** shows testing using sterile CMC eye drops) 3 healthy controls, not enough information on irritant doses.	• Under research[60]	• Oral challenges have been performed using 10 mg, 30 mg oral doses.[61]
Triamcinolone acetonide (contains carboxymethylcellulose)		• 0.1 mg/mL, 1 mg/mL	• 0.1 mg/mL, 1mg/mL of triamcinolone acetonide can be used[47] but not enough evidence on irritant doses.		
Mannitol	• Skin testing has been positive in a few of the published cases with a clear history suggesting allergy to mannitol. • Tests performed using a 1:10 (20 mg/mL) or 1:100 (2 mg/mL) dilution of 200 mg/mL mannitol for intradermal testing. • The severity of clinical reactions, skin test positivity and tryptase increase in one case[64] suggests an IgE-mediated mechanism, and this has been confirmed by the demonstration of mannitol-specific IgE in one report.[63]	• 2 mg/mL, 20 mg/mL[82] • Gentofte Allergy Clinic, Denmark > 400 negative controls on 150 mg/mL	• 2 mg/mL, 20 mg/mL[12,82]	• Under research[63]	• Oral challenges eliciting symptoms have been performed using oral mannitol laxative[12]

Povidone	• Testing can be performed by SPT which has been used safely in several reports. • In the investigators' experience, a commercially available eyedrop containing 50 mg/mL povidone has tested positive in one case and negative in 475 controls. • Intradermal testing and specific IgE against povidone havebeen used.[83,84]	• 50 mg/mL skin prick test has been used[66] • Gentofte Allergy Clinic, Denmark > 400 negative controls	• 50 mg/mL povidone iodine (aqueous solution) diluted 1:100 with normal saline (0.5 mg/mL) has been used, 1 negative control.[84]	• Under research[83]
Protamine	• Skin prick testing to protamine can be performed at concentrations that are similar to NPH insulin (300–350 μg/mL) diluted from stock protamine 10 mg/mL, with intradermal testing in a range of 0.3–30 μg/mL.[14] • Protamine seems nonirritant at 10 mg/mL for skin prick testing and up to 0.01 mg/mL for intradermal testing.[70] • It is important to note that skin sensitization without signs of overt allergy to insulin injections may occur in diabetics, although it is not known whether this poses a risk of anaphylaxis when high-dose intravenous protamine is administered during cardiac surgery. • Antibody testing to detect serum-specific IgG and IgE has also been reported and is commercially available.[85] • Testing strategies that consider the possibility of reactivity to insulin itself along with other insulin ingredients such as meta-Cresol are recommended.	• 10 mg/mL	• 0.01 mg/mL. Potentially irritant at higher concentrations.	• Under research[85] • Commercially available

(continued on next page)

Table 3
(continued)

Excipient	Notes on Testing	Skin Prick Test (SPT)	Intradermal	Blood Testing Modalities	Oral Challenge in Skin Test Negative Patients
Gelatin	• Skin prick testing using commercially available food-grade gelatin diluted with saline to a concentration of 1 g/mL as per current allergy practice parameters (see **Fig. 5**). • Bovine and porcine specific IgE testing can be helpful confirmatory tests. • Patients can sometimes demonstrate specific IgE sensitization to one form of mammalian gelatin but not the other,[29,36] but in practice they should be considered cross-reactive due to lack of information on whether this has clinical significance and labeling that does not report gelatin source.	• 1 g/mL using food-grade gelatin has been used.	• Not typically done, since sterile-grade reagent is preferable.	• Specific IgE testing is com-mercially available • Positivity sometimes varies by gelatin (bovine, porcine)	• Oral challenge can be performed in those with unlikely allergy.
Galactose-alpha-1,3-galactose	• The diagnosis of alpha-gal allergy primarily relies on the presence of serum-specific IgE directed against alpha-gal in patients with a characteristic reaction history. • When trying to determine whether alpha-gal is the culprit behind an individual patient's reaction to a drug, academic centers in endemic areas have used strategies including skin testing, drug alpha-gal IgE binding assays, basophil activation, and drug and food challenges.	• Beef, pork, lamb skin prick tests using standardized reagents at 1:20 wt/vol have been used[85]	• Intradermal tests sometimes used in research setting[86]	• Mainstay of diagnostic testing is positive serum-specific IgE in a patient with likely history.[87,88]	• Oral challenges using sausage patties have been performed to elicit or rule out symptoms.[89] • Pork kidneys have very high content, used in some centers.[90]

Abbreviation: NPH, neutral protamine Hagedorn.

excipient can be labeled. Because generic drugs containing the same active ingredient are frequently manufactured by multiple competing companies, it is also crucial to recognize that inactive ingredients may vary at the level of the manufacturer or even different doses of the same drug preparation. All these barriers are most easily overcome by the use of comprehensive databases on approved drug formulation that can be accessible to the practitioner. In future directions, access to such databases should be standardized within national health care systems, with the possibility of transnational databases of drug formulations over time.

Second, it is important to consider the characteristics of the patient being tested, along with the limitations of the testing modality being used. True excipient allergy patients are rare but patients reporting "allergy" to multiple drugs are common. Standardized skin test protocols and excipient panels are useful in the authors' experience and continuously being refined. Further information on nonirritant concentrations will evolve with time and experience. However, it is also difficult to set up an excipient panel in a small clinic/office. Many practices may not deem that such a panel is needed, as the number of positive tests will be very low, whereas the requirement to perform such testing in specialized centers is higher. Toward that end, skin testing protocols/panels that are validated and readily available are needed in the future. In the meantime, it is recommended that future publications to the literature also provide data on skin testing results from healthy controls. The authors have provided such data, when available, for test protocols suggested in this article (**Table 3**).

Third, there are not many excipient allergies for which ex vivo testing approaches are commercially available or widely used, alpha-gal and gelatin allergy being the key exceptions. Although scientific reports have shown promise in this area for further

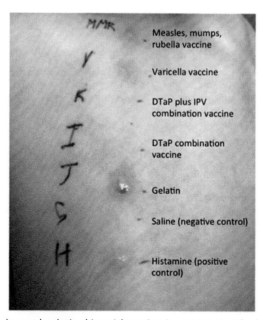

Fig. 5. Positive vaccine and gelatin skin prick testing in a patient with alpha-gal allergy and a reaction to gelatin containing vaccines. (*Modified from* Stone CA Jr, Commins SP, Choudhary S, Vethody C, Heavrin JL, Wingerter J, Hemler JA, Babe K, Phillips EJ, Norton AE. Anaphylaxis after vaccination in a pediatric patient: further implicating alpha-gal allergy. J Allergy Clin Immunol Pract. 2019 Jan;7(1):322-324.e2; with permission.)

excipients, there is a need for scalable collaborations between excipient allergy researchers and the laboratory testing industry to meet this need for confirmatory tests. In future directions, testing modalities that can screen drugs for key allergens before market approval or as a postmarketing safety step will be invaluable. A hope is that in the future, standardized excipient allergy quantification would lead to comprehensive databases that clearly reveal the presence, molecular weight (if applicable), and quantity of key allergens in the drug.

SUMMARY

In conclusion, excipient allergies are uncommon but underrecognized reactions that are potentially fatal; this is due largely to a limited awareness of these ingredients as allergens, the challenges in ascertaining drug ingredients within and across health care systems, the ubiquity of many of these ingredients in otherwise innocuous or important drugs, and the variable nature of allergic responses within sensitized individuals. To answer these challenges, management should focus on increased awareness and recognition, clearly confirming the diagnosis, educating patients and other health care providers about their allergy, teaching patients how to search ingredient lists, and careful avoidance in collaboration with their providers. Knowledge about the sensitization pathways, epidemiology, and host risk is paramount, and international collaboration to obtain large cohorts to study will be essential. The work of such collaborations should focus on standardized skin testing and validation of confirmatory ex vivo tests and encourage readily available access to national drug formularies with information on both active and inactive ingredients.

CONFLICTS OF INTEREST

None to disclose.

CLINICS CARE POINTS

- Cross-reactivity between PEGs, polysorbate 80 and poloxamers, which share long chains of repeating ethylene oxide units can possibly be determined by skin testing, but the clinical relevance of skin test cross-reactivity is currently unknown, and ingestion challenge is considered the gold standard.

- Individuals with parenteral sensitivity to CMC who have demonstrated tolerance to small amounts of oral CMC and other celluloses such as hypromellose can be advised to read labels and avoid injectable medications and high-dose mucosal/enteral drugs containing CMC.

- Because CMC is a common additive to foods and medications, it is recommended that the rare patients who react at lower doses by the oral route should be provided with an epinephrine autoinjector and counseled on strict avoidance.

- In those who are allergic to protamine, avoidance of protamine during cardiac surgery anticoagulation reversal and the use of nonprotamine-containing insulins are the mainstays of management.

- Patients with mammalian gelatin allergy should undergo testing for alpha-gal allergy.

REFERENCES

1. Lukawska J, Mandaliya D, Chan AWE, et al. Anaphylaxis to trometamol excipient in gadolinium-based contrast agents for clinical imaging. J Allergy Clin Immunol Pract 2019;7(3):1086–7.

2. Munk SJ, Heegaard S, Mosbech H, et al. Two episodes of anaphylaxis following exposure to hydroxypropyl methylcellulose during cataract surgery. J Cataract Refract Surg 2013;39(6):948–51.

3. Wenande E, Garvey LH. Immediate-type hypersensitivity to polyethylene glycols: a review. Clin Exp Allergy 2016;46(7):907–22.

4. Medicine USNLo. Daily Med. Daily Med Web site. Published 2021. Accessed 8-17-2021, 2021.

5. Dumortier G, Grossiord JL, Agnely F, et al. A review of poloxamer 407 pharmaceutical and pharmacological characteristics. Pharm Res 2006;23(12):2709–28.

6. Urban-Morlan Z, Castro-Rios R, Chavez-Montes A, et al. Determination of poloxamer 188 and poloxamer 407 using high-performance thin-layer chromatography in pharmaceutical formulations. J Pharm Biomed Anal 2008;46(4):799–803.

7. Singh-Joy SD, McLain VC. Safety assessment of poloxamers 101, 105, 108, 122, 123, 124, 181, 182, 183, 184, 185, 188, 212, 215, 217, 231, 234, 235, 237, 238, 282, 284, 288, 331, 333, 334, 335, 338, 401, 402, 403, and 407, poloxamer 105 benzoate, and poloxamer 182 dibenzoate as used in cosmetics. Int J Toxicol 2008;27(Suppl 2):93–128.

8. Jones MT, Mahler HC, Yadav S, et al. Considerations for the Use of Polysorbates in Biopharmaceuticals. Pharm Res 2018;35(8):148.

9. Stone CA Jr, Rukasin CRF, Beachkofsky TM, et al. Immune-mediated adverse reactions to vaccines. Br J Clin Pharmacol 2019;85(12):2694–706.

10. Badiu I, Geuna M, Heffler E, et al. Hypersensitivity reaction to human papillomavirus vaccine due to polysorbate 80. BMJ Case Rep 2012;2012.

11. Tasneem M, Siddique F, Ahmad A, et al. Stabilizers: indispensable substances in dairy products of high rheology. Crit Rev Food Sci Nutr 2014;54(7):869–79.

12. Calogiuri GF, Muratore L, Nettis E, et al. Immediate-type hypersensitivity reaction to Mannitol as drug excipient (E421): a case report. Eur Ann Allergy Clin Immunol 2015;47(3):99–102.

13. Tenny S, Patel R, Thorell W. Mannitol. Treasure Island (FL): StatPearls; 2021.

14. Lee AY, Chey WY, Choi J, et al. Insulin-induced drug eruptions and reliability of skin tests. Acta Derm Venereol 2002;82(2):114–7.

15. Land MH, Piehl MD, Burks AW. Near fatal anaphylaxis from orally administered gelatin capsule. J Allergy Clin Immunol Pract 2013;1(1):99–100.

16. Khoriaty E, McClain CD, Permaul P, et al. Intraoperative anaphylaxis induced by the gelatin component of thrombin-soaked gelfoam in a pediatric patient. Ann Allergy Asthma Immunol 2012;108(3):209–10.

17. Robbins KA, Keet CA. Intraoperative anaphylaxis likely due to Gelfoam in a pediatric patient undergoing liver biopsy. Ann Allergy Asthma Immunol 2015; 114(6):531–3.

18. Spencer HT, Hsu JT, McDonald DR, et al. Intraoperative anaphylaxis to gelatin in topical hemostatic agents during anterior spinal fusion: a case report. Spine J 2012;12(8):e1–6.

19. Luhmann SJ, Sucato DJ, Bacharier L, et al. Intraoperative anaphylaxis secondary to intraosseous gelatin administration. J Pediatr Orthop 2013;33(5):e58–60.

20. Agarwal N, Spalding C, Nassef M. Life-threatening intraoperative anaphylaxis to gelatin in Floseal during pediatric spinal surgery. J Allergy Clin Immunol Pract 2015;3(1):110–1.

21. Uyttebroek A, Sabato V, Bridts CH, et al. Anaphylaxis to succinylated gelatin in a patient with a meat allergy: galactose-alpha(1, 3)-galactose (alpha-gal) as antigenic determinant. J Clin Anesth 2014;26(7):574–6.

22. Choudhary SK, Karim S, Iweala OI, et al. Tick salivary gland extract induces alpha-gal syndrome in alpha-gal deficient mice. Immun Inflamm Dis 2021;9(3): 984–90.

23. Platts-Mills TAE, Commins SP, Biedermann T, et al. On the cause and consequences of IgE to galactose-alpha-1,3-galactose: A report from the National Institute of Allergy and Infectious Diseases Workshop on Understanding IgE-Mediated Mammalian Meat Allergy. J Allergy Clin Immunol 2020;145(4):1061–71.

24. Schmidle P, Reidenbach K, Kugler C, et al. Recall urticaria-A new clinical sign in the diagnosis of alpha-gal syndrome. J Allergy Clin Immunol Pract 2019;7(2): 685–6.

25. Chung CH, Mirakhur B, Chan E, et al. Cetuximab-induced anaphylaxis and IgE specific for galactose-alpha-1,3-galactose. N Engl J Med 2008;358(11):1109–17.

26. Chitnavis M, Stein DJ, Commins S, et al. First-dose anaphylaxis to infliximab: a case of mammalian meat allergy. J Allergy Clin Immunol Pract 2017;5(5):1425–6.

27. Stone CA Jr, Choudhary S, Patterson MF, et al. Tolerance of porcine pancreatic enzymes despite positive skin testing in alpha-gal allergy. J Allergy Clin Immunol Pract 2020;8(5):1728–1732 e1721.

28. Hawkins RB, Wilson JM, Mehaffey JH, et al. Safety of Intravenous Heparin for Cardiac Surgery in Patients With Alpha-Gal Syndrome. Ann Thorac Surg 2021; 111(6):1991–7.

29. Stone CA Jr, Commins SP, Choudhary S, et al. Anaphylaxis after vaccination in a pediatric patient: further implicating alpha-gal allergy. J Allergy Clin Immunol Pract 2019;7(1):322–324 e322.

30. Caballero ML, Krantz MS, Quirce S, et al. Hidden Dangers: Recognizing Excipients as Potential Causes of Drug and Vaccine Hypersensitivity Reactions. J Allergy Clin Immunol Pract 2021;9(8):2968–82.

31. Mullins RJ, Richards C, Walker T. Allergic reactions to oral, surgical and topical bovine collagen. Anaphylactic risk for surgeons. Aust N Z J Ophthalmol 1996; 24(3):257–60.

32. Takahashi H, Chinuki Y, Tanaka A, et al. Laminin gamma-1 and collagen alpha-1 (VI) chain are galactose-alpha-1,3-galactose-bound allergens in beef. Allergy 2014;69(2):199–207.

33. Vidal C, Mendez-Brea P, Lopez-Freire S, et al. Vaginal Capsules: An Unsuspected Probable Source of Exposure to alpha-Gal. J Investig Allergol Clin Immunol 2016;26(6):388–9.

34. Muglia C, Kar I, Gong M, et al. Anaphylaxis to medications containing meat byproducts in an alpha-gal sensitized individual. J Allergy Clin Immunol Pract 2015; 3(5):796–7.

35. Serrier J, Khoy K, Ollivier Y, et al. Recurrent anaphylaxis to a gelatin-based colloid plasma substitute and to cetuximab following sensitisation to galactose-alpha-1,3-galactose. Br J Anaesth 2021;126(6):e200–2.

36. Stone CA Jr, Hemler JA, Commins SP, et al. Anaphylaxis after zoster vaccine: Implicating alpha-gal allergy as a possible mechanism. J Allergy Clin Immunol 2017;139(5):1710–1713 e1712.

37. Shah S, Prematta T, Adkinson NF, et al. Hypersensitivity to polyethylene glycols. J Clin Pharmacol 2013;53(3):352–5.

38. Gachoka D. Polyethylene Glycol (PEG)-Induced Anaphylactic Reaction During Bowel Preparation. ACG Case Rep J 2015;2(4):216–7.

39. Anton Girones M, Roan Roan J, de la Hoz B, et al. Immediate allergic reactions by polyethylene glycol 4000: two cases. Allergol Immunopathol (Madr) 2008;36(2): 110–2.

40. Pizzimenti S, Heffler E, Gentilcore E, et al. Macrogol hypersensitivity reactions during cleansing preparation for colon endoscopy. J Allergy Clin Immunol Pract 2014;2(3):353–4.

41. Sellaturay P, Nasser S, Ewan P. Polyethylene Glycol-Induced Systemic Allergic Reactions (Anaphylaxis). J Allergy Clin Immunol Pract 2021;9(2):670–5.

42. Sohy C, Vandenplas O, Sibille Y. Usefulness of oral macrogol challenge in anaphylaxis after intra-articular injection of corticosteroid preparation. Allergy 2008;63(4):478–9.

43. Bordere A, Stockman A, Boone B, et al. A case of anaphylaxis caused by macrogol 3350 after injection of a corticosteroid. Contact Dermatitis 2012;67(6):376–8.

44. Wenande EC, Skov PS, Mosbech H, et al. Inhibition of polyethylene glycol-induced histamine release by monomeric ethylene and diethylene glycol: a case of probable polyethylene glycol allergy. J Allergy Clin Immunol 2013; 131(5):1425–7.

45. Brandt N, Garvey LH, Bindslev-Jensen U, et al. Three cases of anaphylaxis following injection of a depot corticosteroid with evidence of IgE sensitization to macrogols rather than the active steroid. Clin Transl Allergy 2017;7:2.

46. Dewachter P, Mouton-Faivre C. Anaphylaxis to macrogol 4000 after a parenteral corticoid injection. Allergy 2005;60(5):705–6.

47. Stone CA Jr, Liu Y, Relling MV, et al. Immediate Hypersensitivity to Polyethylene Glycols and Polysorbates: More Common Than We Have Recognized. J Allergy Clin Immunol Pract 2019;7(5):1533–1540 e1538.

48. Bruusgaard-Mouritsen MA, Johansen JD, Garvey LH. Clinical manifestations and impact on daily life of allergy to polyethylene glycol (PEG) in ten patients. Clin Exp Allergy 2021;51(3):463–70.

49. Krantz MS, Liu Y, Phillips EJ, et al. Anaphylaxis to PEGylated liposomal echocardiogram contrast in a patient with IgE-mediated macrogol allergy. J Allergy Clin Immunol Pract 2020;8(4):1416–1419 e1413.

50. Lu IN, Rutkowski K, Kennard L, et al. Polyethylene glycol may be the major allergen in depot medroxy-progesterone acetate. J Allergy Clin Immunol Pract 2020;8(9):3194–7.

51. Jakubovic BD, Saperia C, Sussman GL. Anaphylaxis following a transvaginal ultrasound. Allergy Asthma Clin Immunol 2016;12:3.

52. Bruusgaard-Mouritsen MA, Jensen BM, Poulsen LK, et al. Optimizing investigation of suspected allergy to polyethylene glycols. J Allergy Clin Immunol 2021; 149(1):168–75.

53. Zhou ZH, Stone CA Jr, Jakubovic B, et al. Anti-PEG IgE in anaphylaxis associated with polyethylene glycol. J Allergy Clin Immunol Pract 2021;9(4):1731–1733 e1733.

54. Carbonell A, Escudero AI, Miralles JC, et al. Anaphylaxis Due to Poloxamer 238. J Investig Allergol Clin Immunol 2018;28(6):419–20.

55. Skanjeti A, Darcissac C, Jaulent C, et al. Grade 3 anaphylactic shock after administration of [(99m)Tc]-labeled nanocolloidal albumin (Nanocoll((R))) for sentinel node scintigraphy. Eur J Nucl Med Mol Imaging 2019;46(6):1214–5.

56. Wenande E, Kroigaard M, Mosbech H, et al. Polyethylene glycols (PEG) and related structures: overlooked allergens in the perioperative setting. A A Case Rep 2015;4(5):61–4.

57. Bergmann KC, Maurer M, Church MK, et al. Anaphylaxis to Mepolizumab and Omalizumab in a Single Patient: Is Polysorbate the Culprit? J Investig Allergol Clin Immunol 2020;30(4):285–7.

58. Steele RH, Limaye S, Cleland B, et al. Hypersensitivity reactions to the polysorbate contained in recombinant erythropoietin and darbepoietin. Nephrology (Carlton). 2005;10(3):317–20.
59. Muroi N, Nishibori M, Fujii T, et al. Anaphylaxis from the carboxymethylcellulose component of barium sulfate suspension. N Engl J Med 1997;337(18):1275–7.
60. Dumond P, Franck P, Morisset M, et al. Pre-lethal anaphylaxis to carboxymethylcellulose confirmed by identification of specific IgE–review of the literature. Eur Ann Allergy Clin Immunol 2009;41(6):171–6.
61. Brockow K, Bauerdorf F, Kugler C, et al. Idiopathic" anaphylaxis caused by carboxymethylcellulose in ice cream. J Allergy Clin Immunol Pract 2021;9(1):555–557 e551.
62. Ohnishi A, Hashimoto K, Ozono E, et al. Anaphylaxis to Carboxymethylcellulose: Add Food Additives to the List of Elicitors. Pediatrics 2019;143(3).
63. Hegde VL, Venkatesh YP. Anaphylaxis to excipient mannitol: evidence for an immunoglobulin E-mediated mechanism. Clin Exp Allergy 2004;34(10):1602–9.
64. Jain SS, Green S, Rose M. Anaphylaxis following intravenous paracetamol: the problem is the solution. Anaesth Intensive Care 2015;43(6):779–81.
65. Gonzalo Garijo MA, Duran Quintana JA, Bobadilla Gonzalez P, et al. Anaphylactic shock following povidone. Ann Pharmacother 1996;30(1):37–40.
66. Bruusgaard-Mouritsen MA, Mortz C, Winther L, et al. Repeated idiopathic anaphylaxis caused by povidone. Ann Allergy Asthma Immunol 2021;126(5):598–600.
67. Liccioli G, Mori F, Barni S, et al. Anaphylaxis to Polyvinylpyrrolidone in Eye Drops Administered to an Adolescent. J Investig Allergol Clin Immunol 2018;28(4):263–5.
68. Gray PE, Katelaris CH, Lipson D. Recurrent anaphylaxis caused by topical povidone-iodine (Betadine). J Paediatr Child Health 2013;49(6):506–7.
69. Kim R. Anaphylaxis to protamine masquerading as an insulin allergy. Del Med J 1993;65(1):17–23.
70. Valchanov K, Falter F, George S, et al. Three Cases of Anaphylaxis to Protamine: Management of Anticoagulation Reversal. J Cardiothorac Vasc Anesth 2019;33(2):482–6.
71. Chu YQ, Cai LJ, Jiang DC, et al. Allergic shock and death associated with protamine administration in a diabetic patient. Clin Ther 2010;32(10):1729–32.
72. Levy JH, Adkinson NF Jr. Anaphylaxis during cardiac surgery: implications for clinicians. Anesth Analg 2008;106(2):392–403.
73. Levy JH, Schwieger IM, Zaidan JR, et al. Evaluation of patients at risk for protamine reactions. J Thorac Cardiovasc Surg 1989;98(2):200–4.
74. Levy JH, Zaidan JR, Faraj B. Prospective evaluation of risk of protamine reactions in patients with NPH insulin-dependent diabetes. Anesth Analg 1986;65(7):739–42.
75. Bollinger ME, Hamilton RG, Wood RA. Protamine allergy as a complication of insulin hypersensitivity: A case report. J Allergy Clin Immunol 1999;104(2 Pt 1):462–5.
76. Mullins RJ, James H, Platts-Mills TA, et al. Relationship between red meat allergy and sensitization to gelatin and galactose-alpha-1,3-galactose. J Allergy Clin Immunol 2012;129(5):1334–1342 e1331.
77. Iglesia EGA, Stone CA Jr, Flaherty MG, et al. Regional and temporal awareness of alpha-gal allergy: An infodemiological analysis using Google Trends. J Allergy Clin Immunol Pract 2020;8(5):1725–1727 e1721.

78. Carter MC, Ruiz-Esteves KN, Workman L, et al. Identification of alpha-gal sensitivity in patients with a diagnosis of idiopathic anaphylaxis. Allergy 2018;73(5): 1131–4.
79. Campbell E, Peebles RJ, Stone C Jr, et al. Evaluation of Alpha Gal in Vaccines and Medications using a Human Monoclonal IgE Antibody. J Allergy Clin Immunol 2021;147(2). AB7.
80. Garcia-Menaya JM, Cordobes-Duran C, Gomez-Ulla J, et al. Successful Desensitization to Cetuximab in a Patient With a Positive Skin Test to Cetuximab and Specific IgE to Alpha-gal. J Investig Allergol Clin Immunol 2016;26(2):132–4.
81. Krantz MS, Bruusgaard-Mouritsen MA, Koo G, et al. Anaphylaxis to the first dose of mRNA SARS-CoV-2 vaccines: Don't give up on the second dose. Allergy 2021; 76(9):2916–20.
82. Biro P, Schmid P, Wuthrich B. [A life-threatening anaphylactic reaction following mannitol]. Anaesthesist 1992;41(3):130–3.
83. Ronnau AC, Wulferink M, Gleichmann E, et al. Anaphylaxis to polyvinylpyrrolidone in an analgesic preparation. Br J Dermatol 2000;143(5):1055–8.
84. Preuss JF, Goddard CE, Clarke RC, et al. Anaphylaxis to intravenous paracetamol containing povidone. A case report and narrative review of excipient allergy related to anaesthesia. Anaesth Intensive Care 2020;48(5):404–8.
85. Weiss ME, Nyhan D, Peng ZK, et al. Association of protamine IgE and IgG antibodies with life-threatening reactions to intravenous protamine. N Engl J Med 1989;320(14):886–92.
86. Commins SP, Satinover SM, Hosen J, et al. Delayed anaphylaxis, angioedema, or urticaria after consumption of red meat in patients with IgE antibodies specific for galactose-alpha-1,3-galactose. J Allergy Clin Immunol 2009;123(2):426–33.
87. Mabelane T, Basera W, Botha M, et al. Predictive values of alpha-gal IgE levels and alpha-gal IgE: Total IgE ratio and oral food challenge-proven meat allergy in a population with a high prevalence of reported red meat allergy. Pediatr Allergy Immunol 2018;29(8):841–9.
88. Brestoff JR, Zaydman MA, Scott MG, et al. Diagnosis of red meat allergy with antigen-specific IgE tests in serum. J Allergy Clin Immunol 2017;140(2): 608–610 e605.
89. Commins SP. Diagnosis & management of alpha-gal syndrome: lessons from 2,500 patients. Expert Rev Clin Immunol 2020;16(7):667–77.
90. Morisset M, Richard C, Astier C, et al. Anaphylaxis to pork kidney is related to IgE antibodies specific for galactose-alpha-1,3-galactose. Allergy 2012;67(5): 699–704.

Mas-Related G Protein–Coupled Receptor-X2 and Its Role in Non-immunoglobulin E–Mediated Drug Hypersensitivity

Chalatip Chompunud Na Ayudhya, DDS, DScD[a],*, Hydar Ali, PhD[b],*

KEYWORDS

- MRGPRX2 • Mast cells • Drug hypersensitivity • Anaphylaxis

KEY POINTS

- Mas-related G protein–coupled receptor-X2 (MRGPRX2) is a receptor expressed predominantly in skin mast cells that functions as a receptor for endogenous ligands such as antimicrobial peptides and defensins. It is also activated by a diverse group of cationic peptides and injectable drugs as well as small molecules such as fluoroquinolones, neuromuscular blocking drugs, and opioids and has been implicated in non-immunoglobulin E (IgE)-mediated drug hypersensitivity reactions.
- Because MRGPRX2 is highly expressed in human skin mast cells, it likely participates in local cutaneous, injection-site reactions. However, whether its activation is capable of triggering systemic reactions to drugs remains unclear.
- Enhanced MRGPRX2 expression and/or function associated with certain conditions (ie, inflammatory skin diseases, mastocytosis, and genetic polymorphisms) may make the receptor more responsive to drug agonists in those individuals.
- Comprehensive analysis of MRGPRX2 polymorphisms, expression, and function could provide a novel standard of care for the diagnosis and prevention of non-IgE–mediated drug hypersensitivity.

INTRODUCTION

Drug hypersensitivity reactions (DHRs) are adverse responses that result from exposure to drugs at therapeutic doses, which pose concerns regarding their safety and potential clinical use.[1–3] Mast cells (MCs) are the main effector cells in allergic reactions. On activation, MCs release a diverse range of biologically active mediators, which contribute to the clinical manifestations of allergy and anaphylaxis.[4,5] It is well

[a] Department of Oral Diagnosis, Faculty of Dentistry, Naresuan University, Phitsanulok 65000, Thailand; [b] Department of Basic and Translational Sciences, University of Pennsylvania, School of Dental Medicine, Philadelphia, PA 19104, USA
* Corresponding authors.
E-mail addresses: chalatipc@nu.ac.th (C.C.N.A.); alih@upenn.edu (H.A.)

Immunol Allergy Clin N Am 42 (2022) 269–284
https://doi.org/10.1016/j.iac.2021.12.003
0889-8561/22/© 2021 Elsevier Inc. All rights reserved.
immunology.theclinics.com

documented that most DHRs involve immunoglobulin E (IgE)/high-affinity IgE receptor (FcεRI)-mediated MC activation. This pathway requires an initial allergen sensitization in order to generate antigen-specific IgE. Reexposure to the same or a cross-reactive antigen results in the cross-linking of specific IgE bound to FcεRI on MC surfaces, which subsequently triggers their degranulation.[6] Interestingly, some individuals develop allergic reactions even without prior exposure to particular allergens. For example, neuromuscular blocking drugs (NMBDs), among the most common drugs responsible for anaphylaxis during general anesthesia, may cause hypersensitivity reactions in NMBD-naïve patients.[7–10] These findings indicate that DHRs can also be mediated via IgE-independent pathways. More recently, IgG-mediated neutrophil activation has been shown to participate in DHRs to certain NMBDs.[11,12]

A novel G protein–coupled receptor (GPCR) known as Mas-related GPCR-X2 (MRGPRX2) has recently been identified as a receptor responsible for non-IgE/IgG-mediated DHRs.[13] It is well documented that MRGPRX2 is expressed at high level in skin and fat MCs with low and variable level of expression in gut and lung MCs.[14–19] Expression of MRGPRX2 has also been reported on basophils and eosinophils but what function they perform remains the subject of controversy.[20,21] Several groups of therapeutic drugs, such as NMBDs, antibiotics, opiates/opioids, and iodinated contrast media, activate MCs via MRGPRX2.[7,13,22,23] More recently, antidepressants clomipramine, paroxetine, and desipramine have been identified as MRGPRX2 agonists.[24] Since the identification of MrgprB2 as the mouse ortholog of human MRGPRX2,[13] there has been an explosion in research related to its potential role in DHRs, providing a paradigm shift in MC biology.

MRGPRX2 is low-affinity receptor, which allows for its interaction with diverse cationic ligands. Skin MCs of all individuals likely express MRGPRX2 but the incidence of DHRs is very low. In this review, the authors first describe the list of drugs that activate MCs via MRGPRX2 and discuss the evidence for and against its role in DHRs. The potential risk factors and evaluation for suspected MRGPRX2-mediated DHRs as well as future directions on MRGPRX2 research are proposed.

DRUGS THAT ACTIVATE HUMAN MAST CELLS VIA MAS-RELATED G PROTEIN–COUPLED RECEPTOR-X2
Antibiotics

Fluoroquinolones
Fluoroquinolones (ie, ciprofloxacin, moxifloxacin, levofloxacin, ofloxacin) are a group of antibiotics that differ according to their spectra of activity based on their side chains. Because of their high potency, favorable bioavailability, and various drug formulations, fluoroquinolones are widely used for treatment of several bacterial infections, especially respiratory and urinary tract infections.[25,26] However, the incidence of hypersensitivity reactions to these antibiotics has been increasing over the past few decades. Currently, they are the second most common antibiotic class associated with new DHRs.[26–28]

Giavina-Bianchi and colleagues[29] reported a case of a patient with systemic mastocytosis who developed several episodes of anaphylaxis to *hymenoptera* venom and ciprofloxacin. Interestingly, specific IgE and skin test results were negative, suggesting that anaphylactic reaction that developed in this patient could be mediated through a non-IgE mechanism. Recently, fluoroquinolones have been shown to activate MCs via MRGPRX2.[13,30–32] They induce Ca^{2+} mobilization in HEK293 cells ectopically expressing MRGPRX2 but not naïve HEK293 cells.[13,30] Fluoroquinolones also trigger degranulation in human MC line LAD2 cells[13,30,31] as well as CD34+-

derived human MCs[32,33] that endogenously express MRGPRX2, and these responses are significantly attenuated in *MRGPRX2* knockdown cells.[13,30–33] Of note, there are differences between the fluoroquinolones in terms of their tendency to cause MRGPRX2 activation. Ciprofloxacin, which is more commonly associated with non-IgE–mediated MC activation, has the lowest EC_{50} value for MRGPRX2 activation (6.8 µg/mL) when compared with others.[13]

Fluoroquinolones induce degranulation of mouse peritoneal MCs (PMCs) via MrgprB2 (mouse ortholog of human MRGPRX2).[13,30] Furthermore, they evoke anaphylactoid reactions, now referred to as non-IgE–mediated MC activation, as measured by increased local vascular permeability and decrease in body temperature in wild-type (WT) but not in MrgprB2$^{-/-}$ mice.[13,30] These findings indicate that MRGPRX2 could participate in fluoroquinolone-induced immediate hypersensitivity reactions.

Vancomycin
Vancomycin is a glycopeptide antibiotic mainly used to treat severe, life-threatening gram-positive bacterial infections that are unresponsive to other antibiotics such as methicillin-resistant *Staphylococcus aureus* infections.[34,35] The most common adverse reaction is vancomycin infusion reaction, manifested as pruritic erythematous rash of the face, neck, and upper torso and are associated with elevated plasma histamine[36]; this was previously known as "red man syndrome" and is caused by rapid infusion of vancomycin (1 g or higher doses infused in <60 min).[37,38] This phenomenon occurs in 4% to 50% of infected patients treated with intravenous vancomycin, with higher risk of severe reactions in patients younger than 40 years.[39]

Vancomycin induces Ca^{2+} mobilization in HEK293 cells stably expressing MRGPRX2 but not in untransfected cells.[40,41] It also causes degranulation in LAD2 cells via MRGPRX2.[7,40] Notably, a recent study demonstrated that the lowest concentration of vancomycin that induces a positive skin response in drug-naïve individuals was 100 µg/mL, whereas all subjects had a positive reaction at the concentration of 1 mg/mL.[42] These findings are consistent with previously reported MC degranulation responses in vitro.[7] Because vancomycin induces IgE-independent degranulation of human skin MCs,[43] which highly express the MRGPRX2,[44] it is likely that positive skin responses to this drug occurs through MRGPRX2 rather than FcεRI. However, skin testing response with vancomycin does not always correlate with the severity of vancomycin infusion reaction following systemic administration[45]: this could reflect low levels of MRGPRX2 expression in lung and gut MCs when compared with skin MCs.[18,44] It is still worth noting that there is variability in the occurrence of the infusion reaction to vancomycin, which is a characteristic of non-IgE–mediated MC activation. Further studies are therefore needed to clarify the relevance of MRGPRX2 activation in vancomycin-induced hypersensitivity reactions.

Neuromuscular Blocking Drugs

Atracurium, cisatracurium, and mivacurium
NMBDs are routinely used in surgery to reduce involuntary muscle movement and to facilitate intratracheal intubation. However, they are responsible for nearly 60% of perioperative anaphylaxis, posing a serious challenge for clinicians.[46] Although thought to be mostly IgE/FcεRI-mediated, some individuals experience allergic reactions even without prior exposure to these drugs, suggesting the involvement of alternative mechanisms.[47,48] Recently, MRGPRX2 has been identified as a target for NMBD-induced MC activation associated with hypersensitivity reactions.[10,13,49]

Atracurium, cisatracurium, and mivacurium provoke Ca^{2+} mobilization in HEK293 cells expressing MRGPRX2 and induce degranulation in LAD2 cells in an MRGPRX2-dependent manner.[7,13,50–52] Furthermore, a recent study demonstrated that atracurium induces degranulation via MRGPRX2 in primary human MCs.[33] All 3 drugs induce degranulation in murine PMCs via MrgprB2.[13,50,51] Intraplantar injection of cisatracurium and mivacurium induces local cutaneous swelling and inflammation in WT mice but these responses are substantially reduced in MrgprB2$^{-/-}$ mice.[50,51] Furthermore, intravenous injection of mivacurium leads to a decrease in body temperature in WT mice but not MrgprB2$^{-/-}$ mice.[51]

Interestingly, despite causing degranulation, cisatracurium and mivacurium do not induce chemokine production in LAD2 cells.[50,51] Therefore, it is possible that wheal and flare reactions to intradermal injection of atracurium, cisatracurium, and mivacurium may reflect degranulation responses of human skin MCs, which express high levels of MRGPRX2.[11,53,54] Patients with chronic spontaneous urticaria (CSU) who displayed increased MRGPRX2 expression on skin MCs showed exaggerated skin reactions to atracurium when compared with those of healthy controls.[55] By contrast, systemic effects of these drugs might in fact be a result of IgE- and IgG-mediated immune cell activation, rather than the activation of MRGPRX2.[11,12]

Rocuronium

Rocuronium is associated with a higher risk of anaphylaxis when compared with other NMBDs.[56–58] Several patients with rocuronium-induced perioperative anaphylaxis displayed positive intradermal skin test result, despite demonstrating both negative drug-specific IgE and basophil activation test (BAT), suggesting non-IgE–mediated mechanisms.[9,59] McNeil and colleagues[13] demonstrated that rocuronium induces Ca^{2+} mobilization in transfected HEK293 cells expressing MRGPRX2 and MrgprB2 with EC_{50} values of 261.3 and 22.2 µg/mL, respectively. They also showed that rocuronium causes degranulation in murine PMCs via MrgprB2.[13] Based on these findings, it was proposed that hypersensitivity to rocuronium may result from an off-target occupancy of MRGPRX2.[9,13] However, a significant difference in the concentration of rocuronium used to activate human MRGPRX2 and mouse MrgprB2 likely reflects the fact that there is only ∼53% sequence homology between these 2 receptors.[13,60] Thus, caution should be exercised when translating data from mice to humans.

Initial studies demonstrated that although rocuronium triggered Ca^{2+} mobilization in LAD2 cells and CD34^{+}-derived human MCs, it failed to induce degranulation.[7,32,52,60] However, more recently, Chompunud Na Ayudhya and colleagues[61] provided the first demonstration that rocuronium induces degranulation in human MCs via MRGPRX2. In LAD2 cells, the minimum concentration rocuronium that induces degranulation is 500 µg/mL, and the maximum response is obtained at a concentration of 2 mg/mL. A high dose of rocuronium (2 mg/mL) also triggered degranulation in primary human skin MCs but the magnitude of this response was much lower than that observed in LAD2 cells, presumably due to the difference in MRGPRX2 expression levels between cell types.[61] These findings suggest that positive skin reactions to irritating concentrations of rocuronium (1 mg/mL and 10 mg/mL) previously reported[9,59] likely represent normal skin MC activation via MRGPRX2 and are unrelated to hypersensitivity reaction.[11,61]

A recent clinical study revealed 3 single nucleotide polymorphisms (SNPs) in MRGPRX2 allele (M196I, L226P, and L237P) of a patient with rocuronium-induced anaphylaxis.[59] The investigators suggested that these mutations would enhance receptor affinity and responsiveness to rocuronium.[59] However, a follow-up study by Chompunud Na Ayudhya and colleagues,[61] failed to demonstrate enhanced response to rocuronium in cells expressing MRGPRX2 variants when compared with cells expressing the normal receptor. Therefore, other mechanisms, possibly involving IgG and neutrophils, could participate in rocuronium hypersensitivity.[11,12,62]

Opiates and Opioids

Opiates (eg, morphine and codeine—of which the active CYP2D6 generated metabolite is morphine) and their synthetic counterparts, opioids, are important analgesics that provide effective and immediate pain relief. However, these drugs induce severe DHRs in susceptible individuals. Local reactions to opiates and opioids are manifested as urticaria, skin rash, and contact dermatitis at the injection site.[63] These signs and symptoms likely result from MC-derived mediators.[64,65] Although IgE/FcεRI pathway may be involved in some rare cases,[66] these drugs were previously thought to trigger direct MC degranulation via an IgE-independent, unknown mechanism.[64,65]

MRGPRX2 has recently been identified as an atypical opioid receptor for both synthetic and endogenous opioids.[7,60,67] Unlike classic opioid receptors, which are preferentially activated by levorotatory ligands, MRGPRX2 displays ~10-fold higher potency to dextro-enantiomers.[60] Opioid agonists (morphine, TAN-67, and dynorphin A(1–13)) induce robust Ca^{2+} mobilization and degranulation in LAD2 cells via MRGPRX2-dependent manner. By contrast, classic opioid agonists (salvinorin A, BW373U86, and DAMGO), which do not activate MRGPRX2, are unable to induce MC degranulation.[60] In addition, naloxone, an opioid antagonist, has no effect on the ability of opioids to activate MRGPRX2.[60] These findings are in line with the clinical observations that morphine and structurally similar analgesics induce pruritus,[68] vasodilation, and hypotension that is poorly reversed by naloxone.[69,70]

Intriguingly, morphine selectively causes degranulation and mediator release from human skin MCs but not from human lung, heart, or intestinal MCs.[16,71,72] Because human skin MCs constitutively express MRGPRX2 but not opioid receptors,[15] it is highly likely that MRGPRX2 mediates opioid-induced MC degranulation and its activation contributes to cutaneous hypersensitivity symptoms. A recent study by Babina and colleagues[22] showed that MRGPRX2 serves as the sole opiate receptor on skin MCs. Codeine also induces human skin MC degranulation via MRGPRX2 and triggers rapid internalization of the receptor. Furthermore, prestimulation with MRGPRX2 agonists (compound 48/80 and codeine) results in unresponsiveness to subsequent stimulation by the same or other MRGPRX2 ligands (cross-desensitization).[22]

Although injection-site reactions following opioid administration are likely due to MRGPRX2-mediated skin MC activation, whether this receptor plays a role in systemic anaphylactic reactions induced by opioids remains unclear. Furthermore, it is noteworthy that some opioid-associated adverse events, such as pruritus, may be mediated via MC-independent mechanism. Evidence suggests that a subset of opioid receptor–expressing neurons in the spinal cord can be activated by opioid agonists to cause pruritus[73]; this might explain why fentanyl, which does not activate MCs nor MRGPRX2,[60,74] still induces pruritus.[75,76]

Antidepressants

Using a high-throughput Ca^{2+} mobilization screening, Wolf and colleagues[24] recently identified a novel class of cationic amphiphilic FDA-approved drugs as MRGPRX2/MrgprB2 agonists. Antidepressants clomipramine, paroxetine, and desipramine induce degranulation in LAD2 cells and primary human skin MCs. The effects of these antidepressants on MCs are MRGPRX2 specific, as CRISPR-Cas9–mediated knock-down of the receptors results in significantly reduced degranulation.[24] Moreover, intradermal injection of clomipramine to 5 healthy volunteers induce wheal-and-flare reaction, which suggests human skin MC activation via MRGPRX2. Interestingly, itch sensation was reported to be highly subjective between each individual.[24]

Clomipramine, paroxetine, and desipramine induce Ca^{2+} mobilization and degranulation in murine PMCs that endogenously express MrgprB2. Furthermore, clomipramine elicits substantial dose-dependent scratching behavior following intradermal injection in WT mice, but this response is reduced in MrgprB2$^{-/-}$ mice.[24]

Iodinated Contrast Media

Iodinated contrast media (ICM) is widely used in X ray–based imaging modalities, including computed tomography (CT) and angiography, to improve imaging resolution between tissues and enhance blood vessel visualization. ICM is administered approximately 75 million times per year globally.[77] The incidence of DHRs to ICM ranges from 0.2% to 3%.[78–80] Although mild cutaneous symptoms represent the most common ICM hypersensitivity reaction, severe anaphylaxis can occur with an estimated death rate of 1 per 100,000 administrations.[77,81]

MC-derived mediators such as histamine and tryptase have been implicated in immediate, anaphylaxis-like reactions caused by ICM.[82] However, specific IgE antibodies to ICM have rarely been detected.[83] In addition, ~30% of patients develop immediate hypersensitivity reactions at the first exposure to ICM, suggesting the involvement of IgE-independent mechanisms.[84,85] Iopamidol, a commonly used ICM, causes histamine and tumor necrosis factor alpha (TNF-α) release in LAD2 cells, but these responses are significantly reduced in cells small interfering RNA–mediated knockdown of MRGPRX2.[23] Furthermore, compared with WT mice, MC-deficient mice and MrgprB2$^{-/-}$ mice exhibit a reduced hindpaw inflammation.[23]

Other ICM such as meglumine amidotrizoate (100 mg/mL) and iomeprol (350 mg/mL) also induce MC degranulation, but the concentrations of the drugs that activate MCs are much higher than those usually administered to patients.[7] In addition, a clinical study in Korean population identified 8 MRGPRX2 SNPs in patients with ICM anaphylaxis.[86] However, there were no statistically significant differences in these SNPs between those with ICM anaphylaxis and the general population.[86] Thus, further studies are required to determine the molecular basis and mechanism of ICM-mediated DHRs.

Other Drugs

Icatibant, a bradykinin B2 receptor antagonist used for the treatment of hereditary angioedema, elicits injection-site erythema and swelling in almost every patient.[87] However, evidence that it induces systemic anaphylactic responses is lacking.[88,89] Icatibant induces degranulation in human and murine MCs via MRGPRX2 and MrgprB2, respectively.[13] Furthermore, icatibant induces paw inflammation in vivo in WT mice but not in MrgprB2$^{-/-}$ mice.[13] These findings suggest that the injection-site reactions to icatibant are mediated via the activation cutaneous MCs through MRGPRX2. Its inability to induce systemic response likely reflects the relatively low level of MRGPRX2 expression in lung and gut MCs.[18,44]

Sinomenine is a natural alkaloid derived from the medicinal plant Sinomenium acutum that is mainly used for the treatment of rheumatoid arthritis.[90,91] However, synovial MCs express MRGPRX2.[92] Evidence shows that sinomenine induces degranulation and cytokine/chemokine secretion (ie, TNF-α, monocyte chemoattractant protein 1, interleukin-8, and macrophage inflammatory protein 1 beta) in LAD2 cells via MRGPRX2 and causes paw edema in mice via MrgprB2.[90]

RISK FACTORS FOR MRGPRX2-MEDIATED DRUG HYPERSENSITIVITY
Combination of cofactors

During general anesthesia, several drugs, including opioids, NMBDs, and antibiotics are administered to the same patient simultaneously. Because these drugs have been described to trigger IgE-independent MC activation via MRGPRX2, it is likely that the combination of cofactors may have a cumulative effect sufficient to activate the receptor to elicit degranulation; this could explain why some individuals develop DHRs during the first administration of the drug. Of note, it should also be noted that certain drugs may cause IgE-mediated anaphylaxis without previous exposure due to cross-reactivity between specific allergenic epitopes, such as substituted ammonium groups.[58,93,94]

Elevated MRGPRX2 expression and function

Upregulation of MRGPRX2 has been reported in patients with chronic inflammatory diseases, such as CSU.[44] Intradermal injection of MRGPRX2 agonists, substance P and vasoactive intestinal peptide, results in significantly larger and longer-lasting wheal reactions in patients with CSU when compared with normal subjects.[44] In addition, CSU patients showed exaggerated skin reactions to icatibant and atracurium when compared with healthy controls, presumably due to higher MRGPRX2 expression.[55] Babina and colleagues[95] recently showed that thymic stromal lymphopoietin selectively enhances MRGPRX2 but not FcεRI-mediated skin MC degranulation via signaling pathway that requires STAT5 activity. Thus, enhanced MRGPRX2 expression and/or its cross-regulation by host-derived factor may increase risk of developing MRGPRX2-mediated DHRs in other inflammatory skin diseases.

Systemic mastocytosis is a proliferative disorder characterized by abnormal accumulation of tissue MCs with or without skin involvement. Patients with systemic mastocytosis have an increased risk of anaphylaxis.[96] Giavina-Bianchi and colleagues[29] reported a case of a systemic mastocytosis patient who developed 5 episodes of anaphylaxis to insect venom and ciprofloxacin. Because mastoparan found in *Hymenoptera* venom and ciprofloxacin activate human MCs via MRGPRX2,[13] it was proposed that anaphylactic reactions found in this patient is mediated through the activation of MRGPRX2.[29] The most common cutaneous manifestation of systemic mastocytosis is termed maculopapular cutaneous mastocytosis (MPCM). Intriguingly, Deepak and colleagues[97] recently demonstrated that the number of MRGPRX2-expressing MCs are increased in cutaneous MCs of patients with MPCM when compared with a healthy subject. Thus, caution should be exercised when prescribing NMBDs and quinolones in patients with mastocytosis[98,99]; this is an emerging topic, and the association between MRGPRX2 upregulation and DHRs requires further evaluation, but it is clear that comorbidities can have a profound influence on allergic reactions.

MRGPRX2 polymorphisms

SNPs are one of the most common genetic variants found among individuals. Analysis of GPCR database (GPCRdb.com) reveals the presence of 107 missense SNPs in MRGPRX2.[100] Some of these naturally occurring missense SNPs in MRGPRX2 have been implicated in the individual differences in responses to the receptor activation.[19,101,102] Therefore, it is possible that certain MRGPRX2 variants could potentially alter the receptor expression, ligand binding affinity, and/or signaling characteristics to promote DHRs. Analysis of MRGPRX2 polymorphisms in the genome of suspected patients together with studies to determine their expression level and susceptibility to degranulation may facilitate the identification of specific MRGPRX2 variants that are involved in DHRs.

EVALUATION OF SUSPECTED MRGPRX2-MEDIATED DRUG HYPERSENSITIVITY

To date, the diagnosis of DHRs is primarily based on medical history and clinical presentation. The medical history should be carefully reviewed to determine any underlying comorbidities that may be associated with enhanced MRGPRX2 expression and/or function. Certain signs and symptoms such as immediate localized erythema, urticaria, and pruritus after receiving a putative MRGPRX2 drug agonist could suggest MRGPRX2-mediated reaction. Notably, MRGPRX2 is a low-affinity receptor. Thus, the involvement of MRGPRX2 in DHRs should be suspected only when events occur at high drug concentrations that are sufficient to activate the receptor.[36,103]

Laboratory investigations are supportive and not confirmatory for most DHRs. Current diagnostic workup for DHRs is mainly based on the detection of specific IgE to relevant causative drugs either in vivo (skin tests) or in vitro (the presence of drug-specific IgE and positive BAT).[104–106] Of these, skin tests are, by far, the most reliable and cost-effective methods for identifying IgE involvement. However, highest nonirritative dilutions recommended for skin testing are not standardized.[104] In case of positive skin reaction to irritating or undiluted concentrations without drug-specific IgE and negative BAT, this could represent an off-target direct MC degranulation via MRGPRX2, which express at high levels on skin MCs. Because basophils are unresponsive to MRGPRX2 agonists,[21,107] it has been speculated that BAT might aid in distinguishing between genuine IgE/FcεRI- and MRGPRX2-mediated DHRs.[108,109]

A novel method of mast cell activation test (MAT) using flow cytometry is a promising diagnostic that allow simultaneous analysis of IgE/FcεRI- and MRGPRX2-dependent DHRs.[110] Using MRGPRX2^{+}- and MRGPRX2^{-}-expressing MCs subpopulations may facilitate the investigation on the role and relevance of MRGPRX2 in IgE-independent DHRs. An integrated approach using skin tests, specific IgE immunoassays, BAT, MAT, and MRGPRX2-silencing experiments may enhance our understanding in the mechanisms of DHRs.

Individuals with increased risks for developing MRGPRX2-mediated DHRs should be tested for MRGPRX2 expression and response to the drugs before drug administration. Antihistamines and corticosteroids have shown some benefits for preventing and treating non-IgE DHRs.[111] Ultimately, utilization of MRGPRX2 antagonists could be favorable for management of MRGPRX2-mediated DHRs.

FUTURE DIRECTIONS

Although MRGPRX2 research has progressed rapidly in recent years and ever-increasing number of agonists have been identified, there remain unmet needs in studying the role of this receptor in DHRs. Addressing these issues will enable physicians to better understand mechanisms of DHRs caused by MRGPRX2 and may improve patient care.

SNPs in MRGPRX2 may enhance the receptor's responsiveness to drugs and thus affect the risk of anaphylactic events mediated via this receptor. However, many MRGPRX2 alleles have yet to be characterized. Also, increased MRGPRX2 expression associated with certain conditions may alter the response mediated by the receptor. Assuming that certain polymorphisms and MRGPRX2 expression levels pose a predisposing factor to DHRs, analyzing MRGPRX2 polymorphisms, expression, and function could be a novel standard of care for diagnosis and prevention of DHRs.

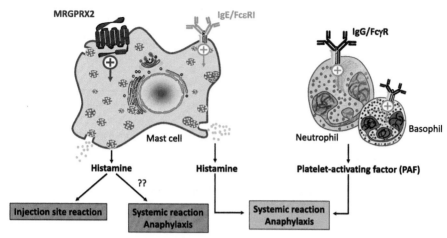

Fig. 1. Activation of skin mast cells (MCs) via MRGPRX2 leads to MC degranulation and the release of mediators including histamine. These contribute to local cutaneous hypersensitivity reactions (erythema, skin rash, and swelling) at the injection site. However, whether this pathway plays an important role in systemic reactions and anaphylaxis remains to be confirmed. Drug-induced anaphylaxis could also reflect immune response involving IgE-mediated histamine release from mast cells and IgG-mediated platelet-activating factor release from neutrophils and basophils.

MrgprB2$^{-/-}$ mice have been extensively used to study the function of MRGPRX2 in vivo. However, the concentrations of agonists needed to activate mouse MrgprB2 markedly differs from human MRGPRX2.[13] For example, although rocuronium at a concentration of 20 μg/mL causes robust degranulation in murine PMCs, ~100-fold higher concentration is needed to induce degranulation in human skin MCs.[61] Moreover, antagonists that inhibit MrgprB2 have no efficacy against MRGPRX2.[112] These antagonists challenge the translatability of animal studies to clinical data and limit our ability to elucidate the underlying mechanisms of DHRs and develop novel therapeutics. Better animal models are needed in order to overcome this issue. A humanized mouse model has been recently developed for studying MRGPRX2-mediated cutaneous DHRs.[113] However, there remain several limitations in the currently available humanized mouse models that prevent full use of these systems.

Several potential MRGPRX2 antagonists, including natural compounds, small molecules, peptides, and DNA aptamers, have been reported.[112,114–119] However, none of them have been tested in clinical trials. Developing a specific MRGPRX2 antagonist could provide a novel approach for the treatment of pseudoallergic reactions.

SUMMARY

The discovery of MRGPRX2 paves a new way to study MC biology and unlock the previous inexplicable puzzles on IgE-independent MC activation. Several FDA-approved drugs have been shown to activate MCs via MRGPRX2, resulting in the release of histamine and other mediators associated with symptoms and signs of DHRs. Although it is likely that MRGPRX2 contributes to local cutaneous reactions due to high receptor expression on skin MCs, whether its activation is capable of triggering systemic anaphylaxis remains unclear. By contrast, IgE- and IgG-mediated immune responses by MCs, basophils, and neutrophils have been implicated in anaphylaxis (**Fig. 1**). Therefore, it is possible that drug-induced anaphylaxis could be initiated by multiple mechanisms, explaining why some people are more susceptible and reactions are inconsistent in severity.

CLINICS CARE POINTS

- Several FDA-approved cationic drugs induce degranulation in human MCs via MRGPRX2, which may contribute to hypersensitivity reactions.
- MRGPRX2 upregulation associated with inflammatory skin conditions may enhance risk and severity of hypersensitivity reactions. Therefore, caution should be exercised when prescribing drugs that activate MRGPRX2 in these patients.
- Analyzing MRGPRX2 polymorphisms, expression, and function could serve as a novel standard-of-care for diagnosis and prevention of drug hypersensitivity in individuals with suspected MRGPRX2-mediated reactions.

ACKNOWLEDGEMENTS

This work was supported by National Institutes of Health grants R01-AI124182, R01-AI143185 and R01-AI149487 to Hydar Ali.

DISCLOSURE OF POTENTIAL CONFLICT OF INTEREST

The authors declare no potential conflicts of interest.

REFERENCES

1. Mayorga C, Fernandez TD, Montañez MI, et al. Recent developments and highlights in drug hypersensitivity. Allergy 2019;74(12):2368–81.
2. Castells M. Diagnosis and management of anaphylaxis in precision medicine. J Allergy Clin Immunol 2017;140(2):321–33.
3. Gomes ESR, Marques ML, Regateiro FS. Epidemiology and Risk Factors for Severe Delayed Drug Hypersensitivity Reactions. Curr Pharm Des 2019;25(36): 3799–812.
4. Metcalfe DD, Peavy RD, Gilfillan AM. Mechanisms of mast cell signaling in anaphylaxis. J Allergy Clin Immunol 2009;124(4):639–46, quiz 647-638.
5. Metz M, Maurer M. Mast cells–key effector cells in immune responses. Trends Immunol 2007;28(5):234–41.
6. Galli SJ, Tsai M. IgE and mast cells in allergic disease. Nat Med 2012;18(5): 693–704.
7. Navinés-Ferrer A, Serrano-Candelas E, Lafuente A, et al. MRGPRX2-mediated mast cell response to drugs used in perioperative procedures and anaesthesia. Sci Rep 2018;8(1):11628.
8. Ebo DG, Clarke RC, Mertes PM, et al. Molecular mechanisms and pathophysiology of perioperative hypersensitivity and anaphylaxis: a narrative review. Br J Anaesth 2019;123(1):e38–49.
9. Spoerl D, D'Incau S, Roux-Lombard P, et al. Non-IgE-Dependent Hypersensitivity to Rocuronium Reversed by Sugammadex: Report of Three Cases and Hypothesis on the Underlying Mechanism. Int Arch Allergy Immunol 2016;169(4):256–62.
10. Porebski G, Kwiecien K, Pawica M, et al. Mas-Related G Protein-Coupled Receptor-X2 (MRGPRX2) in Drug Hypersensitivity Reactions. Front Immunol 2018;9:3027.

11. Ali H. Revisiting the role of MRGPRX2 on hypersensitivity reactions to neuromuscular blocking drugs. Curr Opin Immunol 2021;72:65–71.
12. Jönsson F, de Chaisemartin L, Granger V, et al. An IgG-induced neutrophil activation pathway contributes to human drug-induced anaphylaxis. Sci Transl Med 2019;11(500).
13. McNeil BD, Pundir P, Meeker S, et al. Identification of a mast-cell-specific receptor crucial for pseudo-allergic drug reactions. Nature 2015;519(7542):237–41.
14. Tatemoto K, Nozaki Y, Tsuda R, et al. Immunoglobulin E-independent activation of mast cell is mediated by Mrg receptors. Biochem Biophys Res Commun 2006;349(4):1322–8.
15. Motakis E, Guhl S, Ishizu Y, et al. Redefinition of the human mast cell transcriptome by deep-CAGE sequencing. Blood 2014;123(17):e58–67.
16. Varricchi G, Pecoraro A, Loffredo S, et al. Heterogeneity of Human Mast Cells With Respect to MRGPRX2 Receptor Expression and Function. Front Cell Neurosci 2019;13:299.
17. Manorak W, Idahosa C, Gupta K, et al. Upregulation of Mas-related G Protein coupled receptor X2 in asthmatic lung mast cells and its activation by the novel neuropeptide hemokinin-1. Respir Res 2018;19(1):1.
18. Plum T, Wang X, Rettel M, et al. Human Mast Cell Proteome Reveals Unique Lineage, Putative Functions, and Structural Basis for Cell Ablation. Immunity 2020;52(2):404–416 e405.
19. Chen E, Chuang LS, Giri M, et al. Inflamed Ulcerative Colitis Regions Associated With MRGPRX2-Mediated Mast Cell Degranulation and Cell Activation Modules, Defining a New Therapeutic Target. Gastroenterology 2021;160(5):1709–24.
20. Wedi B, Gehring M, Kapp A. The pseudoallergen receptor MRGPRX2 on peripheral blood basophils and eosinophils: Expression and function. Allergy 2020;75(9):2229–42.
21. Sabato V, Elst J, Van Houdt M, et al. Surface expression of MRGPRX2 on resting basophils: An area of controversy. Allergy 2020;75(9):2421–2.
22. Babina M, Wang Z, Roy S, et al. MRGPRX2 Is the Codeine Receptor of Human Skin Mast Cells: Desensitization through β-Arrestin and Lack of Correlation with the FcεRI Pathway. J Invest Dermatol 2020;141(5):1286–96.e4.
23. Jiang W, Hu S, Che D, et al. A mast-cell-specific receptor mediates Iopamidol induced immediate IgE-independent anaphylactoid reactions. Int Immunopharmacol 2019;75:105800.
24. Wolf K, Kühn H, Boehm F, et al. A group of cationic amphiphilic drugs activates MRGPRX2 and induces scratching behavior in mice. J Allergy Clin Immunol 2021;48(2):506–22.e8.
25. Pham TDM, Ziora ZM, Blaskovich MAT. Quinolone antibiotics. Medchemcomm 2019;10(10):1719–39.
26. Doña I, Moreno E, Pérez-Sánchez N, et al. Update on Quinolone Allergy. Curr Allergy Asthma Rep 2017;17(8):56.
27. McGee EU, Samuel E, Boronea B, et al. Quinolone Allergy. Pharmacy (Basel) 2019;7(3).
28. Blanca-López N, Andreu I, Torres Jaén MJ. Hypersensitivity reactions to quinolones. Curr Opin Allergy Clin Immunol 2011;11(4):285–91.
29. Giavina-Bianchi P, Goncalves DG, Zanandrea A, et al. Anaphylaxis to quinolones in mastocytosis: Hypothesis on the mechanism. J Allergy Clin Immunol Pract 2019;7(6):2089–90.
30. Liu R, Hu S, Zhang Y, et al. Mast cell-mediated hypersensitivity to fluoroquinolone is MRGPRX2 dependent. Int Immunopharmacol 2019;70:417–27.

31. Han S, Lv Y, Kong L, et al. Use of the relative release index for histamine in LAD2 cells to evaluate the potential anaphylactoid effects of drugs. Sci Rep 2017;7(1): 13714.

32. Elst J, Sabato V, Faber MA, et al. MRGPRX2 and Immediate Drug Hypersensitivity: Insights from Cultured Human Mast Cells. J Investig Allergol Clin Immunol 2020;0.

33. Elst J, Maurer M, Sabato V, et al. Novel Insights on MRGPRX2-Mediated Hypersensitivity to Neuromuscular Blocking Agents And Fluoroquinolones. Front Immunol 2021;12:668962.

34. Liu C, Bayer A, Cosgrove SE, et al. Clinical practice guidelines by the infectious diseases society of america for the treatment of methicillin-resistant Staphylococcus aureus infections in adults and children: executive summary. Clin Infect Dis 2011;52(3):285–92.

35. Savoldi A, Azzini AM, Baur D, et al. Is there still a role for vancomycin in skin and soft-tissue infections? Curr Opin Infect Dis 2018;31(2):120–30.

36. McNeil BD. MRGPRX2 and Adverse Drug Reactions. Front Immunol 2021;12: 676354.

37. Rubinstein E, Keynan Y. Vancomycin revisited - 60 years later. Front Public Health 2014;2:217.

38. Alvarez-Arango S, Ogunwole SM, Sequist TD, et al. Vancomycin Infusion Reaction - Moving beyond "Red Man Syndrome". N Engl J Med 2021;384(14): 1283–6.

39. Sivagnanam S, Deleu D. Red man syndrome. Crit Care 2003;7(2):119–20.

40. Azimi E, Reddy VB, Lerner EA. Brief communication: MRGPRX2, atopic dermatitis and red man syndrome. Itch (Phila). 2017;2(1):e5.

41. Grimes J, Desai S, Charter NW, et al. MrgX2 is a promiscuous receptor for basic peptides causing mast cell pseudo-allergic and anaphylactoid reactions. Pharm Res 2019;7(6):e00547.

42. Alvarez-Arango S, Oliver E, Tang O, et al. Vancomycin immediate skin responses in vancomycin-naïve subjects. Clin Exp Allergy 2021;51(7):932–5.

43. Veien M, Szlam F, Holden JT, et al. Mechanisms of nonimmunological histamine and tryptase release from human cutaneous mast cells. Anesthesiology 2000; 92(4):1074–81.

44. Fujisawa D, Kashiwakura J, Kita H, et al. Expression of Mas-related gene X2 on mast cells is upregulated in the skin of patients with severe chronic urticaria. J Allergy Clin Immunol 2014;134(3):622–633 e629.

45. Polk RE, Israel D, Wang J, et al. Vancomycin skin tests and prediction of "red man syndrome" in healthy volunteers. Antimicrob Agents Chemother 1993; 37(10):2139–43.

46. Mertes PM, Alla F, Tréchot P, et al. Anaphylaxis during anesthesia in France: an 8-year national survey. J Allergy Clin Immunol 2011;128(2):366–73.

47. Fisher MM, Munro I. Life-threatening anaphylactoid reactions to muscle relaxants. Anesth Analg 1983;62(6):559–64.

48. Van Gasse AL, Elst J, Bridts CH, et al. Rocuronium Hypersensitivity: Does Off-Target Occupation of the MRGPRX2 Receptor Play a Role? J Allergy Clin Immunol Pract 2019;7(3):998–1003.

49. Subramanian H, Gupta K, Ali H. Roles of Mas-related G protein-coupled receptor X2 on mast cell-mediated host defense, pseudoallergic drug reactions, and chronic inflammatory diseases. J Allergy Clin Immunol 2016;138(3):700–10.

50. Che D, Rui L, Cao J, et al. Cisatracurium induces mast cell activation and pseudo-allergic reactions via MRGPRX2. Int Immunopharmacol 2018;62: 244–50.

51. Che D, Wang J, Ding Y, et al. Mivacurium induce mast cell activation and pseudo-allergic reactions via MAS-related G protein coupled receptor-X2. Cell Immunol 2018;332:121–8.

52. Fernandopulle NA, Zhang SS, Soeding PF, et al. MRGPRX2 activation in mast cells by neuromuscular blocking agents and other agonists: Modulation by sugammadex. Clin Exp Allergy 2020;51(5):685–95.

53. Mertes PM, Moneret-Vautrin DA, Leynadier F, et al. Skin reactions to intradermal neuromuscular blocking agent injections: a randomized multicenter trial in healthy volunteers. Anesthesiology 2007;107(2):245–52.

54. Levy JH, Gottge M, Szlam F, et al. Weal and flare responses to intradermal rocuronium and cisatracurium in humans. Br J Anaesth 2000;85(6):844–9.

55. Shtessel M, Limjunyawong N, Oliver ET, et al. MRGPRX2 Activation Causes Increased Skin Reactivity in Patients with Chronic Spontaneous Urticaria. J Invest Dermatol 2021;141(3):678–81.e672.

56. Petitpain N, Argoullon L, Masmoudi K, et al. Neuromuscular blocking agents induced anaphylaxis: Results and trends of a French pharmacovigilance survey from 2000 to 2012. Allergy 2018;73(11):2224–33.

57. Reddy JI, Cooke PJ, van Schalkwyk JM, et al. Anaphylaxis is more common with rocuronium and succinylcholine than with atracurium. Anesthesiology 2015; 122(1):39–45.

58. Sadleir PH, Clarke RC, Bunning DL, et al. Anaphylaxis to neuromuscular blocking drugs: incidence and cross-reactivity in Western Australia from 2002 to 2011. Br J Anaesth 2013;110(6):981–7.

59. Suzuki Y, Liu S, Kadoya F, et al. Association between mutated Mas-related G protein-coupled receptor-X2 and rocuronium-induced intraoperative anaphylaxis. Br J Anaesth 2020;125(6):e446–8.

60. Lansu K, Karpiak J, Liu J, et al. In silico design of novel probes for the atypical opioid receptor MRGPRX2. Nat Chem Biol 2017;13(5):529–36.

61. Chompunud Na Ayudhya C, Amponnawarat A, Roy S, et al. MRGPRX2 Activation by Rocuronium: Insights from Studies with Human Skin Mast Cells and Missense Variants. Cells 2021;10(1).

62. Bruhns P, Chollet-Martin S. Mechanisms of human drug-induced anaphylaxis. J Allergy Clin Immunol 2021;147(4):1133–42.

63. Golembiewski JA. Allergic reactions to drugs: implications for perioperative care. J Perianesth Nurs 2002;17(6):393–8.

64. Casale TB, Bowman S, Kaliner M. Induction of human cutaneous mast cell degranulation by opiates and endogenous opioid peptides: evidence for opiate and nonopiate receptor participation. J Allergy Clin Immunol 1984;73(6): 775–81.

65. Sheen CH, Schleimer RP, Kulka M. Codeine induces human mast cell chemokine and cytokine production: involvement of G-protein activation. Allergy 2007;62(5):532–8.

66. Harle DG, Baldo BA, Coroneos NJ, et al. Anaphylaxis following administration of papaveretum. Case report: Implication of IgE antibodies that react with morphine and codeine, and identification of an allergenic determinant. Anesthesiology 1989;71(4):489–94.

67. Ali H. Emerging Roles for MAS-Related G Protein-Coupled Receptor-X2 in Host Defense Peptide, Opioid, and Neuropeptide-Mediated Inflammatory Reactions. Adv Immunol 2017;136:123–62.
68. Kumar K, Singh SI. Neuraxial opioid-induced pruritus: An update. J Anaesthesiol Clin Pharmacol 2013;29(3):303–7.
69. Baldo BA, Pham NH. Histamine-releasing and allergenic properties of opioid analgesic drugs: resolving the two. Anaesth Intensive Care 2012;40(2):216–35.
70. Hutchinson MR, Shavit Y, Grace PM, et al. Exploring the neuroimmunopharmacology of opioids: an integrative review of mechanisms of central immune signaling and their implications for opioid analgesia. Pharmacol Rev 2011; 63(3):772–810.
71. Lawrence ID, Warner JA, Cohan VL, et al. Purification and characterization of human skin mast cells. Evidence for human mast cell heterogeneity. J Immunol 1987;139(9):3062–9.
72. Tharp MD, Kagey-Sobotka A, Fox CC, et al. Functional heterogeneity of human mast cells from different anatomic sites: in vitro responses to morphine sulfate. J Allergy Clin Immunol 1987;79(4):646–53.
73. Liu XY, Liu ZC, Sun YG, et al. Unidirectional cross-activation of GRPR by MOR1D uncouples itch and analgesia induced by opioids. Cell 2011;147(2): 447–58.
74. Liu R, Wang J, Zhao T, et al. Relationship between MRGPRX2 and pethidine hydrochloride- or fentanyl citrate-induced LAD2 cell degranulation. J Pharm Pharmacol 2018;70(12):1596–605.
75. Reich A, Szepietowski JC. Opioid-induced pruritus: an update. Clin Exp Dermatol 2010;35(1):2–6.
76. Dinges HC, Otto S, Stay DK, et al. Side Effect Rates of Opioids in Equianalgesic Doses via Intravenous Patient-Controlled Analgesia: A Systematic Review and Network Meta-analysis. Anesth Analg 2019;129(4):1153–62.
77. Brockow K, Ring J. Anaphylaxis to radiographic contrast media. Curr Opin Allergy Clin Immunol 2011;11(4):326–31.
78. Kim MH, Park CH, Kim DI, et al. Surveillance of contrast-media-induced hypersensitivity reactions using signals from an electronic medical recording system. Ann Allergy Asthma Immunol 2012;108(3):167–71.
79. Kim SR, Lee JH, Park KH, et al. Varied incidence of immediate adverse reactions to low-osmolar non-ionic iodide radiocontrast media used in computed tomography. Clin Exp Allergy 2017;47(1):106–12.
80. Christiansen C. X-ray contrast media–an overview. Toxicology 2005;209(2): 185–7.
81. Morales-Cabeza C, Roa-Medellín D, Torrado I, et al. Immediate reactions to iodinated contrast media. Ann Allergy Asthma Immunol 2017;119(6):553–7.
82. Brockow K. Immediate and delayed reactions to radiocontrast media: is there an allergic mechanism? Immunol Allergy Clin N Am 2009;29(3):453–68.
83. Trcka J, Schmidt C, Seitz CS, et al. Anaphylaxis to iodinated contrast material: nonallergic hypersensitivity or IgE-mediated allergy? AJR Am J Roentgenol 2008;190(3):666–70.
84. Dewachter P, Laroche D, Mouton-Faivre C, et al. Immediate reactions following iodinated contrast media injection: a study of 38 cases. Eur J Radiol 2011;77(3): 495–501.
85. Kim MH, Lee SY, Lee SE, et al. Anaphylaxis to iodinated contrast media: clinical characteristics related with development of anaphylactic shock. PLoS One 2014;9(6):e100154.

86. Chung SJ, Kang DY, Lee W, et al. HLA-DRB1*15: 02 Is Associated With Iodinated Contrast Media-Related Anaphylaxis. Invest Radiol 2020;55(5):304–9.

87. Lumry WR, Li HH, Levy RJ, et al. Randomized placebo-controlled trial of the bradykinin B2 receptor antagonist icatibant for the treatment of acute attacks of hereditary angioedema: the FAST-3 trial. Ann Allergy Asthma Immunol 2011; 107(6):529–37.

88. Bas M, Greve J, Stelter K, et al. A randomized trial of icatibant in ACE-inhibitor-induced angioedema. N Engl J Med 2015;372(5):418–25.

89. Sinert R, Levy P, Bernstein JA, et al. Randomized Trial of Icatibant for Angiotensin-Converting Enzyme Inhibitor-Induced Upper Airway Angioedema. J Allergy Clin Immunol Pract 2017;5(5):1402–1409 e1403.

90. Liu R, Che D, Zhao T, et al. MRGPRX2 is essential for sinomenine hydrochloride induced anaphylactoid reactions. Biochem Pharmacol 2017;146:214–23.

91. Huang L, Dong Y, Wu J, et al. Sinomenine-induced histamine release-like anaphylactoid reactions are blocked by tranilast via inhibiting NF-κB signaling. Pharmacol Res 2017;125(Pt B):150–60.

92. Okamura Y, Mishima S, Kashiwakura JI, et al. The dual regulation of substance P-mediated inflammation via human synovial mast cells in rheumatoid arthritis. Allergol Int 2017;66S:S9–20.

93. Rouzaire P, Nosbaum A, Mullet C, et al. Immediate allergic hypersensitivity to quinolones associates with neuromuscular blocking agent sensitization. J Allergy Clin Immunol Pract 2013;1(3):273–279 e271.

94. Baldo BA, Fisher MM, Pham NH. On the origin and specificity of antibodies to neuromuscular blocking (muscle relaxant) drugs: an immunochemical perspective. Clin Exp Allergy 2009;39(3):325–44.

95. Babina M, Wang Z, Franke K, et al. Thymic Stromal Lymphopoietin Promotes MRGPRX2-Triggered Degranulation of Skin Mast Cells in a STAT5-Dependent Manner with Further Support from JNK. Cells 2021;10(1).

96. Schuch A, Brockow K. Mastocytosis and Anaphylaxis. Immunol Allergy Clin North Am 2017;37(1):153–64.

97. Deepak V, Komarow HD, Alblaihess AA, et al. Expression of MRGPRX2 in skin mast cells of patients with maculopapular cutaneous mastocytosis. J Allergy Clin Immunol Pract 2021;9(10):3841–3.e1.

98. Hermans MAW, Arends NJT, Gerth van Wijk R, et al. Management around invasive procedures in mastocytosis: An update. Ann Allergy Asthma Immunol 2017;119(4):304–9.

99. Doña I, Blanca-López N, Boteanu C, et al. Clinical Practice Guidelines for Diagnosis and Management of Hypersensitivity Reactions to Quinolones. J Investig Allergol Clin Immunol 2021;31(4):292–307.

100. Roy S, Chompunud Na Ayudhya C, Thapaliya M, et al. Multifaceted MRGPRX2: New insight into the role of mast cells in health and disease. J Allergy Clin Immunol 2021;148(2):293–308.

101. Alkanfari I, Gupta K, Jahan T, et al. Naturally Occurring Missense MRGPRX2 Variants Display Loss of Function Phenotype for Mast Cell Degranulation in Response to Substance P, Hemokinin-1, Human beta-Defensin-3, and Icatibant. J Immunol 2018;201(2):343–9.

102. Chompunud Na Ayudhya C, Roy S, Alkanfari I, et al. Identification of Gain and Loss of Function Missense Variants in MRGPRX2's Transmembrane and Intracellular Domains for Mast Cell Activation by Substance P. Int J Mol Sci 2019; 20(21).

103. McNeil BD. Minireview: Mas-related G protein-coupled receptor X2 activation by therapeutic drugs. Neurosci Lett 2021;751:135746.

104. Ansotegui IJ, Melioli G, Canonica GW, et al. IgE allergy diagnostics and other relevant tests in allergy, a World Allergy Organization position paper. World Allergy Organ J 2020;13(2):100080.

105. Broyles AD, Banerji A, Castells M. Practical Guidance for the Evaluation and Management of Drug Hypersensitivity: General Concepts. J Allergy Clin Immunol Pract 2020;8(9s):S3–15.

106. Mayorga C, Celik G, Rouzaire P, et al. In vitro tests for drug hypersensitivity reactions: an ENDA/EAACI Drug Allergy Interest Group position paper. Allergy 2016;71(8):1103–34.

107. Elst J, Sabato V, Hagendorens MM, et al. Measurement and Functional Analysis of the Mas-Related G Protein-Coupled Receptor MRGPRX2 on Human Mast Cells and Basophils. Methods Mol Biol 2020;2163:219–26.

108. Ebo DG, Elst J, Van Gasse A, et al. Basophil Activation Experiments in Immediate Drug Hypersensitivity: More Than a Diagnostic Aid. Methods Mol Biol 2020; 2163:197–211.

109. Ebo DG, Van der Poorten ML, Elst J, et al. Immunoglobulin E cross-linking or MRGPRX2 activation: clinical insights from rocuronium hypersensitivity. Br J Anaesth 2020;126(1):e27–9.

110. Elst J, van der Poorten MM, Van Gasse AL, et al. Mast cell activation tests by flow cytometry: A new diagnostic asset? Clin Exp Allergy 2021;51(11): 1482–500.

111. Drug allergy: an updated practice parameter. Ann Allergy Asthma Immunol 2010;105(4):259–73.

112. Azimi E, Reddy VB, Shade KC, et al. Dual action of neurokinin-1 antagonists on Mas-related GPCRs. JCI Insight 2016;1(16):e89362.

113. Mencarelli A, Gunawan M, Yong KSM, et al. A humanized mouse model to study mast cells mediated cutaneous adverse drug reactions. J Leukoc Biol 2020; 107(5):797–807.

114. Ogasawara H, Furuno M, Edamura K, et al. Novel MRGPRX2 antagonists inhibit IgE-independent activation of human umbilical cord blood-derived mast cells. J Leukoc Biol 2019;106(5):1069–77.

115. Suzuki Y, Liu S, Ogasawara T, et al. A novel MRGPRX2-targeting antagonistic DNA aptamer inhibits histamine release and prevents mast cell-mediated anaphylaxis. Eur J Pharmacol 2020;878:173104.

116. Callahan BN, Kammala AK, Syed M, et al. Osthole, a Natural Plant Derivative Inhibits MRGPRX2 Induced Mast Cell Responses. Front Immunol 2020;11:703.

117. Kumar M, Singh K, Duraisamy K, et al. Protective Effect of Genistein against Compound 48/80 Induced Anaphylactoid Shock via Inhibiting MAS Related G Protein-Coupled Receptor X2 (MRGPRX2). Molecules 2020;25(5).

118. Ding Y, Che D, Li C, et al. Quercetin inhibits Mrgprx2-induced pseudo-allergic reaction via PLCγ-IP3R related Ca(2+) fluctuations. Int Immunopharmacol 2019;66:185–97.

119. Wang J, Zhang Y, Li C, et al. Inhibitory function of Shikonin on MRGPRX2-mediated pseudo-allergic reactions induced by the secretagogue. Phytomedicine 2020;68:153149.

Hypersensitivity Reactions and Immune-Related Adverse Events to Immune Checkpoint Inhibitors: Approaches, Mechanisms, and Models

Benjamin C. Park, BS[a], Cosby A. Stone Jr, MD, MPH[b,1],
Anna K. Dewan, MD[c,2], Douglas B. Johnson, MD[b,3],*

KEYWORDS

- Immune checkpoint inhibitor • PD-1 • CTLA-4 • Toxicity • Hypersensitivity • Allergy
- PD-L1 • Colitis

KEY POINTS

- Immune checkpoint inhibitors (ICI) cause toxicities related to removing negative regulators on T cells that may affect any organ.
- Traditional immune toxicities occur more commonly and in a dose-dependent manner when CTLA-4 inhibitors are used compared with anti-PD-1/PD-L1 agents, which are also not dose dependent.
- The management of these toxicities involves withholding therapy, supportive management, and usually high-dose glucocorticoid treatment.
- ICI may also uncommonly cause infusion reactions and other hypersensitivity reactions, which are largely manageable reactions.

INTRODUCTION

Immune checkpoint inhibitors (ICIs) are novel immunomodulatory oncologic therapies that have distinct mechanisms of action, activity profiles, and toxicities from traditional

---

[a] Vanderbilt University School of Medicine, Office of Enrollment Services, PMB 407939224 Eskind Biomedical Library and Learning Center, Nashville, TN 37240-7939, USA; [b] Department of Medicine, Vanderbilt University Medical Center, Nashville, TN 37232, USA; [c] Department of Dermatology, Vanderbilt University Medical Center, Nashville, TN 37232, USA
[1] Present address: 1161 21st Avenue South, T-1218, MCN, Nashville, TN 37232-2650.
[2] Present address: One Hundred Oaks, Department of Dermatology, 719 Thompson Lane, Suite 26300, Nashville, TN 37204.
[3] Present address: 777 PRB, 2220 Pierce Avenue, Nashville, TN 37232.
* Corresponding author. 2220 Pierce Ave, 777 PRB, Nashville, TN 37232.
E-mail address: douglas.b.johnson@vumc.org

Immunol Allergy Clin N Am 42 (2022) 285–305
https://doi.org/10.1016/j.iac.2021.12.006   immunology.theclinics.com
0889-8561/22/© 2021 Elsevier Inc. All rights reserved.

cancer treatments. These drugs improve survival for numerous cancers with previously poor prognoses by reinvigorating stalled immune responses to target neoplastic cells. ICIs augment the adaptive immune response of the host by stimulating T cells rather than by directly targeting cancer cells. Three major classes of ICIs have been developed against cytotoxic T lymphocyte-associated antigen 4 (CTLA-4), programmed cell death protein 1 (PD-1), and its ligand, programmed cell death ligand-1 (PD-L1).

When T cells contact antigens that are expressed on major histocompatibility complexes (MHCs) of foreign or target cells, activation of CD4+ T cells leads to release of cytokines and an inflammatory cascade response. Activated CD8+ T cells can perform direct cytolysis using perforin and granzyme.[1] To prevent this immune response from damaging nontarget cells, PD-L1 is expressed in native tissues, activating the PD-1 protein on activated T cells and promoting immune tolerance. Cancer cells hijack this pathway by presenting PD-L1, inducing T-cell exhaustion and immune evasion.[2] This class of immunomodulators therefore restores the ability of the immune system to target and destroy tumor cells.[3,4]

Since 2011, when the first checkpoint inhibitor, ipilimumab, was approved by the US Food and Drug Administration (FDA) to treat melanoma, there has been rapid development and approval of ICIs. Although the development of ipilimumab was a key "proof-of-principle" advance, its activity was limited to modest (albeit durable) response rates of 15% to 20% in metastatic melanoma.[5] Since then, anti-PD-1/PD-L1 agents have

Table 1
Immune checkpoint inhibitors approved by the Food and Drug Administration[9,10]

Target	Drug Name	Indications
PD-1	Nivolumab	Melanoma, non–small cell lung cancer, small cell lung cancer, renal cell carcinoma, classic Hodgkin lymphoma, squamous cell carcinoma of head and neck, urothelial carcinoma, colorectal cancer, hepatocellular cancer, and esophageal squamous cell carcinoma[11]
	Pembrolizumab	Melanoma, non–small cell lung cancer, small cell lung cancer, head and neck squamous cell cancer, classic Hodgkin lymphoma, primary mediastinal large B-cell lymphoma, urothelial carcinoma, microsatellite instability-high cancer, mismatch repair-deficient colorectal cancer, gastric cancer, esophageal cancer, cervical cancer, hepatocellular carcinoma, Merkel cell carcinoma, renal cell carcinoma, endometrial carcinoma, tumor mutational burden-high cancer, cutaneous squamous cell carcinoma, and triple-negative breast cancer[12]
	Cemiplimab	Metastatic cutaneous squamous cell carcinoma or advanced cutaneous squamous cell carcinoma, basal cell carcinoma, non–small cell lung cancer[13]
	Dostarlimab	deficient DNA mismatch repair (dMMR) recurrent or advanced endometrial cancer[14]
PD-L1	Avelumab	Merkel cell carcinoma, advanced or metastatic urothelial carcinoma, advanced renal cell carcinoma[15]
	Durvalumab	Advanced or metastatic urothelial carcinoma, stage III non–small cell lung cancer, small cell lung cancer[16]
	Atezolizumab	Urothelial carcinoma, non–small cell lung cancer, triple-negative breast cancer, small cell lung cancer, hepatocellular carcinoma, and melanoma[17]
CTLA-4	Ipilimumab	Melanoma, renal cell carcinoma, colorectal cancer, hepatocellular carcinoma, non–small cell lung cancer, and mesothelioma[11]

Table 2
Immune-related adverse events and drug hypersensitivity reactions: clinical presentations and management

Organ System	irAE and Drug Hypersensitivity Reactions[a]	Specific irAE Management	Drug Hypersensitivity Reaction Management
Dermatologic	Maculopapular rash, bullous pemphigoid eruptions, vitiligo, psoriasiform rash, lichenoid eruptions, SCARs (Steven's Johnson syndrome/TEN, DRESS, etc), Grover disease, mucositis, erythroderma, neutrophilic dermatosis, inflammatory dermatitis[20–23]	Most irAEs are manageable without discontinuation of ICIs. Treatment is based on their classic dermatoses with agents such as vitamin D analogues and dupulimab[24]	General principles include prompt discontinuation of the offending drug and supportive treatment[18,19] **Immediate reactions** Mild reactions can be treated with antihistamines Suspicion for anaphylaxis should be treated with intramuscular epinephrine and adjunctive antihistamines[25] **Nonimmediate reactions** Mild reactions can be treated with antihistamines Serious reactions can be treated with systemic corticosteroids and other immunosuppressive measures such as IVIG, cyclophosphamide, and plasmapheresis as needed on a case-by-case basis[26] **SCARs** Early withdrawal of the offending agent, supportive treatment (IV fluid resuscitation, pain control, nutrition, etc.), systemic corticosteroids as needed, and SCAR-specific management.[27] Most are managed in the ICU or burn unit[28] **Drug desensitization:** Indicated in IgE-mediated drug allergy and select non-IgE-mediated drug allergies.[18,29,30] Several protocols exist; however, the BWH 12-step RDD protocol is considered the safest and most effective.[29,31–33] DD to ICIs has been reported through case reports with the
Renal	Acute interstitial nephritis, minimal change disease, immune complex glomerulonephritis, pauci-immune glomerulonephritis, membranous nephropathy, IgA nephropathy, acute tubular necrosis[23,34,35]	Monitor creatinine routinely for treatment efficacy[36]	
Neurologic	Encephalitis, aseptic meningitis, Guillain-Barré syndrome, myasthenia gravis, myasthenic Lambert-Eaton syndrome, peripheral neuropathy, autonomic neuropathy, transverse myelitis[23,37,38]	Corticosteroids are first line; however, high-dose IV corticosteroids and ICI discontinuation is used with higher-grade events. Additional immunosuppressive therapy is often required such as IVIG, plasmapheresis, rituximab, and cyclosporine[39–41]	
Cardiac	Pericarditis, valvular disease, Takotsubo syndrome, cardiomyopathy, heart failure, cardiac arrest, myocardial infarction, arrhythmias, vasculitis, myocarditis, venous thromboembolism[23,38,42,43]	Hold and permanently discontinue ICIs after any grade toxicity. Manage specific cardiac complications according to American College of Cardiology/AHA guidelines[36]	
GI	Diarrhea, colitis, enterocolitis, gastritis, hepatitis, and microscopic colitis[23,38,44]	Grade 2 toxicities and greater may be offered esophagogastroduodenoscopy/colonoscopy, endoscopy, as well as infliximab in addition to corticosteroids based on severity[36]	
Endocrine	Hypothyroidism, hyperthyroidism, hyperglycemia, thyroiditis, primary adrenal insufficiency, hypophysitis, type I	Monitor thyroid function for both diagnosis and monitoring. Thyroid hormone supplementation and other hormone replacement therapy as needed.	

(continued on next page)

Table 2
(continued)

Organ System	irAE and Drug Hypersensitivity Reactions[a]	Specific irAE Management	Drug Hypersensitivity Reaction Management
	diabetes, pancreatitis, hypogonadism, hypopituitarism[23,38,45,46]	Symptoms of hyperthyroidism may be managed with β-blockers and supportive care[36]	following agents: nivolumab, pembrolizumab, and atezolizumab.[23]
Respiratory	Interstitial lung disease including pneumonitis, pulmonary fibrosis, pulmonary hemorrhage[23,38,47,48]	Hold ICIs with radiographic evidence of pneumonitis progression and resume with improvement. Grade 3/4 toxicities require permanent ICI discontinuation and empirical antibiotics and methylprednisolone[36]	
Rheumatologic	Inflammatory arthritis, myositis, vasculitis, myalgias, rheumatoid arthritis, polymyalgia rheumatica, sicca symptoms, Sjögren syndrome[49,50]	Initiate analgesia such as NSAIDs for pain control. Synthetic (methotrexate, leflunomide) or biologic DMARDs (TNF-α, IL-6 inhibitors) may be offered in addition to prednisone depending on the condition[36]	
Other	Hemolytic anemia, acquired thrombotic thrombocytopenic purpura, hemolytic uremic syndrome, aplastic anemia, acquired hemophilia, leukopenia, immune thrombocytopenia, uveitis, iritis, conjunctivitis, blepharitis, optic neuritis, ocular myasthenia, autoimmune retinopathy, inflammatory arthritis, myositis, polymyalgialike syndrome[23,38,51–53]	For hematologic toxicities, discontinue with grade 2 toxicities and greater. Red blood transfusion as needed. Severe cases with bone marrow involvement may require bone marrow transplantation. Additional immunosuppressive agents such as rituximab, IVIG, cyclosporin A, and mycophenolate mofetil as needed[36]	
Immediate reactions	Back or neck pains; chills or shaking; dizziness; fever; flushing; itching; rash; dyspnea; wheezing; swelling of face, lips, or throat; dysphagia; muscle and joint pain; bronchospasm; anaphylaxis[38,54]		

Abbreviations: AHA, American Heart Association; BWH, Brigham and Women's Hospital; DD, drug desensitization; DMARD, disease modifying anti-rheumatic drug; DRESS, drug reaction with eosinophilia and systemic symptoms; ICU, intensive care unit; IV, intravenous; IVIG, intravenous immunoglobulin; NSAID, nonsteroidal anti-inflammatory drug; RDD, rapid drug desensitization; SCARs, severe cutaneous adverse reactions; TEN, toxic epidermal necrolysis; TNF-α, tumor necrosis factor-α.

[a] Likely, a significant overlap exists between these categories, although this is one way to conceptualize differences between categories.

demonstrated often durable response rates of 15% to 80% in a wide variety of both solid and hematologic cancers.[6] The indications and combinations for ICIs have been rapidly expanding as these therapies are shifting to first-line use for many advanced cancers, as well as being used in adjuvant (postsurgical) settings; nearly half of all patients with advanced cancer are eligible for ICI therapy.[7,8] At present, the FDA has approved 8 checkpoint inhibitors for the treatment of approximately 20 different types of cancers as shown in **Tables 1** and **2**. By virtue of their ability to activate the immune system, these drugs also have unique, autoimmunelike toxicities (termed immune-related adverse events [irAEs]), some of which can be fatal.[55] Managing these side effects can represent a clinical challenge in the patient who needs immune-based therapies for the treatment of cancer. ICIs may also cause other less common adverse drug reactions (ADRs).

In this review, we summarize the current knowledge of irAEs and hypersensitivity reactions (HRs) caused by ICIs that have emerged to date.

MECHANISM OF ACTION OF IMMUNE CHECKPOINT INHIBITORS
Pathways and Targets

The targets of ICI, the so-called immune checkpoint proteins, function to maintain immune homeostasis but are hijacked by cancer cells. PD-1 is a receptor expressed on the surface of activated T cells and other immune cells. PD-L1 is a ligand commonly expressed by normal tissues including the placenta, heart, lung, and liver, and on resting B cells, T cells, macrophages, and dendritic cells.[56] CTLA-4 is a receptor induced in response to TCR/CD28 costimulation, normally on Treg cells.[57] Two signals are required for T-cell activation: recognition of peptide antigen presented by MHC (**signal 1**) and costimulation through CD28 following binding to CD80 or CD86 expressed by APCs (**signal 2**). Both CD28 and CTLA-4 are homodimers that bind the ligands CD80/CD86. Contrary to CD28, which is expressed on both resting and activated cells, CTLA-4 is induced in response to TCR/CD28 costimulation. Both CTLA-4 and PD-1 on T cells produce inhibitory effects when bound to CD80/86 and PD-L1, respectively. CTLA-4 competes with CD28 for binding to B7 ligands with higher affinity, thus inhibiting T-cell activation. Pharmacologic blockade of CTLA-4, therefore, allows for CD28 and CD80 binding, resulting in T-cell activation. Similarly, blockade of either PD-1 or PD-L1 prevents their binding and thus precludes the exhausted T-cell state induced by this interaction.

ICI-associated toxicities: More than half of patients who receive ICIs experience at least one irAE.[58,59] Clinically, irAEs are autoimmunelike syndromes that affect nearly any organ system (**Fig. 1**).[60] These toxicities stem from blockade of key negative regulators of T-cell activation (PD-1, PD-L1, CTLA-4), resulting in organ-specific inflammation. Given the crucial context in which the mechanism of these drugs is disinhibition of the host's immune system, such toxicities could be roughly considered as type A ADRs, although with agent-based variability in dose dependence[61,62]; they may also be considered as "off-target," in that the unleashing was intended for the purpose of cancer eradication, but was permissive of autoimmunity directed at other tissues. Although this general intuitive framework is at least theoretically understood, specific mechanisms have not been fully elucidated (eg, why specific patients develop off-target organ involvement). Studies have suggested that potential mechanisms include increasing immune activation against a common antigen in both tumor and inflamed organs, increasing levels of preexisting autoantibodies, enhanced proinflammatory cytokines, microbial or other environmental factors, or complement-mediated inflammation through direct binding of ICI antibodies to target organs.[63-70] For example, CTLA-4 is expressed in various normal tissues such as the

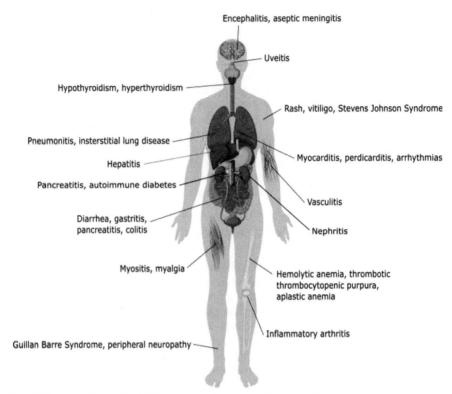

Fig. 1. Organs affected by irAEs and drug hypersensitivity reactions.

pituitary gland.[71,72] T-cell-mediated mechanisms are thought to be the primary cause of these toxicities, although B cell and macrophages also seem to play some role.[73]

OVERLAP BETWEEN ANTITUMOR AND AUTOIMMUNE RESPONSES

Several studies and meta-analyses have reported increased survival outcomes such as overall survival and progression-free survival in patients who develop irAEs.[74–76] In particular, several studies have shown that the development of vitiligo as a cutaneous irAE is associated with survival benefits in patients with melanoma.[77–79] Early evidence suggests that irAEs may be triggered due to a common antigen in both tumor and inflamed organs, creating both an antitumor and an autoimmune response[60]; this also raises the concern of whether the treatment of irAEs affects the antitumor response; although patients with irAEs have superior outcomes, evidence is conflicting whether immunosuppressive treatments such as corticosteroids may in turn blunt the antitumor response and impact outcome and survival.[80,81]

MANAGEMENT FOR IMMUNE-RELATED ADVERSE EVENTS CAUSED BY IMMUNE CHECKPOINT INHIBITORS

Several guidelines have been developed for general and organ-specific management approaches.[36,82,83] General strategies include holding immunotherapy and using corticosteroids.[39] In general, ICI therapy is continued for most grade 1 toxicities with supportive measures (eg, hormone replacement for endocrinopathies, pain relievers for arthritis). Grade 2 events are generally managed with either initial observation with escalation to high-dose steroids (prednisone 1 mg/kg/d or equivalent) or upfront steroids. Grade 3 to 4 events are managed with upfront high-dose steroids and potential escalation to other immunosuppressants on an individual case basis.[39] Dose adjustments are generally not recommended with ICIs. Rechallenge after an irAE is possible assessing each case individually depending on the risk-reward ratio, which is often acceptable based on several factors including use of systemic corticosteroids or immunomodulatory agents, speed of irAE resolution, occurrence of concomitant irAEs, current and expected tumor response, duration of previous course of immunotherapy, organ system effected, and alternative treatment options.[84,85] Multidisciplinary, systems-based care is important due to the unpredictable and diagnostically challenging presentations associated with irAEs.[86]

DERMATOLOGIC IMMUNE-RELATED ADVERSE EVENTS OF IMMUNE CHECKPOINT INHIBITOR THERAPY

Cutaneous irAEs (cirAEs) are the most common irAEs with ICIs, occurring in up to 30% to 50% of patients, and more often with anti-CTLA-4 than anti-PD-1.[87–89] Most events are self-limiting, readily managed, and occur relatively early in the course of therapy, although there is a wide spectrum of dermatologic manifestations.[90,91] Classification is based on clinical morphology into the following categories: inflammatory dermatoses, bullous eruptions, pruritus with or without rash, pigmentary disorders, severe cutaneous adverse reactions (SCARs)/life-threatening drug reactions, and miscellaneous skin manifestations.[92] Morbilliform eruptions, lichenoid reactions, pruritus, and vitiligo are the most common. Vitiligo is primarily seen in patients with melanoma and has a positive association with survival.[89] Rare SCARs resemble known clinical phenotypes such as Stevens-Johnson syndrome/toxic epidermal necrolysis, other immunobullous disorders such as bullous pemphigoid, and drug reaction with eosinophilia and systemic symptoms.[20,21] Pharmacovigilance data suggest that ICIs have a significantly higher proportion of fatal SCARs compared with other anticancer agents.[93,94] Cancer type is an independent risk factor with lung cancer, melanoma, and renal cell carcinoma associated with more cirAEs.[89] Workup and management includes thorough review of prior skin conditions and other potential causes, total body skin examination evaluating body surface area (BSA) and mucosal involvement, and determining the need for dermatology consult and biopsy.[24,95] Treatment of cirAEs consists of topical corticosteroids and antihistamines for low-grade events, with systemic steroids given in more severe cases. Treatment of cirAEs should be based on treatment of the idiopathic version of the skin disease. For example, a low-grade psoriasis flare triggered by ICIs can be treated with topical corticosteroids and vitamin D analogues, and bullous disease may benefit from dupilumab.[24] Pruritus associated with ICI may have a strong neurogenic component and respond more favorably to combination approaches such as antihistamines combined with agents such as gabapentin, doxepin or other antidepressants, NK-1 receptor antagonists (aprepitant), or corticosteroids for higher-grade reactions.

NEUROLOGIC IMMUNE-RELATED ADVERSE EVENTS

Neurologic events may affect the central nervous system (encephalitis, aseptic meningitis), peripheral nervous system (sensory or motor neuropathy, including Guillain-Barré syndrome), and neuromuscular junctions (myasthenia gravis or myasthenic Lambert-Eaton syndrome).[37] Estimated incidence of any grade neurologic irAEs (nAEs) is 1% to 6% with monotherapy and up to 12% to 14% with combination therapy.[96] Rates of nAEs are greater with CTLA-4 agents compared with PD-1 agents.[97] nAEs have high fatality rates compared with other irAEs.[98] First-line management includes corticosteroids, with high-dose intravenous corticosteroids and ICI discontinuation for high-grade events. For steroid-refractory cases (and for initial treatment of myasthenia gravis and Guillain-Barré syndrome) intravenous immunoglobulins (IVIGs) and plasmapheresis should be considered in conjunction with neurology consultation.[97]

CARDIAC IMMUNE-RELATED ADVERSE EVENTS

Myocarditis is the most common cardiac irAE with incidence reported up to 1.14%,[99,100] higher in anti-PD-1/L1 and combination regimens compared with anti-CTLA-4 agents. Myocarditis has a median time to onset of 30 days following ICI treatment and has a mortality rate as high as 50%.[42,101] The clinical presentation of myocarditis is variable from asymptomatic cardiac biomarker elevation to sudden death.[99,102] Patients often present with concurrent skeletal muscle involvement, with either myositis or a myasthenia gravis-like syndrome.[101,103] Diagnosis may be complex given the difficulty of obtaining myocardial biopsy and the relative lack of sensitivity and specificity of cardiac imaging, but workup may include cardiac biomarkers, electrocardiography, echocardiography, cardiac MRI, and cardiology consultation.[102,104] The mainstay of management includes discontinuing ICIs and pulse-dose glucocorticoids (methylprednisolone 1 g/d associated with lower mortality compared with lower doses).[105] If refractory to steroids, or in severe initial presentations, other immune modulators such as mycophenolate mofetil, abatacept, or IVIG can be considered.[102,106] ICIs can also be associated with several potential other cardiac events such as pericarditis, valvular disease, Takotsubo syndrome, cardiomyopathy, arrhythmias, and vasculitis.[42,43]

GASTROINTESTINAL IMMUNE-RELATED ADVERSE EVENTS

Gastrointestinal irAEs are among the most common and severe ICI-induced toxicities, more common with anti-CTLA-4 compared with anti-PD-1/L1; these may affect any region of the gastrointestinal system, but most often affect the colon.[44] Upper gastrointestinal (GI) involvement may include symptoms of nausea, vomiting, dysphagia, and epigastric pain. Lower GI involvement, the most common presentation, includes symptoms of diarrhea and less often abdominal pain or hematochezia.[107,108] Endoscopic biopsy is the gold standard for diagnosis, particularly for enterocolitis, although patients are often treated empirically in situations with less diagnostic uncertainty.[108,109] Treatment strategies, similar to other irAEs, include systemic steroids and biologics such as infliximab and vedolizumab in steroid-refractory cases.[107,108]

PNEUMONITIS

Pneumonitis occurs in 3.5% to 19%, with higher rates of pneumonitis with combination immunotherapy and PD-1/PD-L1 inhibitors versus CTLA-4 inhibitors, and in non–small cell lung cancer and renal cell carcinoma.[110,111] Time to onset is widely variable with median onset of approximately 2.5 months.[111,112] Pneumonitis presents as interstitial lung disease in 4 patterns: organizing pneumonia, nonspecific interstitial pneumonia, hypersensitivity pneumonitis, and diffuse alveolar damage. Common symptoms include cough and dyspnea, and less commonly with fever or productive cough.[47,48] Clinical suspicion of ICI-induced pneumonitis should prompt an evaluation with a chest computed tomographic (CT) and infectious workup. Diagnostic bronchoscopy with bronchoalveolar lavage may be considered when diagnostic uncertainty exists. Asymptomatic cases identified only with imaging are generally managed by holding ICI. Moderate and severe cases should receive oral or intravenous corticosteroids, with additional immunosuppression such as infliximab or IVIG in steroid-refractory cases.[39]

ENDOCRINE IMMUNE-RELATED ADVERSE EVENTS

Endocrine irAEs occur in up to 40% of patients treated with ICIs.[113] Hypothyroidism is the most common and is often preceded by transient thyrotoxicosis.[45,46] Other less common irAEs include adrenal insufficiency, type I diabetes, hypophysitis, and hypo-pituitarism.[46] Hypophysitis is more common with anti-CTLA-4 agents, whereas thyroid dysfunction and type 1 diabetes mellitus are more prevalent with anti-PD-1 agents.[45] Time of onset is unpredictable, from weeks to months, but usually occurs within 6 months of ICI initiation.[45,114] Diagnosis may be difficult because symptoms of thyroid dysfunction often overlap with generalized symptoms of cancer or nonspecific fatigue from ICIs. Pituitary and adrenal irAEs may present with symptoms related to neurocompression such as headache, nausea, visual field defects (when pituitary inflammation is present), hypotension, or adrenal crisis. Thyroid function tests are important in diagnosing thyroid dysfunction and should be monitored at least every other treatment cycle; however, routine monitoring of adrenal and pituitary function (in the absence of symptoms) is less common in clinical practice.[46,115] Thyroid irAEs are treated with levothyroxine ± β-blockers; steroids have little to no role. Pituitary and adrenal irAEs are treated with replacement glucocorticoids and other hormone replacement therapy (testosterone, estrogen, and mineralocorticoids) as needed.[114] ICI therapy may be continued with endocrine toxicity, because recovery of gland function is uncommon and independent of continuation of therapy.[115]

Rheumatologic Immune-Related Adverse Events

The most common rheumatologic irAEs (Rh-irAEs) are inflammatory arthritis and myositis. Some rarer Rh-irAEs include polymyalgia rheumatica, sicca symptoms, and vasculitis.[49] In contrast with many other irAEs, many Rh-irAEs continue to persist in an inflammatory phase even after stopping therapy in up to half of patients, requiring long-term treatment.[50] General treatment guidelines include continuing immunotherapy and using supportive management (eg, nonsteroidal anti-inflammatory drugs) for grade 1 events. For grade 2 or higher events, corticosteroids and other immunomodulatory agents may be indicated, with ICI discontinuation for more severe events.[50]

RENAL

ICI-induced acute kidney injury (AKI) is uncommon (1%–2% for monotherapy and up to 5% for combination) but tends to present as acute interstitial nephritis.[34] There are several other rarer histologic types including minimal change disease, immune complex glomerulonephritis, pauci-immune glomerulonephritis, membranous nephropathy, IgA nephropathy, and acute tubular necrosis.[35] The onset of renal irAEs ranges from 21 days to 12 months after the first ICI dose.[116] The clinical presentation of ICI-induced AKIs are relatively nonspecific, with variable proteinuria and leukocyturia.[35] Management is variable, but systemic corticosteroids and ICI discontinuation are mainstays of treatment.[116] Other potential contributing medications (eg, concurrent proton pump inhibitors) should also be discontinued.

OCULAR

The incidence of uveitis is approximately 1% to 2.8% of patients with onset within weeks to months of ICI initiation and may present with blurred vision or eye pain.[117]

Less common irAEs include optic neuritis, ocular myasthenia, and autoimmune reti-nopathy.[118] Management includes topical, periocular, and systemic corticosteroids depending on the area affected, and discontinuation should be considered in the case of potential irreversible damage.[36,117]

DRUG HYPERSENSITIVITY REACTIONS RELATED TO IMMUNE CHECKPOINT INHIBITORS

Adverse reactions associated with ICIs are most common irAEs related to their under-lying mechanism of action and typically not related to an HR to the specific structure of the drug or its excipient. Drug hypersensitivity classification and mechanisms have been described to explain how drugs activate T cells that largely relate to small mole-cule drugs, and relevance to large molecule drugs and ICIs is unknown.[119,120] (Fig. 2); DHRs are also classified into immediate reactions (IR) if symptoms occur within 6 hours or nonimmediate reactions (NIR) if symptoms appear greater than 6 hours after drug intake. IRs can present with the classic symptoms of pruritus, rash, urticaria, angioedema, or anaphylaxis, whereas NIRs can induce rarer and potentially more dangerous symptoms. Immediate HRs are mediated by more than just IgE-antigen in-teractions; several endotypes are possible including non-IgE mast cell mediated, IgG mediated, and other mechanisms leading to a spectrum of potential clinical pheno-types.[127] Beyond classic presentations, rarer clinical presentations are also possible.

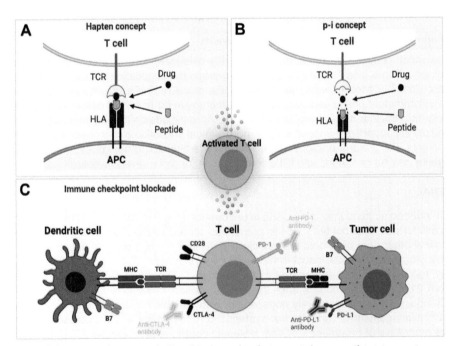

Fig. 2. (A) Drug or drug metabolites bind covalently to proteins or antigen to create new hapten-protein complexes that can activate T cells. (B) Drug or drug metabolites my bind via noncovalent bonds directly to T-cell receptor leading to T-cell activation.[121–126] (C) Im-mune checkpoint inhibitors can directly bind PD-1, PD-L1, and CTLA-4 to activate T cells. APC, Antigen presenting cell; HLA, Human leukocyte antigen; TCR, T cell receptor. (Created with BioRender.com.)

Mast cell-mediated endotypes may see systems-based presentations that include naso-ocular, cardiovascular, lower airway, gastrointestinal, and cutaneous symptoms.[127] The clinical presentation of these NIRs can be similar to that of irAEs in that they can affect any organ system in the body including cutaneous, gastrointestinal, respiratory, cardiovascular systems, and so forth.[23]

IMMUNE CHECKPOINT INHIBITOR-MEDIATED DRUG HYPERSENSITIVITY REACTIONS

The risk of developing drug hypersensitivity reactions (DHRs) to ICIs depends on the extent of humanization of the agent, with fully human monoclonal antibodies (mABs) being less immunogenic than chimeric mABs.[128] IRs can be mediated by cytokines or by IgE. Most mAB infusion reactions are IRs due to cytokine release rather than T-cell activation. Common manifestations of immediate HRs include nonspecific symptoms such as flushing, dyspnea, throat tightness, dizziness/hypotension, GI symptoms, headache, hypertension, fever. Reactions thought to be IgE-mediated usually occur after having a prior exposure and include symptoms ranging from skin symptoms to anaphylactic shock.[128,129] In this regard, ICIs may be similar to other mAbs, which comprise a rapidly increasing portion of all reported anaphylactic reactions.[130] NIRs to mABs commonly include a serum sickness-like reaction with additional symptoms such as fever, malaise, arthralgia/arthritis, jaw pain, skin eruption, purpura, and hyperemia typically 5 to 7 days after infusion.[128] NIRs occur more commonly after a prior exposure than at first exposure.[131]

Type 1 HRs of varying severity, up to anaphylaxis, have been rarely reported and are thought to be Type I IgE-mediated HRs.[38,132] More rarely, type IV HRs to specific ICIs, particularly nivolumab and atezolizumab have been reported.[133–135] Beyond that, immediate infusion reactions as well as cytokine release reactions have also been reported, which can typically be differentiated from IgE-mediated immediate hypersensitivity by the transient self-limited nature of these events.[23]

Infusion reactions occur in 1% to 6% of patients, although these events tend to be mild and less than 1% of events are grade 3 or above.[46,136,137] Notably, avelumab, an anti-PD-L1 mAb, has a higher risk of infusion reaction (approximately 25%), although these are also uncommonly severe (0%–3% grade 3) and nearly always subside after the first infusion.[46,136–138] These events tend to occur during the infusion and may include "typical" infusion reaction symptoms, including rash, cough, wheezing, angioedema, hypotension, and even anaphylaxis.

MANAGEMENT FOR DRUG HYPERSENSITIVITY REACTIONS TO IMMUNE CHECKPOINT INHIBITORS

True IgE-mediated reactions manifest by anaphylaxis are extremely uncommon. Where suspected, changing to a different ICI or desensitization could be considered.

Infusion reactions should be managed according to existing guidelines, which involve holding the infusion and antihistamines or steroids with premedication considered for future infusion.[83]

Potential Biomarkers for Immune-Related Adverse Events and Hypersensitivities

Biomarkers for the prediction, early diagnosis, risk stratification, and management of irAEs is an area of active investigation with currently limited clinical applicability. With the large number of potential irAEs and organ systems involved, the list of potential biomarkers is expansive. Relative cell counts and circulating cytokine levels have modestly correlated with irAEs.[139–141] Studies have suggested that circulating autoantibodies could be predictive, including antithyroid antibodies (thyroid), anti-BP180 IgG (skin disorders, including bullous pemphigoid), anti-GNAL (hypophysitis), and anti-CD74 (pneumonitis).[142] Genetics have long been considered to play a part in the multifactorial causes of autoimmunity. There are reports of several single nucleotide polymorphisms, microRNA expression, specific genes involved with T-cell activation, and human leukocyte antigen profiles associated with irAEs.[143–152] For IHRs, there are several potential biomarkers including skin testing, serum drug-specific IgE, basophil activation testing, secreted markers (tryptase, histamine, platelet-activating factor, tumor necrosis factor-α, interleukin-6, and interleukin-1b), markers of complement activation (sC5b-9, C4d, Bb, C3a, C5a), and genetics (deleterious BRCA mutations), although these are largely nonoverlapping with irAE candidate biomarkers.[127]

COMPARISON BETWEEN IMMUNE-RELATED ADVERSE EVENTS AND DRUG HYPERSENSITIVITY REACTIONS AND MANAGEMENT STRATEGIES

Management strategies differ between irAEs and DHRs, because one is based on immune suppression and the other is based on prevention. irAEs are generally managed with corticosteroids and potentially withholding ICI.[39,83,85] DHRs are generally managed with strategies that define the implicated small molecule structure driving the HRs, avoidance of that drug and all structurally related drugs, sequential drug rechallenges when the benefit outweighs the risk, and desensitization for a subset of reactions.[23,127] Rechallenge is possible in both irAEs and DHRs after treatment and drug desensitization, respectively, on a case-by-case basis.[153–157]

SUMMARY

As ICIs become first-line therapy for advanced malignancies, side effects that may limit treatment have becoming increasingly important. Among side effects, irAEs are particularly challenging to clinicians because they are very common and have diverse, potentially overlapping clinical presentations. However, most of these toxicities are reversible and the risk of fatal ICI-associated adverse events is lower than that of traditional cancer therapies.[113] True DHRs related to the structure of the ICI are extremely uncommon. With the addition of new indications and treatment combinations for ICIs, evidence-based guidelines must be developed to differentiate these distinct entities. Mechanistic differences make translational research into biomarkers and risk factors a promising future direction in developing models for diagnosis and management. Multidisciplinary involvement will be necessary to support appropriate diagnosis and optimize therapeutic outcomes.

CLINICS CARE POINTS

- When treating patients with ICI, monitor for organ dysfunction with history and physical, thyroid, liver, and kidney laboratory monitoring.
- When patients experience endocrinopathies or low-grade (grade 1) toxicities, treat with supportive management and continue ICI
- When patients experience high-grade toxicities, treat with high-dose systemic corticosteroids and hold ICI.
- When patients experience HRs (ie, infusion reactions), manage as with existing guidelines, including antihistamines, steroids, and premedications.

DISCLOSURE

D.B. Johnson is on advisory boards or consults for BMS, Catalyst, Iovance, Jansen, Merck, Mosaic ImmunoEngineering, Novartis, Oncosec, Pfizer, and Targovax and receives research funding from BMS and Incyte.

REFERENCES

1. Eun Y, Kim IY, Sun J-M, et al. Risk factors for immune-related adverse events associated with anti-PD-1 pembrolizumab. Sci Rep 2019;9(1):14039.
2. Iwai Y, Ishida M, Tanaka Y, et al. Involvement of PD-L1 on tumor cells in the escape from host immune system and tumor immunotherapy by PD-L1 blockade. Proc Natl Acad Sci U S A 2002;99(19):12293–7.
3. Alsaab HO, Sau S, Alzhrani R, et al. PD-1 and PD-L1 checkpoint signaling inhibition for cancer immunotherapy: mechanism, combinations, and clinical outcome. Front Pharmacol 2017;8:561.
4. Gassmann D, Weiler S, Mertens JC, et al. Liver allograft failure after nivolumab treatment—a case report with systematic literature research. Transplant Direct 2018;4(8). https://doi.org/10.1097/TXD.0000000000000814.
5. Hodi FS, O'Day SJ, McDermott DF, et al. Improved survival with ipilimumab in patients with metastatic melanoma. N Engl J Med 2010;363(8):711.
6. Yarchoan M, Hopkins A, Jaffee EM. Tumor mutational burden and response rate to PD-1 inhibition. N Engl J Med 2017;377(25):2500.
7. Haslam A, Gill J, Prasad V. Estimation of the percentage of US patients with cancer who are eligible for immune checkpoint inhibitor drugs. JAMA Netw Open 2020;3(3):e200423.
8. Vilgelm AE, Johnson DB, Richmond A. Combinatorial approach to cancer immunotherapy: strength in numbers. J Leukoc Biol 2016;100(2):275.
9. Twomey JD, Zhang B. Cancer immunotherapy update: FDA-approved checkpoint inhibitors and companion diagnostics. AAPS J 2021;23(2):1–11.
10. Vaddepally RK, Kharel P, Pandey R, et al. Review of Indications of FDA-Approved Immune Checkpoint Inhibitors per NCCN guidelines with the Level of Evidence. Cancers (Basel) 2020;12(3). https://doi.org/10.3390/CANCERS12030738.
11. fda, cder. Highlights of prescribing information. Available at: www.fda.gov/medwatch. Accessed August 12, 2021.
12. Fda. Highlights of prescribing information these highlights do not include all the information needed to use KEYTRUDA safely and effectively. See full prescribing information for KEYTRUDA. KEYTRUDA ® (pembrolizumab) for injection, for intravenous use KEYTRUDA ® (pembrolizumab) injection, for intravenous use. Available at: www.fda.gov/medwatch. Accessed August 12, 2021.
13. fda, cder. Highlights of prescribing information. 2021. Available at: www.fda.gov/medwatch. Accessed August 12, 2021.
14. Highlights of prescribing information. Available at: www.fda.gov/medwatch. Accessed August 12, 2021.
15. And Warnings, Precautions. Highlights of Prescribing Information. Available at: www.fda.gov/medwatch. Accessed August 12, 2021.
16. Fda, Cder. Highlights of prescribing information. Available at: www.fda.gov/medwatch. Accessed July 27, 2021.
17. Fda, Cder. Highlights of prescribing information full prescribing information: contents* 1 indications and usage 1.1 locally advanced or metastatic urothelial carcinoma 1.2 metastatic non-small cell lung cancer 2 dosage and

administration 2.1 recommended dosing 2.2 dose modifications 2.3 preparation and administration 3 dosage forms and strengths 4 contraindications 5 warnings and precautions.. 2016. Available at: www.fda.gov/medwatch. Accessed July 27, 2021.

18. Warrington R, Silviu-Dan F, Wong T. Drug allergy. Allergy, Asthma. Clin Immunol 2018;14(2):60.

19. Krantz MS, Stone CA Jr, Yu R, et al. Criteria for intradermal skin testing and oral challenge in patients labeled as fluoroquinolone allergic. J Allergy Clin Immunol Pract 2021;9(2):1024–8.e3.

20. Coleman EL, Olamiju B, Leventhal JS. The life-threatening eruptions of immune checkpoint inhibitor therapy. Clin Dermatol 2020;38(1):94–104.

21. Tattersall IW, Leventhal JS. Focus: skin: cutaneous toxicities of immune checkpoint inhibitors: the role of the dermatologist. Yale J Biol Med 2020;93(1):123. Available at: /pmc/articles/PMC7087048/. Accessed July 27, 2021.

22. Geisler AN, Phillips GS, Barrios DM, et al. Immune checkpoint inhibitor–related dermatologic adverse events. J Am Acad Dermatol 2020;83(5):1255–68.

23. Labella M, Castells M. Hypersensitivity reactions and anaphylaxis to checkpoint inhibitor–monoclonal antibodies and desensitization. Ann Allergy Asthma Immunol 2021;126(6):623–9.

24. He C, Qu T. Immune checkpoint inhibitor-related cutaneous adverse events. Asia Pac J Clin Oncol 2020;16(5):e149–53.

25. Dykewicz MS, Lam JK. Drug Hypersensitivity Reactions. Med Clin North Am 2020;104(1):109–28.

26. Drug Allergies|World Allergy Organization. Available at: https://www.worldallergy.org/education-and-programs/education/allergic-disease-resource-center/professionals/drug-allergies. Accessed August 10, 2021.

27. Cho Y-T, Chu C-Y. Treatments for severe cutaneous adverse reactions. J Immunol Res 2017;2017. https://doi.org/10.1155/2017/1503709.

28. Mustafa SS, Ostrov D, Yerly D. Severe cutaneous adverse drug reactions: presentation, risk factors, and management. Curr Allergy Asthma Rep 2018; 18(4):1–9.

29. Cernadas JR, Brockow K, Romano A, et al. General considerations on rapid desensitization for drug hypersensitivity – a consensus statement. Allergy 2010;65(11):1357–66.

30. Mirakian R, Ewan PW, Durham SR, et al. BSACI guidelines for the management of drug allergy. Clin Exp Allergy 2009;39(1):43–61.

31. Castells M. Drug desensitization in oncology: chemotherapy agents and monoclonal antibodies. Drug Hypersensitivity 2007;413–25. https://doi.org/10.1159/000104218.

32. Bavbek S, Kendirlinan R, Çerçi P, et al. Rapid drug desensitization with biologics: a single-center experience with four biologics. Int Arch Allergy Immunol 2016;171(3–4):227–33.

33. del Carmen Sancho M, Breslow R, Sloane D, et al. Desensitization for hypersensitivity reactions to medications. Chem Immunol Allergy 2012;97:217–33.

34. Shingarev R, Glezerman IG. Kidney complications of immune check point inhibitors: a review. Am J Kidney Dis 2019;74(4):529.

35. Espi M, Teuma C, Novel-Catin E, et al. Renal adverse effects of immune checkpoints inhibitors in clinical practice: ImmuNoTox study. Eur J Cancer 2021;147: 29–39.

36. Brahmer JR, Lacchetti C, Schneider BJ, et al. Management of immune-related adverse events in patients treated with immune checkpoint inhibitor therapy:

American Society of Clinical Oncology Clinical Practice Guideline. J Clin Oncol 2018;36(17):1714.

37. Johnson DB, Manouchehri A, Haugh AM, et al. Neurologic toxicity associated with immune checkpoint inhibitors: a pharmacovigilance study. J Immunother Cancer 2019;7(1). https://doi.org/10.1186/S40425-019-0617-X.

38. Gülsen A, Wedi B, Jappe U. Hypersensitivity reactions to biologics (part I): allergy as an important differential diagnosis in complex immune-derived adverse events. Allergo J Int 2020;29(4):97.

39. Thompson JA, Schneider BJ, Brahmer J, et al. Management of immunotherapy-related toxicities, Version 1.2019. J Natl Compr Canc Netw 2019;17(3):255–89.

40. Touat M, Talmasov D, Ricard D, et al. Neurological toxicities associated with immune-checkpoint inhibitors. Curr Opin Neurol 2017;30(6):659–68.

41. Williams TJ, Benavides DR, Patrice KA, et al. Association of autoimmune encephalitis with combined immune checkpoint inhibitor treatment for metastatic cancer. JAMA Neurol 2016;73(8):928–33.

42. Ball S, Ghosh RK, Wongsaengsak S, et al. Cardiovascular toxicities of immune checkpoint inhibitors: JACC review topic of the week. J Am Coll Cardiol 2019; 74(13):1714–27.

43. Agostinetto E, Eiger D, Lambertini M, et al. Cardiotoxicity of immune checkpoint inhibitors: a systematic review and meta-analysis of randomised clinical trials. Eur J Cancer 2021;148:76–91.

44. de Malet A, Antoni G, Collins M, et al. Evolution and recurrence of gastrointestinal immune-related adverse events induced by immune checkpoint inhibitors. Eur J Cancer 2019;106:106–14.

45. Chang L-S, Barroso-Sousa R, Tolaney SM, et al. Endocrine toxicity of cancer immunotherapy targeting immune checkpoints. Endocr Rev 2019;40(1):17–65.

46. Wang Y, Zhou S, Yang F, et al. Treatment-related adverse events of PD-1 and PD-L1 inhibitors in clinical trials: a systematic review and meta-analysis. JAMA Oncol 2019;5(7):1008.

47. Jain A, Shannon VR, Sheshadri A. Immune-related adverse events: pneumonitis. Adv Exp Med Biol 2018;995:131–49.

48. Kalisz KR, Ramaiya NH, Laukamp KR, et al. Immune checkpoint inhibitor therapy–related pneumonitis: patterns and management 2019;39(7):1923–37.

49. Sebastiani GD, Scirocco C, Galeazzi M. Rheumatic immune related adverse events in patients treated with checkpoint inhibitors for immunotherapy of cancer. Autoimmun Rev 2019;18(8):805–13.

50. Calabrese LH, Calabrese C, Cappelli LC. Rheumatic immune-related adverse events from cancer immunotherapy. Nat Rev Rheumatol 2018;14(10):569–79.

51. Zhang HC, Luo W, Wang Y. Acute liver injury in the context of immune checkpoint inhibitor-related colitis treated with infliximab. J Immunother Cancer 2019;7(1). https://doi.org/10.1186/S40425-019-0532-1.

52. Peeraphatdit TB, Wang J, Odenwald MA, et al. Hepatotoxicity from immune checkpoint inhibitors: a systematic review and management recommendation. Hepatology 2020;72(1):315–29.

53. Kramer R, Zaremba A, Moreira A, et al. Hematological immune related adverse events after treatment with immune checkpoint inhibitors. Eur J Cancer 2021; 147:170–81.

54. Gülsen A, Wedi B, Jappe U. Hypersensitivity reactions to biologics (part II): classifications and current diagnostic and treatment approaches. Allergo J Int 2020;29(5):139–54.

55. Johnson DB, Chandra S, Sosman JA. Immune checkpoint inhibitor toxicity in 2018. JAMA 2018;320(16):1702–3.
56. Okazaki T, Honjo T. PD-1 and PD-1 ligands: from discovery to clinical application. Int Immunol 2007;19(7):813–24.
57. Rudd CE, Taylor A, Schneider H. CD28 and CTLA-4 coreceptor expression and signal transduction. Immunol Rev 2009;229(1):12–26.
58. Kottschade LA. Incidence and management of immune-related adverse events in patients undergoing treatment with immune checkpoint inhibitors. Curr Oncol Rep 2018;20(3):1–8.
59. Chen TW, Razak AR, Bedard PL, et al. A systematic review of immune-related adverse event reporting in clinical trials of immune checkpoint inhibitors. Ann Oncol 2015;26(9):1824–9.
60. Das S, Johnson DB. Immune-related adverse events and anti-tumor efficacy of immune checkpoint inhibitors. J Immunother Cancer 2019;7(1):1–11.
61. Sen S, Hess KR, Hong DS, et al. Impact of immune checkpoint inhibitor dose on toxicity, response rate, and survival: A pooled analysis of dose escalation phase 1 trials 2018;36(15_suppl):3077.
62. Feng Y, Roy A, Masson E, et al. Exposure-response relationships of the efficacy and safety of ipilimumab in patients with advanced melanoma. Clin Cancer Res 2013;19(14):3977–86.
63. Berner F, Bomze D, Diem S, et al. Association of checkpoint inhibitor–induced toxic effects with shared cancer and tissue antigens in non–small cell lung cancer. JAMA Oncol 2019;5(7):1.
64. Johnson DB, Balko JM, Compton ML, et al. Fulminant myocarditis with combination immune checkpoint blockade. N Engl J Med 2016;375(18):1749.
65. de Moel EC, Rozeman EA, Kapiteijn EH, et al. Autoantibody development under treatment with immune-checkpoint inhibitors. Cancer Immunol Res 2019;7(1):6–11.
66. Lim SY, Lee JH, Gide TN, et al. Circulating cytokines predict immune-related toxicity in melanoma patients receiving Anti-PD-1-based immunotherapy. Clin Cancer Res 2019;25(5):1557–63.
67. Dubin K, Callahan MK, Ren B, et al. Intestinal microbiome analyses identify melanoma patients at risk for checkpoint-blockade-induced colitis. Nat Commun 2016;7. https://doi.org/10.1038/NCOMMS10391.
68. Andrews MC, Duong CPM, Gopalakrishnan V, et al. Gut microbiota signatures are associated with toxicity to combined CTLA-4 and PD-1 blockade. Nat Med 2021;1–10. https://doi.org/10.1038/s41591-021-01406-6.
69. Johnson DB, McDonnell WJ, Ericsson-Gonzalez PI, et al. A case report of clonal EBV-like memory CD4+ T cell activation in fatal checkpoint inhibitor-induced encephalitis. Nat Med 2019;25(8):1243.
70. Iwama S, Remigis A De, Callahan MK, et al. Pituitary expression of CTLA-4 mediates hypophysitis secondary to administration of CTLA-4 Blocking Antibody. Sci Transl Med 2014;6(230):230ra45.
71. Postow MA, Sidlow R, Hellmann MD. Immune-related adverse events associated with immune checkpoint blockade. N Engl J Med 2018;378(2):158–68.
72. König D, Läubli H. Mechanisms of immune-related complications in cancer patients treated with immune checkpoint inhibitors. Pharmacology 2021;106(3–4):123–36.
73. Das R, Bar N, Ferreira M, et al. Early B cell changes predict autoimmunity following combination immune checkpoint blockade. J Clin Invest 2018;128(2):715–20.

74. Shankar B, Zhang J, Naqash AR, et al. Multisystem immune-related adverse events associated with immune checkpoint inhibitors for treatment of non–small cell lung cancer. JAMA Oncol 2020;6(12):1952–6.

75. Ricciuti B, Genova C, De Giglio A, et al. Impact of immune-related adverse events on survival in patients with advanced non-small cell lung cancer treated with nivolumab: long-term outcomes from a multi-institutional analysis. J Cancer Res Clin Oncol 2019;145(2):479–85.

76. Zhou X, Yao Z, Yang H, et al. Are immune-related adverse events associated with the efficacy of immune checkpoint inhibitors in patients with cancer? A systematic review and meta-analysis. BMC Med 2020;18(1):1–14.

77. Hua C, Boussemart L, Mateus C, et al. Association of vitiligo with tumor response in patients with metastatic melanoma treated with pembrolizumab. JAMA Dermatol 2016;152(1):45–51.

78. Boasberg PD, Hoon DSB, Piro LD, et al. Enhanced survival associated with vitiligo expression during maintenance biotherapy for metastatic melanoma. J Invest Dermatol 2006;126(12):2658–63.

79. Gogas H, Ioannovich J, Dafni U, et al. Prognostic significance of autoimmunity during treatment of melanoma with interferon. N Engl J Med 2006;354(7):709–18.

80. Faje AT, Lawrence D, Flaherty K, et al. High-dose glucocorticoids for the treatment of ipilimumab-induced hypophysitis is associated with reduced survival in patients with melanoma. Cancer 2018;124(18):3706–14.

81. Arbour KC, Mezquita L, Long N, et al. Impact of baseline steroids on efficacy of programmed cell death-1 and programmed death-ligand 1 blockade in patients with non–small-cell lung cancer 2018;36(28):2872–8.

82. Thompson JA, Schneider BJ, Brahmer J, et al. NCCN Guidelines Insights: Management of Immunotherapy-Related Toxicities, Version 1.2020: Featured Updates to the NCCN Guidelines. J Natl Compr Cancer Netw 2020;18(3):230–41.

83. Brahmer JR, Abu-Sbeih H, Ascierto PA, et al. Society for Immunotherapy of Cancer (SITC) clinical practice guideline on immune checkpoint inhibitor-related adverse events. J Immunother Cancer 2021;9(6):e002435.

84. Simonaggio A, Michot JM, Voisin AL, et al. Evaluation of readministration of immune checkpoint inhibitors after immune-related adverse events in patients with cancer. JAMA Oncol 2019;5(9):1310–7.

85. Michot JM, Lappara A, Le Pavec J, et al. The 2016–2019 ImmunoTOX assessment board report of collaborative management of immune-related adverse events, an observational clinical study. Eur J Cancer 2020;130:39–50.

86. Johnson DB, Reynolds KL, Sullivan RJ, et al. Immune checkpoint inhibitor toxicities: systems-based approaches to improve patient care and research. Lancet Oncol 2020;21(8):e398–404.

87. Tattersall IW, Leventhal JS. Cutaneous toxicities of immune checkpoint inhibitors: The role of the dermatologist. Yale J Biol Med 2020;93(1):123–32. Available at: /pmc/articles/PMC7087048/?report=abstract. Accessed January 3, 2021.

88. Muntyanu A, Netchiporouk E, Gerstein W, et al. Cutaneous immune-related adverse events (irAEs) to immune checkpoint inhibitors: a dermatology perspective on management. J Cutan Med Surg 2020. https://doi.org/10.1177/1203475420943260.

89. Wongvibulsin S, Pahalyants V, Kalinich M, et al. Epidemiology and risk factors for the development of cutaneous toxicities in patients treated with immune-checkpoint inhibitors: A United States population-level analysis. J Am Acad Dermatol 2021. https://doi.org/10.1016/J.JAAD.2021.03.094.

90. Sibaud V. Dermatologic reactions to immune checkpoint inhibitors. Am J Clin Dermatol 2017;19(3):345–61.
91. Belum VR, Benhuri B, Postow MA, et al. Characterization and management of dermatologic adverse events to agents targeting the PD-1 receptor. Eur J Cancer 2016;60:12.
92. Apalla Z, Papageorgiou C, Lallas A, et al. Cutaneous adverse events of immune checkpoint inhibitors: a literature review. Dermatol Pract Concept 2021;11(1): e2021155.
93. Raschi E, Antonazzo IC, La Placa M, et al. Serious cutaneous toxicities with immune checkpoint inhibitors in the U.S. Food and drug administration adverse event reporting system. Oncologist 2019;24(11):e1228.
94. Han Y, Wang J, Xu B. Cutaneous adverse events associated with immune checkpoint blockade: A systematic review and meta-analysis. Crit Rev Oncol Hematol 2021;163. https://doi.org/10.1016/J.CRITREVONC.2021.103376.
95. Darnell EP, Mooradian MJ, Baruch EN, et al. Immune-Related Adverse Events (irAEs): diagnosis, management, and clinical pearls. Curr Oncol Rep 2020; 22(4):1–11.
96. Pan PC, Haggiagi A. Neurologic immune-related adverse events associated with immune checkpoint inhibition. Curr Oncol Rep 2019;21(12):1–11.
97. Möhn N, Beutel G, Gutzmer R, et al. Neurological immune related adverse events associated with nivolumab, ipilimumab, and pembrolizumab therapy— review of the literature and future outlook. J Clin Med 2019;8(11):1777.
98. Guidon AC, Burton LB, Chwalisz BK, et al. Consensus disease definitions for neurologic immune-related adverse events of immune checkpoint inhibitors. J Immunother Cancer 2021;9:2890.
99. Tajiri K, Ieda M. Cardiac complications in immune checkpoint inhibition therapy. Front Cardiovasc Med 2019;6(3). https://doi.org/10.3389/FCVM.2019.00003.
100. Salem JE, Manouchehri A, Moey M, et al. Cardiovascular toxicities associated with immune checkpoint inhibitors: an observational, retrospective, pharmacovigilance study. Lancet Oncol 2018;19(12):1579–89.
101. Moslehi JJ, Salem JE, Sosman JA, et al. Increased reporting of fatal immune checkpoint inhibitor-associated myocarditis. Lancet (London, England) 2018; 391(10124):933.
102. Palaskas N, Lopez-Mattei J, Durand JB, et al. Immune checkpoint inhibitor myocarditis: pathophysiological characteristics, diagnosis, and treatment. J Am Heart Assoc 2020;9(2). https://doi.org/10.1161/JAHA.119.013757.
103. Allenbach Y, Anquetil C, Manouchehri A, et al. Immune checkpoint inhibitor-induced myositis, the earliest and most lethal complication among rheumatic and musculoskeletal toxicities. Autoimmun Rev 2020;19(8). https://doi.org/10.1016/J.AUTREV.2020.102586.
104. Bonaca MP, Olenchock BA, Salem JE, et al. Myocarditis in the setting of cancer therapeutics: proposed case definitions for emerging clinical syndromes in cardio-oncology. Circulation 2019;140(2):80–91.
105. Mahmood SS, Fradley MG, Cohen JV, et al. Myocarditis in patients treated with immune checkpoint inhibitors. J Am Coll Cardiol 2018;71(16):1755–64.
106. Salem J-E, Allenbach Y, Vozy A, et al. Abatacept for severe immune checkpoint inhibitor–associated myocarditis 2019;380(24):2377–9.
107. Choi J, Lee SY. Clinical characteristics and treatment of immune-related adverse events of immune checkpoint inhibitors. Immune Netw 2020;20(1). https://doi.org/10.4110/IN.2020.20.E9.

108. Dougan M. Gastrointestinal and hepatic complications of immunotherapy: current management and future perspectives. Curr Gastroenterol Rep 2020; 22(4):1–11.

109. Shivaji UN, Jeffery L, Gui X, et al. Immune checkpoint inhibitor-associated gastrointestinal and hepatic adverse events and their management. Therap Adv Gastroenterol 2019;12. https://doi.org/10.1177/1756284819884196.

110. Nishino M, Giobbie-Hurder A, Hatabu H, et al. Incidence of programmed cell death 1 inhibitor–related pneumonitis in patients with advanced cancer: a systematic review and meta-analysis. JAMA Oncol 2016;2(12):1607–16.

111. Cadranel J, Canellas A, Matton L, et al. Pulmonary complications of immune checkpoint inhibitors in patients with nonsmall cell lung cancer. Eur Respir Rev 2019;28(153). https://doi.org/10.1183/16000617.0058-2019.

112. Gomatou G, Tzilas V, Kotteas E, et al. Immune Checkpoint Inhibitor-Related Pneumonitis. Respiration 2020;99(11):932–42.

113. Martins F, Sofiya L, Sykiotis GP, et al. Adverse effects of immune-checkpoint inhibitors: epidemiology, management and surveillance. Nat Rev Clin Oncol 2019; 16(9):563–80.

114. Wright JJ, Powers AC, Johnson DB. Endocrine toxicities of immune checkpoint inhibitors. Nat Rev Endocrinol 2021;17(7):389–99.

115. Del Rivero J, Cordes LM, Klubo-Gwiezdzinska J, et al. Endocrine-related adverse events related to immune checkpoint inhibitors: proposed algorithms for management. Oncologist 2020;25(4):290.

116. Murakami N, Motwani S, Riella LV. Renal complications of immune checkpoint blockade. Curr Probl Cancer 2017;41(2):100.

117. Fortes BH, Liou H, Dalvin LA. Ophthalmic adverse effects of immune checkpoint inhibitors: the Mayo Clinic experience. Br J Ophthalmol 2020. https://doi.org/10.1136/BJOPHTHALMOL-2020-316970.

118. Shahzad O, Thompson N, Clare G, Welsh S, Damato E, Corrie P. Ocular adverse events associated with immune checkpoint inhibitors: a novel multidisciplinary management algorithm: Ther Adv Med Oncol 2021; 12;13:1758835921992989.

119. Dispenza MC. Classification of hypersensitivity reactions. Allergy Asthma Proc 2019;40:470–3.

120. Franceschini F, Bottau P, Caimmi S, et al. Mechanisms of hypersensitivity reactions induced by drugs. Acta Biomed 2019;90(Suppl 3):44–51.

121. Pichler WJ. Immune pathomechanism and classification of drug hypersensitivity. Allergy Eur J Allergy Clin Immunol 2019;74(8):1457–71.

122. Chen CB, Abe R, Pan RY, et al. An updated review of the molecular mechanisms in drug hypersensitivity. J Immunol Res 2018;2018. https://doi.org/10.1155/2018/6431694.

123. Elst J, Maurer M, Sabato V, et al. Novel insights on MRGPRX2-mediated hypersensitivity to neuromuscular blocking agents and fluoroquinolones. Front Immunol 2021;12. https://doi.org/10.3389/FIMMU.2021.668962.

124. Yuan F, Zhang C, Sun M, et al. MRGPRX2 mediates immediate-type pseudo-allergic reactions induced by iodine-containing iohexol. Biomed Pharmacother 2021;137. https://doi.org/10.1016/J.BIOPHA.2021.111323.

125. Subramanian H, Gupta K, Ali H. Roles of mas-related G protein-coupled receptor X2 on mast cell-mediated host defense, pseudoallergic drug reactions, and chronic inflammatory diseases. J Allergy Clin Immunol 2016;138(3):700–10.

126. Grimes J, Desai S, Charter NW, et al. MrgX2 is a promiscuous receptor for basic peptides causing mast cell pseudo-allergic and anaphylactoid reactions. Pharmacol Res Perspect 2019;7(6). https://doi.org/10.1002/PRP2.547.

127. Jakubovic BD, Vecillas LL, Jimenez-Rodriguez TW, et al. Drug hypersensitivity in the fast lane: What clinicians should know about phenotypes, endotypes, and biomarkers. Ann Allergy Asthma Immunol 2020;124(6):566–72.

128. Picard M, Galvão VR. Current knowledge and management of hypersensitivity reactions to monoclonal antibodies. J Allergy Clin Immunol Pract 2017;5(3): 600–9.

129. Sloane D, Govindarajulu U, Harrow-Mortelliti J, et al. Safety, costs, and efficacy of rapid drug desensitizations to chemotherapy and monoclonal antibodies. J Allergy Clin Immunol Pract 2016;4(3):497–504.

130. Yu R, Krantz MS, Phillips EJ, et al. Emerging causes of drug-induced anaphylaxis: a review of anaphylaxis-associated reports in the FDA adverse event reporting system (FAERS). J Allergy Clin Immunol Pract 2021;9(2):819–29.e2.

131. Cheifetz A. The incidence and management of infusion reactions to infliximab: a large center experience. Am J Gastroenterol 2003;98(6):1315–24.

132. Bian LF, Zheng C, Shi XL. Atezolizumab-induced anaphylactic shock in a patient with hepatocellular carcinoma undergoing immunotherapy: a case report. World J Clin Cases 2021;9(16):4110–5.

133. Kumari S, Yun J, Soares JR, et al. Severe infusion reaction due to nivolumab: A case report. Cancer Rep 2020;3(3). https://doi.org/10.1002/cnr2.1246.

134. Choi B, McBride A, Scott AJ. Treatment with pembrolizumab after hypersensitivity reaction to nivolumab in a patient with hepatocellular carcinoma. Am J Heal Pharm 2019;76(21):1749–52.

135. Lu J, Thuraisingam T, Chergui M, et al. Nivolumab-associated DRESS syndrome: a case report. JAAD Case Rep 2019;5(3):216–8.

136. Momtaz P, Park V, Panageas KS, et al. Safety of infusing ipilimumab Over 30 minutes. J Clin Oncol 2015;33(30):3454–8.

137. El Osta B, Hu F, Sadek R, et al. Not all immune-checkpoint inhibitors are created equal: Meta-analysis and systematic review of immune-related adverse events in cancer trials. Crit Rev Oncol Hematol 2017;119:1–12.

138. Kelly K, Infante JR, Taylor MH, et al. Safety profile of avelumab in patients with advanced solid tumors: a pooled analysis of data from the phase 1 JAVELIN solid tumor and phase 2 JAVELIN Merkel 200 clinical trials. Cancer 2018; 124(9):2010–7.

139. Michailidou D, Khaki AR, Morelli MP, et al. Association of blood biomarkers and autoimmunity with immune related adverse events in patients with cancer treated with immune checkpoint inhibitors. Sci Rep 2021;11(1):1–10.

140. Diehl A, Yarchoan M, Hopkins A, et al. Relationships between lymphocyte counts and treatment-related toxicities and clinical responses in patients with solid tumors treated with PD-1 checkpoint inhibitors. Oncotarget 2017;8(69): 114268.

141. Fujisawa Y, Yoshino K, Otsuka A, et al. Fluctuations in routine blood count might signal severe immune-related adverse events in melanoma patients treated with nivolumab. J Dermatol Sci 2017;88(2):225–31.

142. Tahir SA, Gao J, Miura Y, et al. Autoimmune antibodies correlate with immune checkpoint therapy-induced toxicities. Proc Natl Acad Sci U S A 2019; 116(44):22246–51.

143. Jing Y, Liu J, Ye Y, et al. Multi-omics prediction of immune-related adverse events during checkpoint immunotherapy. Nat Commun 2020;11(1):1–7.

144. Stamatouli AM, Quandt Z, Perdigoto AL, et al. Collateral damage: insulin-dependent diabetes induced with checkpoint inhibitors. Diabetes 2018;67(8): 1471–80.

145. Shahabi V, Berman D, Chasalow SD, et al. Gene expression profiling of whole blood in ipilimumab-treated patients for identification of potential biomarkers of immune-related gastrointestinal adverse events. J Transl Med 2013;11(1):75.
146. Hommes JW, Verheijden RJ, Suijkerbuijk KPM, et al. Biomarkers of checkpoint inhibitor induced immune-related adverse events—a comprehensive review. Front Oncol 2021;0:2916.
147. Itzstein MS von, Khan S, Gerber DE. Investigational biomarkers for checkpoint inhibitor immune-related adverse event prediction and diagnosis. Clin Chem 2020;66(6):779.
148. Johnson DB, Jakubovic BD, Sibaud V, et al. Balancing cancer immunotherapy efficacy and toxicity. J Allergy Clin Immunol Pract 2020;8(9):2898.
149. Thong BY, Tan TC. Epidemiology and risk factors for drug allergy. Br J Clin Pharmacol 2011;71(5):684–700.
150. Drug allergies|World Allergy Organization. Available at: https://www.worl dallergy.org/education-and-programs/education/allergic-disease-resource-cent er/professionals/drug-allergies. Accessed July 28, 2021.
151. Demoly P, Adkinson NF, Brockow K, et al. International Consensus on drug allergy. Allergy 2014;69(4):420–37.
152. Khan DA, Solensky R. Drug allergy. J Allergy Clin Immunol 2010;125(2 Suppl 2). https://doi.org/10.1016/J.JACI.2009.10.028.
153. Scherer K, Brockow K, Aberer W, et al. Desensitization in delayed drug hypersensitivity reactions – an EAACI position paper of the Drug Allergy Interest Group. Allergy 2013;68(7):844–52.
154. de Las Vecillas Sánchez L, Alenazy LA, Garcia-Neuer M, et al. Drug hypersensitivity and desensitizations: mechanisms and new approaches. Int J Mol Sci 2017;18(6). https://doi.org/10.3390/IJMS18061316.
155. Watanabe H, Kubo T, Ninomiya K, et al. The effect and safety of an immune checkpoint inhibitor rechallenge in non-small cell lung cancer 2018;36(15_Suppl):e21147.
156. Mohamed AA, Zhang S, Faust G. The efficacy and safety of rechallenge with an alternative immune checkpoint inhibitor in metastatic malignant melanoma. Ann Oncol 2018;29:x19–20.
157. Picard M, Pur L, Caiado J, et al. Risk stratification and skin testing to guide re-exposure in taxane-induced hypersensitivity reactions. J Allergy Clin Immunol 2016;137(4):1154–64.e12.

Skin Testing Approaches for Immediate and Delayed Hypersensitivity Reactions

Annick Barbaud, MD, PhD[a],*, Antonino Romano, MD, PhD[b]

KEYWORDS

- Diagnosis • Delayed hypersensitivity • Drugs • Immediate hypersensitivity
- Intradermal tests • Patch tests • Prick tests • Provocation tests

KEY POINTS

- Drug patch tests are well tolerated and have a good sensitivity in assessing acute generalized exanthematous pustulosis and drug rash with eosinophilia and systemic symptoms.
- Skin prick tests are used for immediate hypersensitivity reactions and can be done with all drugs except opiates.
- Intradermal tests (IDTs) are performed by injecting 0.02 mL of the appropriately diluted suspected drug to evaluate immediate (with immediate readings) and delayed hypersensitivity reactions (with delayed readings).
- For IDTs, appropriate dilutions—summarized in this paper—have to be respected in order to avoid irritant false-positive reactions.
- A negative drug skin test does not exclude the responsibility of a drug in the occurrence of an adverse drug reaction.

Abbreviations	
ADR	adverse drug reaction
AGEP	acute generalized exanthematous pustulosis
BLs	beta-lactam antibiotics
CADRs	cutaneous adverse drug reactions
DHR	delayed hypersensitivity reaction
DPT	drug provocation test
DRESS	drug reaction with systemic symptoms
EAACI	european Academy of Allergy and Clinical Immunology
ICM	iodinated contrast media

[a] département de Dermatologie et Allergologie, Sorbonne Université, INSERM, Institut Pierre Louis d'Epidémiologie et de Santé Publique, AP-HP.Sorbonne Université, Hôpital Tenon, Paris F75020, France; [b] Oasi Research Institute-IRCCS, Troina, Italy
* Corresponding author.
E-mail address: annick.barbaud@aphp.fr

Immunol Allergy Clin N Am 42 (2022) 307–322
https://doi.org/10.1016/j.iac.2022.01.003
0889-8561/22/© 2022 Elsevier Inc. All rights reserved.

IDTs	intradermal tests
IgE	immunoglobulin E
IHR	immediate hypersensitivity reaction
MPE	maculopapular exanthema
PEG	polyethylene glycol
PTs	patch tests
SDRIFE	symmetric drug-related intertriginous and flexural exanthema
SJS/TEN	stevens-Johnson syndrome/toxic epidermal necrolysis
STs	skin tests
UV	ultraviolet
W20	papule (wheal) measured after 20 minutes
Wi	injection papule (wheal) measured immediately after injection

Patch tests (PTs) and skin tests (STs), namely skin prick tests (SPTs) and intradermal tests (IDTs), are useful tools for diagnosing drug hypersensitivity. They can be used to demonstrate the responsibility of a drug in the occurrence of an adverse drug reaction (ADR), as well as to assess cross-reactivity among drugs and find safe alternatives.

In performing these tests, however, there is a lack of standardized methodological approaches and particularly inconsistency with regard to the drug concentrations,[1] which makes comparisons between centers difficult. Moreover, there are differences between Europe and North America in the approach to the diagnosis of drug hypersensitivity reactions.[2]

In this article, we considered international guidelines and relevant reviews,[3–5] especially more recent ones,[6,7] summarizing the data concerning the diagnostic value of both STs and PTs and providing information for their adequate indication and correct performance. In any case, the reference standard to confirm or exclude drug hypersensitivity is the drug provocation test (DPT), which consists in the controlled administration of a therapeutic dose of the suspected drug.[6,8,9]

In nonsevere ADRs, negative STs and/or PTs can be followed by an ingestion challenge or DPTs. There is a broad consensus on the indication of direct DPTs (ie, not preceded by skin testing) in children with benign nonimmediate) reactions to beta-lactam antibiotics (BLs), especially in those with mild maculopapular exanthema (MPE).[10–14] Direct DPTs with BLs were also carried out in adults assessed as low risk for true BL allergy.[13,15] However, this approach was not recommended in a recent review on STs[7] because it was evaluated in a limited number of patients and the indication for direct DPTs did not agree with that of the European Academy of Allergy and Clinical Immunology (EAACI) guidelines on the diagnosis of BL allergy.[12] In the latter, only adults with palmar exfoliative exanthema can be candidates for direct DPTs. Regarding immediate reactions (ie, occurring within 1–6 hours after the last administered dose)[16,17] to BLs, there is no consensus on which subjects reporting such nonanaphylactic reactions are low risk. In this connection, recently, Sabato and colleagues[17] demonstrated that urticarial reactions to BLs that appear within one 1 hour after the first dose and subside within 1 day (ie, meeting the "1-1-1" criterion) are highly predictive of positive allergy testing.

In this article, we mainly referred to a recent review[7] on STs and PTs in the workup of cutaneous adverse drug reactions (CADRs).

Regarding the timing of their performance, in general, it is recommended to carry out STs and PTs at least 4 weeks and within 1 year after the ADR.[3,4] In drug reaction with systemic symptoms (DRESS), they must be done at least 6 months after the disappearance of the CADR and in the absence of high virus replication.[18] Note that immunoglobulin E (IgE)-mediated hypersensitivity to BLs can wane over time.[19] Some studies[20,21] followed-up patients with such hypersensitivity prospectively over 5 years and found that more than 60% of the participants who completed the studies and were initially skin test positive reverted to skin test negative with the implicated drug. Consequently, to avoid false-negative results, it is crucial to evaluate these subjects within a few months.[22] On the other hand, T-cell–mediated hypersensitivity to antibiotics, including BLs, seems to be a long-lasting condition.[23]

Some drugs or ultraviolet (UV) exposure can diminish the skin reactivity to drug STs. In immediate hypersensitivity reactions (IHRs), the use of β-blockers is considered as a relative contraindication to skin testing. However, a study by Fung and colleagues[24] demonstrated the safety of administrating SPTs to patients on β-blocker treatment.

Topical corticosteroids should be stopped the week before on the site of any drug ST.[3,4,7] Systemic corticosteroids have no inhibitory impact on SPTs but have to be stopped 1 month before PTs or IDTs.[25] Immunosuppressive drugs can affect the skin reactivity for any drug ST and should be stopped 1 month before testing if possible. UV exposure should be avoided up to 4 weeks before STs and PTs.

In IHRs, antihistamines should be stopped 4 days (7 days for loratadine and desloratadine and tricyclic antidepressants with antihistaminic activity) before STs, but they have no impact on PT results.[3,4,7] Concerning psychotropic drugs, imipramine and phenothiazines that have antihistaminic activity, but not escitalopram, fluoxetine, and sertraline,[25] can diminish skin reactivity to SPTs.[26]

DRUG PATCH TESTS

PTs reproduce a delayed hypersensitivity reaction (DHR). PTs are applied to the upper back on unaffected and untreated skin, using IQ chambers (Chemotechnique, Velinge, Sweden) or an equivalent fixed with a "hypoallergic" tape. They are left for 2 days, then read on day 2 (30 minutes after removing the test material) and on day 4 or 5, and until after 1 week for those with corticosteroids. Reading result's criteria are identical to those used for contact allergy (ie, negative, irritant, + to +++).[27] At least 10 negative controls are necessary to assess the specificity of a positive PT. Negative controls have been published for PTs with many drugs.[7,28] PTs are particularly useful for evaluating DHRs to noninjectable drugs such as most anticonvulsants and nonvitamin K antagonist oral anticoagulants.[29,30] However, only a limited number of molecules marketed by Chemotechnique (Velinge, Sweden) or SmartPractice Canada are available as ready-to-use material, in which most drugs, either the trade or reagent grade product, are diluted at 10% in petrolatum. In most cases, it is necessary to prepare the test material by diluting the drugs in their marketed form provided by the patients themselves. As the stability of PT material has not been validated or established for most drugs, it should be prepared just before testing. PTs with the drug in its commercially available oral form can be prepared by diluting it at 30%[3] or 20%[4] in petrolatum. Ideally, a concentration of 10% of the active ingredient should be obtained. Brajon and colleagues[28] showed that the exact amount of the active ingredient in the PT material prepared by diluting commercial forms of the drugs concerned at 30% in petrolatum varied widely and 25% of that material had an active ingredient's concentration of less than 2%. From a practical point of view, because it is impossible to obtain a 10% active ingredient's concentration for each drug tested, we recommend that studies using PTs with drugs provide the exact concentration of active ingredient, so that the results obtained by different centers can be compared.[28]

When the active ingredient is in pure form (eg, lyophilized powder), it is recommended to dilute it at 10% in petrolatum.[3]

Some drugs, such as captopril (at 1% in pet.), celecoxib (if tested >10% in pet.), chloroquine (at 30% in pet.), misoprostol (if tested > 1% in pet.), and sodium valproate (at 1% in pet.), have been reported as irritant.[7] Some centers have pharmacy services that dilute drugs for PTs. Assier and colleagues[31] demonstrated that material prepared by physicians led to results equivalent to those obtained with the ready-to-use products commercialized by Chemotechnique.

A control PT has to be done with the vehicle (eg, petrolatum, alcohol) used to dilute the drug for the preparation of the PT material.

DRUG SKIN PRICK TESTS

SPTs can be done with any form of commercialized drug, usually, in undiluted form: pills reduced to very fine powder, capsule contents, liquid, or injectable solutions.[1] In SPTs, a small drop of reagent is applied on volar forearm skin, and a standardized 1-mm-tipped lancet (pricker) is passed through the drop and perpendicularly inserted into the skin..[3,4,7,26] Reactions to SPTs are considered positive when the diameter of the wheal is at least 3 mm greater than that of the negative control and is surrounded by erythema, 20 minutes after the prick. A positive control is done with histamine at 10 mg/mL. As a negative control, normal saline and/or any other solvent used to dilute are used. SPTs can be performed with all drugs except opiates. If there is a global shortage of a drug (eg, biologicals, COVID 19 vaccines), it could be possible to perform a prick-to-prick test by dipping the lancet in the drug solution residual of the vials already used and then carrying out the skin puncture with it.

Nonspecific degranulation is observed in SPTs with certain antibiotics or anesthetic drugs at the usual concentrations. The highest nonirritating concentrations for SPTs are reported in **Table 1**. SPTs are useful for evaluating IHRs. In effect, although they have a sensitivity of 6.9%, they have a very good specificity (98.8%) and a good negative predictive value (85.7%).[32]

Seldom late positive responses to SPTs have been reported in MPE, DRESS, and acute generalized exanthematous pustulosis (AGEP).[7,18] A SPT causes a delayed positive reaction when there is erythema and infiltration at the puncture site after 1 or 2 days.[3,4]

SPTs with additives can be done by diluting them as follows: polyethylene glycol (PEG) 3000 at 50% water/volume, PEG 6000 at 50% water/volume, and polysorbate 80 at 20% water/volume.[33]

DRUG INTRADERMAL TESTS

IDTs are performed and interpreted differently in drug allergy centers. Recently, a multicenter study standardized an IDT method that helped reduce variability, allowing for a more reliable comparison of results between physicians and centers.[34] According to this study,[34] the recommended volume to be injected intradermally on the volar forearm is 0.02 mL. It produces a small superficial bleb approximately 5 mm in diameter. For intradermal administrations, a tuberculin syringe is used, which contains only 0.02 mL of the reagent solution and has a flat-ended plunger.

The diameter of the injection papule (wheal) should be measured immediately after injection (Wi) and then at 20 minutes (W20). At that time, the IDT is considered positive if the diameter of the measured wheal (W20) is greater than or equal to the diameter of the Wi + 3 mm and if there is surrounding erythema that has also to be measured.

In subjects with DHRs, IDTs can be positive on delayed readings (eg, after 1–3 days). Any late responses to IDT should be documented by the diameter of the erythema and the infiltration, as well as a morphologic description. Patients are advised

Table 1
Highest nonirritating concentrations recommended for drug prick and intradermal testing (According to published literature, mainly form Brockow et al.,[5] EAACI position papers,[12,35,36] and a recent update on drug skin tests[7]). If nothing is written in "skin prick tests" column, the same concentration as those of IDT can be used.

	Intradermal Tests	Skin Prick Tests[a]
ANTIBIOTICS		
Beta-lactams		
Amoxicillin, ampicillin, and other semisynthetic penicillins	20 mg/mL	—
Aztreonam	2–20 mg/mL	—
Benzylpenicilloyl-poly-L-lysine	6×10^{-5} mol/L	—
Benzylpenicilloyl-octa-L-lysine	8.64×10^{-5} mol/L	—
Sodium benzylpenilloate	1.5×10^{-3} mol/L	—
Benzylpenicillin	10,000 IU/mL	—
Cefepime	2 mg/mL	—
Cephalosporins other than cefepime	20 mg/mL	—
Clavulanic acid	20 mg/mL	—
Imipenem-cilastatin	0.5 mg/mL–0.5 mg/mL	—
Ertapenem and meropenem	1 mg/mL	—
Quinolones		
Ciprofloxacin	0.006 mg/mL	—
Levofloxacin	0.025 mg/mL	—
Ofloxacin	0.05 mg/mL	—
Pefloxacin	No IDT	0.32 mg/mL
Rifampicin	2 mcg/mL	—
Macrolides		
Azithromycin	0.01 mg/mL	—
Clarithromycin	0.05 mg/mL	—
Erythromycin	0.01–0.05 mg/mL	5 mg/mL
Rovamycin	37.5 U/mL	37,500 IU/mL
Others		
Clindamycin	15 mg/mL	—
Cotrimoxazole	0.8 mg/mL	—
Gentamycin	4 mg/mL	—
Rifampicin	0.002 mg/mL	—
Tobramycin	4 mg/mL	—
Vancomycin	0.005–0.05 mg/mL	—
PERIOPERATIVE DRUGS		
Neuromuscular blocking agents		
Atracurium	0.01 mg/mL	1 mg/mL
Cisatracurium	0.02 mg/mL	2 mg/mL
Mivacurium	0.002 mg/mL	0.2 mg/mL
Pancuronium	0.02 mg/mL	2 mg/mL

(continued on next page)

Table 1
(*continued*)

	Intradermal Tests	Skin Prick Tests[a]
Rocuronium	0.05 mg/mL	10 mg/mL
Suxamethonium	0.1 mg/mL	10 mg/mL
Vecuronium	0.04 mg/mL	4 mg/mL
Anesthetic agents		
Etomidate	0.2 mg/mL	2 mg/mL
Ketamine	0.1 mg/mL	100 mg/mL
S-Ketamine	0.25 mg/mL	25 mg/mL[b]
Midazolam	0.05 mg/mL	5 mg/mL
Propofol	1 mg/mL	10 mg/mL
Thiopental	2.5 mg/mL	25 mg/mL
Reversal agents		
Sugammadex	10 mg/mL	—
Opiates		
Alfentanil	0.05 mg/mL	0.5 mg/mL
Fentanyl	0.0005 mg/mL	0.05 mg/mL
Morphine	0.005 mg/mL	1.0 mg/mL[b]
Remifentanil	0.005 mg/mL	0.05 mg/mL
Sufentanil	0.0005 mg/mL	0.005 mg/mL
Local anesthetics		
Articaine	2 mg/mL	—
Bupivacaine	0.25 mg/mL	—
Chloroprocaine (ester derivative)	1 mg/mL	—
Levobupivacaine	0.75 mg/mL	—
Lidocaine	1 mg/mL	—
Mepivacaine	2 mg/mL	—
Prilocaine	2 mg/mL	—
Ropivacaine	1 mg/mL	—
CHEMOTHERAPEUTIC DRUGS		
Paclitaxel	0.03 mg/mL	—
Docetaxel	0.1 mg/mL	—
Platinum salts	1 mg/mL[c]	—
Carboplatin	1 mg/mL	—
Cisplatin	0.1 mg/mL	—
Cisplatin	1 mg/mL	—
Oxaliplatin	0.5 mg/mL	—
Oxaliplatin	1 mg/mL	—
CORTICOSTEROIDS		
Betamethasone	0.4 mg/mL	—
Cortivazol	2.5 mg/mL	—
Dexamethasone	0.4 mg/mL	—
Hydrocortisone	1 mg/mL	—

(*continued on next page*)

Table 1 (continued)	Intradermal Tests	Skin Prick Tests[a]
Hydrocortisone hemisuccinate	5 mg/mL	—
Triamcinolone	4 mg/mL	—
Methylprednisolone	4 mg/mL	—
Prednisolone	2.5 mg/mL	—
HEPARINS	Diluted 1:10	—
INSULINS	Diluted 1:10	—
CYTOKINES, BIOLOGICAL AGENTS		
Anti-TNF		
Adalimumab	50 mg/mL	—
Etanercept	5 mg/mL	—
Infliximab	2 mg/mL	—
Infliximab	10 mg/mL	—
Omalizumab	1.25 mcg/mL	—
Rituximab	10 mg/mL (7 negative controls)	—
Tocilizumab	0.2 mg/mL or 20 mg/mL (10 negative controls) 1.62 mg/mL	—
Interferons	Undiluted	—
Nonsteroidal antiinflammatory drugs (NSAIDs)		
Diclofenac	2.5 mg/mL	—
Ketoprofen	2 mg/mL	—
Piroxicam	2 mg/mL	—
Pyrazolones and other injectable NSAIDs	0.1 mg/mL	—
CONTRAST MEDIA		
Iodinated contrast media	Diluted 1:10 for immediate reactions, maybe undiluted for delayed reactions	—
Gadolinium derivatives	Diluted 1:10	—
PROTON PUMP INHIBITORS		
Esomeprazole	0.4 or 4 mg/mL	—
Omeprazole	0.4 or 4 mg/mL	—
Pantoprazole	0.4 or 4 mg/mL.	—
MISCELLANEOUS DRUGS, EXCIPIENTS, DYES		
Paracetamol/Acetaminophen	1 mg/mL	—
Chlorhexidine	0.002 mg/mL (sterile uncolored alcohol-free solution)	—
Fluorescein	Diluted 1:10 (10 mg/mL in our experience)	—
Carboxymethylcellulose	0.01 mg/mL	—
Hydroxyethyl starch	6 mg/mL	—
Methylene blue	0.1 mg/mL	—
Patent blue	0.25 mg/mL	—

(continued on next page)

	Intradermal Tests	Skin Prick Tests[a]
Table 1 *(continued)*		
Polyethylene glycol (PEG)/Macrogol		
PEG 300	—	Undiluted
PEG 3000	—	50% water/volume
PEG 2000	—	50% water/volume
PEG 6000	—	50% water/volume
Polysorbate 80	—	20% water/volume

[a] Highest nonirritating concentrations when undiluted drugs can be irritant.
[b] Possibly irritant.
[c] Can induce false-positive results on delayed readings.[56]

to return to show any positive responses appearing within 1 week after IDT, as well as to take pictures of positive or doubtful IDTs.[12]

For IDTs, sterile injectable solutions are obligatory. In most cases, dilutions of reagents are done in normal saline. Performing a positive control with histamine at 1 mg/mL is not mandatory if a positive control SPT is performed. As a negative control, normal saline and/or any other solvent used to dilute are used.

The initial dilution of the IDT reagents depends on the severity of the index reaction. In IHRs, IDTs should be performed after ensuring the negativity of SPTs. As in the diagnosis of IHRs to BLs,[12] the suggested sequence of STs is as follows: (1) SPT (1/10 and the highest nonirritating concentrations) at intervals of 20 minutes, and if SPTs are negative (2) IDTs (1/100 of the highest nonirritating concentration, 1/10, and the highest nonirritating concentration) at intervals of 20 minutes. The procedure is stopped when a positive ST is found. In evaluating subjects who suffered severe anaphylactic reactions, starting concentrations of ST reagents should be at least 10^{-3} of the highest nonirritating ones to avoid systemic reactions.[2] In any case, it is advisable to perform IDTs in a hospital setting.

In low-risk patients, the workup can be simplified by performing SPTs and IDTs directly with the highest nonirritating concentrations.

IDTs can induce false-positive results mainly due to irritating reagent concentrations. An EAACI position paper provided information on drug concentrations for skin testing.[5] **Table 1** shows the highest nonirritating concentrations for drug prick and IDTs recommended in this and other EAACI position papers,[5,12,35] as well as in practice parameters[36] and relevant reviews.[7] Note that these concentrations were determined in studies where IDTs were performed using many different techniques. Moreover, these concentrations were defined only regarding IHRs.[5] For IDTs, the highest nonirritating concentration of many drugs might not be similar to that which evokes a T-cell response after 6 to 24 hours. This is particularly true for drugs such as fluoroquinolones and vancomycin, which intrinsically cause direct release of histamine and in which the sensitivity of IDTs using the lowest concentrations to avoid non–IgE-mediated mast cell activation by IDTs is very poor.

Regarding STs with the main drugs, amoxicillin, amoxicillin-clavulanic acid, and ampicillin can be tested at concentrations up to 20 mg/mL, similar to other semisynthetic penicillins, aztreonam, and all cephalosporins except cefepime.[12,37,38] macrolides,[39,40] rifampicin,[39] or quinolones[39,41] can be very irritant. IDTs with diluted solutions are of interest with glycopeptides.[42] They could be of value in IHRs to proton pump inhibitors.[43]

IHRs to iodinated contrast media (ICM) can be assessed by SPTs with undiluted products and by IDTs with dilutions 1:10.[36,44,45] In DHRs, PTs can be useful and delayed-reading IDTs can be done with undiluted ICM.[36] For STs with gadolinium derivatives, dilutions 1:10[46] or undiluted products[47] can be used.

Heparin and heparinoids can be tested diluted 1:10 or undiluted.[48] Nevertheless, STs are contraindicated in subjects with an index reaction of necrosis at the site of heparin injection. Because the positive reaction is often delayed, readings should also be performed after 72 hours or later.

Corticosteroids can be tested diluted 1:10.[49–51] STs with corticosteroids at high concentrations, mainly with those with long-lasting effects, can induce skin atrophy.[49] Allergy to excipients, mainly carboxymethylcellulose or polysorbate, should be considered and investigated. Carboxymethylcellulose can be tested by SPTs and IDTs at a concentration of 10 mcg/mL.[52,53] Insulins are tested diluted at 1:10.[54] Immediate-reading IDTs with platinum salts at concentrations from 0.1 to 1 mg/mL, depending on the salt, are specific[55]; however, a nonspecific erythematous infiltration can occur at 24 hours with these IDTs. Therefore, their delayed readings do not seem to be specific, as published with carboplatin at 1 mg/mL[56] and observed with oxaliplatin.[7]

IDTs with biologicals and cytokines are of little use.[57] For STs with antitumor necrosis factors, specificity thresholds have been reported at the following concentrations: infliximab less than or equal to 2 mg/mL, adalimumab less than or equal to 50 mg mL, and etanercept less than or equal to 5 mg/mL.[7] Some articles have reported studies in which IDTs were performed with rituximab[57,58] or tocilizumab.[57,59,60] IDTs with interferons were thought to be nonspecific, but they seem to be interesting, with good positive and negative predictive value (NPV)[61] in evaluating generalized exanthemas due to these molecules. The thresholds for the specificity of IDTs are reported in **Table 1**.

For IDTs with general anesthetics, the same method should be adopted. Some guidelines recommended an injection of 0.03 mL,[62] others a volume of 0.03 mL to 0.05 mL[63] or 0.02 mL to 0.05 mL,[64] but a recent EAACI position paper recommended a volume of 0.02 mL, as for other IDTs.[35]

STs with some drugs are irritating and can induce false-positive results. STs with vaccines are not standardized, and their specificity is discussed. False-positive results are frequent in delayed readings and should not be considered. In case of IHRs, SPTs or prick-to-prick tests with the undiluted vaccine and, when available, its excipients (eg, gelatin, egg, PEG) can be done. However, IDTs with vaccines diluted 1:10 and even 1:100, mainly with influenzae vaccine, frequently induce irritative reactions.[65] False-positive results have also been reported with IDTs performed with glatiramer acetate at a concentration of 200 mcg/mL and in some cases at that of 20 mcg/mL. For STs with this molecule, the specificity threshold has not yet been determined.[66] Finally, a recent practical guidance for the evaluation and management of drug hypersensitivity[6] provided information on STs with a huge number of drugs, including antivirals, antifungals, and antimalarials.

NEGATIVE PREDICTIVE VALUE OF DRUG SKIN TESTS

Because STs and DPTs are not standardized, it is difficult to compare the results regarding the NPV of STs across the literature. For BLs, the NPV of STs is around 90%, depending on the type of hypersensitivity and the method used for DPTs.[12] For ICM, the NPV varies from 80% to 97.3%.[36]

Table 2
Use of skin prick tests, intradermal tests, and/or patch tests in immediate or delayed drug reactions

	Patch Tests	Prick Tests	IDT	Provocation Tests
Urticaria/angioedema, anaphylaxis	Not useful, can be dangerous	Useful (immediate reading)	Useful (immediate reading)	Adapted to the low- or high-risk profile of the patient[12]
Maculopapular exanthema	Useful	Limited value (DR)	Useful (DR)	After negative skin tests with delayed readings in low-risk subjects[12] NPV of 90%
Generalized eczema (contact reaction)	Useful	Limited value (DR)	Useful (DR)	After negative delayed skin test with delayed readings. NPV unknown
SDRIFE	Useful (positive in 36%–82%)	Limited value (DR)	Useful (DR)	After negative skin tests with delayed readings. NPV unknown
Fixed drug eruption	Useful if applied on the area of eruption[68,69]	Not useful	Not useful	At full dose when patch tests or repeated application tests are negative. NPV unknown.
Generalized bullous fixed drug eruption	Maybe useful	Contraindicated	Contraindicated	Contraindicated
Acute generalized exanthematous pustulosis (AGEP)	Useful, sensitivity up to 58%[18]	Limited value (DR)	Potentially useful (DR)	Contraindicated with suspected drugs and cross-reactive ones
Drug reaction with eosinophilia and systemic symptoms (DRESS)	Useful, sensitivity 32%–64% depending on the tested drug[18,67] Advised 6 mo after disappearance of DRESS	Limited value (DR)	Delayed reading at 24 h [18,74]	Contraindicated with highly suspected drug and cross-reactive ones[1,77]
SJS/TEN	Low sensitivity (<30%)	Unknown value (DR)	Contraindicated with the suspected drugs	Contraindicated.
Photosensitivity	Photo patch tests with a 5 J/cm² UVA irradiation	No value	No value	No value without exposure to UV
Vasculitis	No value	No value	No value	Contraindicated

Abbreviations: DR, delayed reading (ie, after 24–48 h); SDRIFE, symmetric drug-related intertriginous and flexural exanthema; SJS/TEN, Stevens-Johnson syndrome/toxic epidermal necrolysis.

DRUG SKIN TESTS AND PATCH TESTS HAVE TO BE ADAPTED ACCORDING TO THE CLINICAL FEATURES AND THE DRUG INVOLVED

The diagnostic value of STs and PTs depends on the ADR clinical features and the drug tested. STs are useful for identifying the responsible drug only in IgE- or T-cell–mediated reactions. They are not useful in some ADRs such as those to nonsteroidal antiinflammatory drugs with a cross-reactivity pattern, bradykinin-induced angioedema due to angiotensin-converting enzyme inhibitors, and sartans, as well as reactions to dipeptidyl peptidase-4 inhibitors, as such reactions are not caused by allergic hypersensitivity. Moreover, STs have no diagnostic value in drug-induced autoimmune diseases or pruritus.

In IHRs, as for BLs,[12] STs have to be adapted to the risk profile of the patient. STs have been reported as useful with many drugs but mainly with BLs, ICM, gadoterate meglumine, general anesthetics, insulins, proton pump inhibitors, corticosteroids, and platinum salts. PTs are not recommended. In case of anaphylactic shock, PTs are absolutely contraindicated, as they have a poor value in IHRs, but mainly because they can reinduce the shock. Anaphylactic shocks induced by PTs have been reported with BLs, neomycin, gentamicin, bacitracin, and diclofenac.[7]

Regarding DHRs, recently, an international consensus on their diagnosis was reached,[1] and its adapted conclusions are summarized in **Table 2**. Drug PTs have a lower sensibility than IDTs and are of value for evaluating MPE, systemic contact dermatitis, symmetric drug-related intertriginous and flexural exanthema, or flexural exanthema, eczematous reactions at injection sites, AGEP, DRESS, and Stevens-Johnson syndrome/toxic epidermal necrolysis (SJS/TEN).[1,7] Many drugs have been reported to have positive results when evaluated by PTs, but PTs performed with allopurinol, salazopyrin, or paracetamol are mostly or ever negative.[18,67]

In MPE, delayed-reading IDTs have the highest sensitivity. Delayed positive IDT results have been reported mainly with BLs, glycopeptides, heparins, ICM, and corticosteroids.

In fixed drug eruptions (FDEs), PTs are applied in duplicate on the back but also on the site of eruption (residual sometimes pigmented lesion; ie, "in situ PTs") and read at day 1 or 2.[68,69] If in situ PTs are negative, an in situ repeated open application test can be done.[69] The preparation for the in situ PT is given to the patient and applied to a surface of 2 cm × 2 cm, once a day for 1 week. In case of negative STs, a DPT can be done in benign FDE, but it is absolutely contraindicated in generalized bullous FDE.

In investigating a drug-induced photosensitivity, both PTs and photo patch tests with the suspected drug have to be performed. It is recommended to test with a 1% concentration of an active ingredient, but only at 0.1% for phenothiazines.[70] The irradiation for drug photo patch tests is performed at day 2 with a 5 J/cm^2 UVA.[70] A nonirradiated control PT is also applied. The reading is done 2 days after the irradiation. Criteria for positive results are identical to those used for PTs with haptens (ie, negative, irritant, + to +++).[27]

Regarding severe DHRs, such as SJS/TEN, DRESS, AGEP, and bullous exanthemas, as stated in some European guidelines,[3,4,12,71,72] PTs with the suspected drugs should be used as the first line of investigation (ie, before STs). In the case of positive responses to PTs, STs should be avoided, whereas in the case of negative results, IDTs might be performed, starting with a lower concentration of the drug concerned (eg, 1 mg/mL for semisynthetic penicillins). In some studies,[18,73] this approach proved to be safe and useful not only for identifying the responsible drugs[18] but also for detecting any cross-reactivity and finding safe alternatives.[73] Specifically, in the 72 patients with DRESS, 45 with AGEP, and 17 with SJS/TEN of a multicenter study,[18] PT sensitivity was 64%, 58%, and 24%, respectively. Of the 11 patients with AGEP and 4 with DRESS associated with BLs who were negative to PTs, 4 and 3 were positive to delayed-reading IDTs, respectively. Nevertheless, the use of IDTs in evaluating severe DHRs to drugs remains controversial, even though recent studies on subjects with such reactions confirmed and emphasized their safety and usefulness, in particular, for exploring cross-reactivity and cosensitization in DRESS.[74–77]

For an alternative or suspected low-imputable drug, if irreplaceable and negative to STs, a graded DPT can be discussed by specialists involved in severe cutaneous ADRs.[77]

In conclusion, in order to compare the results from one center with another, it is time to consider standardizing drug skin testing methods. For PTs, it is essential to report results with reference to the concentration of the active ingredient. For IDTs, the only way is to work on a known allergen dose and not on injection-wheal diameters. Therefore, a controlled volume injected in IDTs seems to be the best method. We always have to keep in mind that a negative ST does not exclude the responsibility of a drug in the occurrence of a CADR.

CLINICS CARE POINTS

- In case of positive drug skin tests, in order to ensure specific results, please give 10 negative control results from your experience or literature.

- In nonsevere adverse reactions, drug STs have to be done before DPTs but can be avoided before provocation in children with nonsevere delayed reactions or in adults with palmar exfoliative exanthema.

- Drug patch tests reproduce a delayed hypersensitivity reaction; use it for delayed cutaneous ADRs and not in case of anaphylaxis (not useful and able to reinduce an anaphylactic shock).

- Drug patch tests are applied on the back, but in FDE they also have to be applied in duplicate on the site of eruption (residual sometimes pigmented lesion; ie, "in situ PTs")

- In immediate hypersensitivity reactions, as for BL antibiotics, STs have to be adapted to the risk profile of the patient.

- For IDTs, sterile injectable solutions are obligatory; do not use crushed pills even with filtration of the solution.

- IDTs have to be done with a controlled volume of 0.02 mL, not based on a given diameter of the injection wheal (bleb).

- A negative drug skin test does not exclude the responsibility of a drug in the occurrence of an ADR.

REFERENCES

1. Phillips EJ, Bigliardi P, Bircher AJ, et al. Controversies in drug allergy: Testing for delayed reactions. J Allergy Clin Immunol 2019;143:66–73.
2. Torres MJ, Romano A, Celik G, et al. Approach to the diagnosis of drug hypersensitivity reactions: similarities and differences between Europe and North America. Clin Transl Allergy 2017;7:7.
3. Barbaud A, Gonçalo M, Bruynzeel D, et al. Guidelines for performing skin tests with drugs in the investigation of cutaneous adverse drug reactions. Contact Dermatitis 2001;45:321–8.
4. Brockow K, Romano A, Blanca M, et al. General considerations for skin test procedures in the diagnosis of drug hypersensitivity. Allergy 2002;57:45–51.

5. Brockow K, Garvey LH, Aberer W, et al. ENDA/EAACI drug allergy interest group. Skin test concentrations for systemically administered drugs – an ENDA/EAACI drug allergy interest group position paper. Allergy 2013;68:702–12.
6. Broyles AD, Banerji A, Barmettler S, et al. Practical Guidance for the Evaluation and Management of Drug Hypersensitivity: Specific Drugs. J Allergy Clin Immunol Pract 2020;8(9S):S16–116.
7. Barbaud A, Castagna J, Soria A. Skin tests in the work-up of cutaneous adverse drug reactions - A review and update. Contact Dermatitis 2022. https://doi.org/10.1111/cod.14063.
8. Aberer W, Bircher A, Romano A, et al. European Network for Drug Allergy (ENDA); EAACI interest group on drug hypersensitivity. Drug provocation testing in the diagnosis of drug hypersensitivity reactions: general considerations. Allergy 2003;58:854–63.
9. Joint Task Force on Practice Parameters, American Academy of Allergy, Asthma and Immunology, American College of Allergy, Asthma and Immunology, Joint Council of Allergy, Asthma and Immunology. Drug allergy: an updated practice parameter. Ann Allergy Asthma Immunol 2010;105:259–73.
10. Banks TA, Tucker M, Macy E. Evaluating penicillin allergies without skin testing. Curr Allergy Asthma Rep 2019;19:27.
11. Khan DA. Proactive management of penicillin and other antibiotic allergies. Allergy Asthma Proc 2020;41:82–9.
12. Romano A, Atanaskovic-Markovic M, Barbaud A, et al. Towards a more precise diagnosis of hypersensitivity to beta-lactams - an EAACI position paper. Allergy 2020;75:1300–15.
13. Cooper L, Harbour J, Sneddon J, et al. Safety and efficacy of de-labelling penicillin allergy in adults using direct oral challenge: a systematic review. JAC Antimicrob Resist 2021;3:123.
14. Iammatteo M, Lezmi G, Confino-Cohen R, et al. Direct Challenges for the Evaluation of Beta-Lactam Allergy: Evidence and Conditions for Not Performing Skin Testing. J Allergy Clin Immunol Pract 2021;9:2947–56.
15. Ramsey A, Mustafa SS, Holly AM, et al. Direct challenges to penicillin-based antibiotics in the inpatient setting. J Allergy Clin Immunol Pract 2020;8:2294–301.
16. Demoly P, Adkinson NF, Brockow K, et al. International consensus on drug allergy. Allergy 2014;69:420–37.
17. Sabato V, Gaeta F, Valluzzi RL, et al. Urticaria: The 1-1-1 criterion for optimized risk stratification in β-lactam allergy delabeling. J Allergy Clin Immunol Pract 2021;9:3697–704.
18. Barbaud A, Collet E, Milpied B, et al. A multicenter study to determine the value and safety of drug patch tests for the three main classes of severe cutaneous adverse drug reactions. Br J Dermatol 2013;168:555–62.
19. Castells M, Khan DA, Phillips EJ. Penicillin allergy. N Engl J Med 2019;381:2338–51.
20. Blanca M, Torres MJ, García JJ, et al. Natural evolution of skin test sensitivity in patients allergic to beta-lactam antibiotics. J Allergy Clin Immunol 1999;103(5 Pt1):918–24.
21. Romano A, Gaeta F, Valluzzi RL, et al. Natural evolution of skin-test sensitivity in patients with IgE-mediated hypersensitivity to cephalosporins. Allergy 2014;69:806–9.
22. Romano A, Valluzzi RL, Caruso C, et al. Evaluating immediate reactions to cephalosporins: time is of the essence. J Allergy Clin Immunol Pract 2021;9:1648–16457.e1.

23. Pinho A, Marta A, Coutinho I, et al. Long-term reproducibility of positive patch test reactions in patients with non-immediate cutaneous adverse drug reactions to antibiotics. Contact Dermatitis 2017;76:204–9.

24. Fung IN, Kim HL. Skin prick testing in patients using beta-blockers: a retrospective analysis. Allergy Asthma Clin Immunol 2010;6:2.

25. Isik SR, Celikel S, Karakaya G, et al. The effects of antidepressants on the results of skin prick tests used in the diagnosis of allergic diseases. Int Arch Allergy Immunol 2011;154:63–8.

26. Bousquet J, Heinzerling L, Bachert C, et al. Practical guide to skin prick tests in allergy to aeroallergens. Allergy 2012;67:18–24.

27. Johansen JD, Aalto-Korte K, Agner T, et al. European society of contact dermatitis guideline for diagnostic patch testing - recommendations on best practice. Contact Dermatitis 2015;73:195–221.

28. Brajon D, Menetre S, Waton J, et al. Non-irritant concentrations and amounts of active ingredient in drug patch tests. Contact Dermatitis 2014;71:170–5.

29. Romano A, Viola M, Gaeta F, et al. Patch testing in non-immediate drug eruptions. Allergy Asthma Clin Immunol 2008;4:66–74.

30. Cortellini G, Carli G, Franceschini L, et al. Evaluating nonimmediate cutaneous reactions to non-vitamin K antagonist oral anticoagulants via patch testing. J Allergy Clin Immunol Pract 2020;8:3190–3.

31. Assier H, Valeyrie-Allanore L, Gener G, et al. Patch testing in non-immediate cutaneous adverse drug reactions: value of extemporaneous patch tests. Contact Dermatitis 2017;77:297–302.

32. Indradat S, Veskitkul J, Pacharn P, et al. Provocation proven drug allergy in Thai children with adverse drug reactions. Asian Pac J Allergy Immunol 2016;34:59–64.

33. Bruusgaard-Mouritsen MA, Jensen BM, Poulsen LK, et al. Optimizing investigation of suspected allergy to polyethylene glycols. J Allergy Clin Immunol.149(1):168-175.e4.

34. Barbaud A, Weinborn M, Garvey LH, et al. Intradermal tests with drugs: an approach to standardization. Front Med (Lausanne) 2020;7:156.

35. Garvey LH, Ebo DG, Mertes PM, et al. An EAACI position paper on the investigation of perioperative immediate hypersensitivity reactions. Allergy 2019;74:1872–84.

36. Torres MJ, Trautmann A, Böhm I, et al. Practice parameters for diagnosing and managing iodinated contrast media hypersensitivity. Allergy 2021;76:1325–39.

37. van der Poorten MM, Van Gasse AL, Hagendorens MM, et al. Nonirritating skin test concentrations for ceftazidime and aztreonam in patients with a documented beta-lactam allergy. J Allergy Clin Immunol Pract 2021;9:585–8.e1.

38. van der Poorten MM, Hagendorens MM, Faber MA, et al. Nonirritant concentrations and performance of ceftaroline skin tests in patients with an immediate β-lactam hypersensitivity. J Allergy Clin Immunol Pract 2021;9:4486–8.e2.

39. Brož P, Harr T, Hecking C, et al. Nonirritant intradermal skin test concentrations of ciprofloxacin, clarithromycin, and rifampicin. Allergy 2012;67:647–52.

40. Kuyucu S, Mori F, Atanaskovic-Markovic M, et al. Hypersensitivity reactions to non-betalactam antibiotics in children: an extensive review. Pediatr Allergy Immunol 2014;25:534–43.

41. Lobera T, Audícana MT, Alarcón E, et al. Allergy to quinolones: low cross-reactivity to levofloxacin. J Investig Allergol Clin Immunol 2010;20:607–11.

42. Perrin-Lamarre A, Petitpain N, Trechot P, et al. Toxidermies aux glycopeptides. Résultats du bilan immuno-allergologique dans une série de huit cas. Ann Dermatol Venereol 2010;137:101–5.

43. Bonadonna P, Lombardo C, Bortolami O, et al. Hypersensitivity to proton pump inhibitors: Diagnostic accuracy of skin tests compared to oral provocation test. J Allergy Clin Immunol 2012;130:547–9.

44. Brockow K, Romano A, Aberer W, et al. Skin testing in patients with hypersensitivity reactions to iodinated contrast media - a European multicenter study. Allergy 2009;64:234–41.

45. Lerondeau B, Trechot P, Waton J, et al. Analysis of cross-reactivity among radiocontrast media in 97 hypersensitivity reactions. J Allergy Clin Immunol 2016;137: 633–5.

46. Rosado Ingelmo A, Doña Diaz I, Cabañas Moreno R, et al. Clinical practice guidelines for diagnosis and management of hypersensitivity reactions to contrast media. J Investig Allergol Clin Immunol 2016;26:144–55.

47. Clement O, Dewachter P, Mouton-Faivre C, et al. Immediate hypersensitivity to contrast agents: the french 5-year CIRTACI study. EClinicalMedicine 2018;1: 51–61.

48. Scherer K, Tsakiris DA, Bircher AJ. Hypersensitivity reactions to anticoagulant drugs. Curr Pharm Des 2008;14:2863–73.

49. Soria A, Baeck M, Goossens A, et al. Patch, prick or intradermal tests to detect delayed hypersensitivity to corticosteroids? Contact Dermatitis 2011;64:313–24.

50. Patel A, Bahna SL. Immediate hypersensitivity reactions to corticosteroids. Ann Allergy Asthma Immunol 2015;115:178–82.

51. Barbaud A, Waton J. Systemic allergy to corticosteroids: clinical features and cross reactivity. Curr Pharm Des 2016;22:6825–31.

52. Dumond P, Franck P, Morisset M, et al. Pre-lethal anaphylaxis to carboxymethylcellulose confirmed by identification of specific IgE–review of the literature. Eur Ann Allergy Clin Immunol 2009;41:171–6.

53. Barbaud A. Place of excipients in systemic drug allergy. Immunol Allergy Clin North Am 2014;34:671–9.

54. Shuster S, Borici-Mazi R, Awad S, et al. Rapid desensitization with intravenous insulin in a patient with diabetic ketoacidosis and insulin allergy. AACE Clin Case Rep 2020;6:e147–50.

55. Pasteur J, Favier L, Pernot C, et al. Low cross-reactivity between cisplatin and other platinum salts. J Allergy Clin Immunol Pract 2019;7:1894–900.

56. Guyot-Caquelin P, Granel F, Kaminsky MC, et al. False positive results can occur on delayed reading of intradermal tests with cisplatin. J Allergy Clin Immunol 2010;125:1410–1.

57. Bavbek S, Pagani M, Alvarez-Cuesta E, et al. Hypersensitivity reactions to biologicals: an EAACI position paper. Allergy.;77(1):39-54.

58. Novelli S, Soto L, Caballero A, et al. Assessment of confirmed clinical hypersensitivity to rituximab in patients affected with B-Cell Neoplasia. Adv Hematol 2020; 2020:4231561.

59. Rocchi V, Puxeddu I, Cataldo G, et al. Hypersensitivity reactions to tocilizumab: role of skin tests in diagnosis. Rheumatology (Oxford) 2014;53:1527–9.

60. Tétu P, Hamelin A, Moguelet P, et al. Management of hypersensitivity reactions to Tocilizumab. Clin Exp Allergy 2018;48:749–52.

61. Poreaux C, Bronowicki JP, Debouverie M, et al. Managing generalized interferon-induced eruptions and the effectiveness of desensitization. Clin Exp Allergy 2014;44:756–64.

62. Ewan PW, Dugué P, Mirakian R, et al. BSACI guidelines for the investigation of suspected anaphylaxis during general anaesthesia. Clin Exp Allergy 2010;40: 15–31.

63. Mertes PM, Laxenaire MC, Lienhart A, et al. Reducing the risk of anaphylaxis during anaesthesia: guidelines for clinical practice. J Investig Allergol Clin Immunol 2005;15:91–101.

64. Mertes PM, Malinovsky JM, Jouffroy L, Working Group of the SFAR and SFA, Aberer W, Terreehorst I, Brockow K, Demoly P, ENDA. EAACI Interest Group on Drug Allergy. Reducing the risk of anaphylaxis during anesthesia: 2011 updated guidelines for clinical practice. J Investig Allergol Clin Immunol 2011;21:442–53.

65. Dreskin SC, Halsey NA, Kelso JM, et al. International consensus (ICON): allergic reactions to vaccines. World Allergy Organ J 2016;9:32.

66. Amsler E, Autegarden JE, Gaouar H, et al. Management of immediate hypersensitivity reaction to glatiramer acetate. Eur J Dermatol 2017;27(1):92–5.

67. Santiago F, Gonçalo M, Vieira R, et al. Epicutaneous patch testing in drug hypersensitivity syndrome (DRESS). Contact Dermatitis 2010;62:47–53.

68. Andrade P, Brinca A, Gonçalo M. Patch testing in fixed drug eruptions–a 20-year review. Contact Dermatitis 2011;65:195–201.

69. Barbaud A, Groupe FISARD de la SFD. Investigations allergologiques dans les érythèmes pigmentés fixes. Méthode recommandée par le groupe FISARD de la SFD [Allergological investigations in fixed pigmented erythema. Method recommended by the FISARD (drug eruptions) group of the French Dermatology Society]. Ann Dermatol Venereol 2018;145:210–3.

70. Gonçalo M, Ferguson J, Bonevalle A, et al. Photopatch testing: recommendations for a European photopatch test baseline series. Contact Dermatitis 2013;68: 239–43.

71. Romano A, Blanca M, Torres MJ, et al, ENDA, EAACI. Diagnosis of nonimmediate reactions to beta-lactam antibiotics. Allergy 2004;59:1153–60.

72. Blanca M, Romano A, Torres MJ, et al. Update on the evaluation of hypersensitivity reactions to betalactams. Allergy 2009;64:183–93.

73. Romano A, Gaeta F, Valluzzi RL, et al. Cross-reactivity and tolerability of aztreonam and cephalosporins in subjects with a T cell-mediated hypersensitivity to penicillins. J Allergy Clin Immunol 2016;138:179–86.

74. Soria A, Hamelin A, de Risi Pugliese T, et al. Are drug intradermal tests dangerous to explore cross-reactivity and co-sensitization in DRESS? Br J Dermatol 2019;181:611–2.

75. Trubiano JA, Chua KYL, Holmes NE, et al. Safety of cephalosporins in penicillin class severe delayed hypersensitivity reactions. J Allergy Clin Immunol Pract 2020;8:1142–6.e4.

76. Copaescu A, Mouhtouris E, Vogrin S, et al. Australasian registry of severe cutaneous adverse reactions (AUS-SCAR). The role of in vivo and ex vivo diagnostic tools in severe delayed immune-mediated adverse antibiotic drug reactions. J Allergy Clin Immunol Pract 2021;9:2010–5.e4.

77. Desroche T, Poreaux C, Waton J, et al. Can we allow a further intake of drugs poorly suspected as responsible in drug reaction with eosinophilia and systemic symptoms (DRESS)? A study of practice. Clin Exp Allergy 2019;49:924–8.

Telemedicine in Drug Hypersensitivity

Deva Wells, MD[a],*, Katherine L. DeNiro, MD[a], Allison Ramsey, MD[b]

KEYWORDS

- Telemedicine • Penicillin allergy • Severe cutaneous adverse reaction
- Electronic consult • Telehealth • Drug allergy • Adverse drug reaction

KEY POINTS

- Telemedicine is being used to risk-stratify patients with drug hypersensitivity reactions between those who should be seen in person versus those who may be seen completely by telemedicine.
- Inpatient telemedicine consultation for penicillin allergies and severe cutaneous adverse reactions is a promising development.
- Electronic consults have emerged as a tool for physician-to-physician guidance for drug hypersensitivity reactions.

INTRODUCTION

Telemedicine is defined as "the remote diagnosis and treatment of patients by means of telecommunications technology."[1] In the past several years, and especially during the COVID-19 pandemic, the use of telemedicine as a means to deliver health care has expanded dramatically. Similarly, the types of telemedicine delivery systems and the terminology used to describe them have grown. Telemedicine can be conducted by telephone, virtual video connection (eg, Zoom audio/video conferencing or Vsee Clinic), or text-based care chat. Telemedicine can take place between the clinician and patient directly or between the clinician and consultant. Telemedicine may also include a review of laboratory data, studies, and/or images; physical examination elements may be captured in real time by live interactive video or review of previously stored images ("store-and-forward"). Numerous specialties of medicine are now providing remote care through telemedicine, including allergy and immunology and dermatology. For the purposes of this review, the authors focus on the ways telemedicine is being used to risk-stratify and triage for in-clinic visits in order to diagnose and treat drug hypersensitivity reactions.

[a] Division of Dermatology, University of Washington, 1959 Northeast Pacific Street, Box 356524, Seattle, WA 98195, USA; [b] Division of Allergy/Immunology, Rochester Regional Health, University of Rochester, 222 Alexander Street, Suite 3000, Rochester, NY 14607, USA
* Corresponding author.
E-mail address: devaw@uw.edu

Immunol Allergy Clin N Am 42 (2022) 323–333
https://doi.org/10.1016/j.iac.2021.12.007
0889-8561/22/© 2022 Elsevier Inc. All rights reserved.
immunology.theclinics.com

Adverse drug reactions (ADRs) are defined as any noxious, unintended, or undesired effect of a drug that occurs at a standard dose.[2] Drug hypersensitivity reactions are a subset of ADRs and are the results of immune or inflammatory cell stimulation by the medication. The most common drug hypersensitivity reactions result from either type I or type IV hypersensitivity reactions. Type I hypersensitivity reactions occur within minutes to hours of exposure to an allergen, manifest as urticaria and/or angioedema and anaphylaxis, and are mediated by immunoglobulin E (IgE) with resulting activation of mast cells and/or basophils. An acute reaction to penicillin is a prototypical example of a type 1 hypersensitivity. Type IV hypersensitivity reactions are T cell mediated and occur within days to weeks of antigen exposure. Type IV hypersensitivity reactions typically present with cutaneous symptoms, including morbilliform drug rashes as well as severe cutaneous adverse reactions (SCARs), such as Stevens-Johnson syndrome/toxic epidermal necrolysis (SJS/TEN) and drug-induced hypersensitivity syndrome (DIHS), also known as drug rash with eosinophilia and systemic symptoms (DRESS).

ADRs are commonly encountered in inpatient and outpatient medicine. One meta-analysis of adult inpatient prospective studies found the incidence of ADRs to be 15%.[3] Similarly, 18% of outpatients reported an ADR from a prescribed medicine within the past year.[4] Telemedicine has served as a convenient and effective platform for triaging, diagnosing, and treating ADRs either labeled as or suspicious for drug hypersensitivity reactions. This review focuses on current applications of telemedicine for drug hypersensitivity reactions with a focus on emerging tools during the COVID-19 pandemic.

Telemedicine for Risk Stratification of Drug Hypersensitivity Reactions

Some of the first data regarding the use of telemedicine for evaluation of drug hypersensitivity reactions in allergy/immunology were presented by Waibel.[5] In this report of 112 synchronous allergy/immunology encounters in Germany, there were 6 encounters for drug allergy. Of these 6 drug allergy encounters, 3 were recommended to present for an in-person appointment because of the need for an oral challenge, and this was statistically significantly less as compared with other diagnoses. This report illustrates that telemedicine may not obviate an in-person appointment owing to the need for testing or clinical or logistical challenges, but that it may allow for risk stratification to identify those whereby an in-clinic visit should be prioritized.

A subsequent analysis in pediatric outpatients further supported the utility of telemedicine for risk stratification in drug hypersensitivity. Allen and colleagues[6] analyzed the feasibility of delabeling low-risk penicillin allergy in a primary care setting. This study used predefined criteria for low-risk penicillin allergy (history negative for anaphylaxis, angioedema/urticaria, symptoms suggestive of SCAR, poorly controlled asthma, reaction to parenteral penicillin, AND history including a nonimmediate cutaneous reaction, family history of penicillin allergy, or gastrointestinal disturbance). With this approach, 118/140 patients were classified as "low risk," and 102/118 underwent a challenge with supervision by a pediatrician with allergy/immunology training and were delabeled. The risk-stratification approach illustrated in this article afforded full delabeling of low-risk patients by telemedicine, thus saving an in-person visit. A minority of this patient population was deemed high risk and would have required an in-person appointment.

Anstey and colleagues[7] looked at the use of telemedicine for patients with cystic fibrosis, a group at high risk for antibiotic hypersensitivity. In the 115 adult patients studied, 60.1% had at least 1 documented drug allergy, and there were 32 patients prioritized for a drug allergy evaluation. The allergy evaluations were initially completed in person as part of a multidisciplinary clinic but were transitioned to telemedicine visits after the allergy/immunology clinic changed physical office space. There were 6 telemedicine visits, but none of the prioritized drug allergies were able to be cleared without an in-person visit. The investigators were encouraged by a potential role for telemedicine but noted the need for further study of telemedicine as a means to evaluate drug allergies among patients with cystic fibrosis.

One study out of Ireland examined the cost-effectiveness of using telemedicine for pediatric penicillin allergy delabeling. The study used telemedicine to risk-stratify patients based on reaction history, with low-risk patients undergoing an outpatient challenge. This telemedicine approach successfully delabeled 99 children, and cost 56,456 USD compared with an estimated total cost of 146,242 USD with the usual practice of an outpatient evaluation followed by a challenge on a hospital day ward. The investigators concluded that telemedicine is a helpful risk-stratification tool that can optimize health care resource use,[8] and this approach is likely scalable to care settings with varying patient volumes. The cost estimate in this approach was still relatively high and could potentially be greater depending on the type of penicillin allergy evaluation completed after risk stratification by telemedicine.

The use of telemedicine to identify and risk-stratify SCARs with the goal of earlier diagnosis and management appears promising. Wong and colleagues[9] reported adopting a telemedicine triaging system in collaboration with a regional burn center and transfer center that is still in use. The process flow involves the following steps: (1) a requesting provider suspicious for SJS/TEN contacts the transfer center, who assists with procuring store-and-forward photographs of the skin and mucosal findings; (2) the photographs are forwarded for collaborative review by the on-call dermatologist and burn surgeon, who then speak directly with the requesting provider for pertinent historical information; and (3) a decision is made by the dermatologist and burn surgeon on likelihood of SJS/TEN, or similar dermatoses that can cause extensive mucocutaneous denuding, and need for intensive care, and acceptance for transfer is arranged accordingly. The investigators report a significant improvement in the positive predictive value of SJS/TEN spectrum disease after implementing the telemedicine triage system, as well as a reduction in the number of patients transferred for uncomplicated drug rashes who did not require intensive care.[9] At least one other institution has reported using a telemedicine triaging system for evaluating possible SJS/TEN.[10] This application of telemedicine may allow for timely care for severe cases of SCARs.

Telemedicine for Inpatient Penicillin Allergy Evaluations

Staicu and colleagues[11] used telemedicine for use in the hospital setting to evaluate penicillin allergy. The investigators' approach included an advanced practice provider (APP) who was available to travel to the hospital, perform skin prick and intradermal testing to penicillin, and then connect with the allergy/immunology physician synchronously by video for the physician to examine skin testing results and to counsel the patient. The investigators delabeled 46 of 50 patients' penicillin allergy and also demonstrated that this approach maintained patient satisfaction, with most patients reporting a "good" or "excellent" impression of penicillin sensitivity testing with consultation using telemedicine. This approach proved to be timesaving for the allergy/immunology physician, allowing them to continue seeing allergy/immunology outpatients.[11] Although the investigators used an APP as part of their telemedicine approach, illustrating a way to use telemedicine regardless of historical reaction risk, a risk-stratification approach could also be used for inpatients not requiring penicillin skin testing. After this study publication, data regarding direct challenges to penicillin have become more widely accepted.[12–15]

Telemedicine for Assessing Severe Adverse Cutaneous Reactions

Although most cutaneous adverse reactions are benign, there are numerous SCARs that may pose a risk of high morbidity and/or mortality.[16–19] These typically include SJS/TEN, DIHS/DRESS, anticoagulant-induced skin necrosis, acute generalized exanthematous pustulosis, generalized fixed drug eruption, and immunobullous reactions with extensive involvement, such as drug-induced bullous pemphigoid or linear IgA bullous dermatosis.[18,20–22] In addition to causing severe discomfort, SCARs can cause serious systemic illness through impaired homeostasis and electrolyte balances, increased risk of infection and sepsis, and multiorgan dysfunction,[18,20,21] and thus critically must be differentiated from uncomplicated drug rashes, such as morbilliform and acneiform eruptions.

Drug eruptions are a common reason for dermatology consultation in the acute care setting; several studies estimate that 8% to 10% of inpatient dermatology consults are attributable to drug eruptions among specific dermatologic diagnoses.[23–26] Drug eruptions with systemic symptoms are also a frequent reason for dermatology consult in the hospitalized pediatric population.[27] There are few reports of telemedicine specifically applied for diagnosis and management of acute drug eruptions. Charlston and Siller[28] reported a retrospective analysis of telemedicine consults for drug eruptions among patients receiving antiviral medications for treatment of hepatitis C infections using store-and-forward photographs. The average time to establish a diagnosis and treatment plan was approximately 2 hours, but about one-quarter of consults required additional photographs because of insufficient quality of the first submission. The referring providers were surveyed and reported a high level of satisfaction with the service. Phang and colleagues[29] described a virtual, real-time telemedicine clinic for titrating allopurinol for treatment of gout with monitoring of pertinent laboratory tests and for adverse reactions, although oversight was provided by rheumatologists rather than by dermatologists. There were 2 cases of adverse cutaneous reactions, with 1 patient developing DIHS and another patient with oral ulcers. The coordinated telemedicine care enabled early detection and swift cessation of the medication in both instances.

Gordon[30] reported a small pilot study using real-time, remote-controlled technology for telemedicine consultation, with the goal of eventually using this system for evaluation of cutaneous adverse effects related to chemotherapy and biologic medications. Patients scheduled for in-person dermatology visits were sent to an offsite infusion center where they participated in a video-based consultation with a teledermatologist initiated and coordinated by the site-based nurse; the teledermatologist then remotely controlled a "total body assessment camera" in real time during the video visit for visual examination. Participating patients and providers expressed a high level of satisfaction with the technology. As previously discussed, Wong and colleagues[9] implemented a telemedicine triaging system using store-and-forward technology to evaluate possible drug eruptions suspicious for SJS/TEN spectrum disease and clinical mimickers. Although that triaging system, used by 2 of the authors here, focuses on SJS/TEN for the purposes of transfer needs, the dermatology and burns specialists frequently evaluate other complicated drug eruptions, such as DIHS/DRESS and severe immunobullous reactions as well as uncomplicated morbilliform or exanthematous eruptions, raising the possibility for the use of telemedicine for these conditions.

Importantly, several recent studies have demonstrated generally high concordance between in-person dermatology consultative assessments and recommendations and those rendered through telemedicine.[31–33] One prospective study evaluated interrater reliability of store-and-forward telemedicine care with in-person dermatology consultation of hospitalized patients and found fair concordance of single, primary suspected diagnosis and substantial and near-perfect agreement for expanded differential diagnoses and management recommendations. Six of 41 of the patients included in this study had a final diagnosis of drug hypersensitivity reactions, suggesting telemedicine evaluation is an acceptable alternative to in-person evaluation.[32] Barbieri and colleagues[30,34] described a study comparing triaging and biopsy decisions between in-person and smartphone-based dermatology consultations. Drug hypersensitivity reactions were the most common diagnosis in this cohort. There was moderate concordance of triaging patients to be seen the same day, next day, within several days, or as an outpatient; concordance on the decision to biopsy was found to be fair to moderate. With respect to cases deemed more urgent, Barbieri and colleagues reported that "the teledermatologists rarely failed to triage a consultation to be seen the same day when the in-person dermatologist believed it was necessary (<10% of cases)."[30,34]

Electronic Consults and Drug Allergy

Electronic consults (E-consults) have also emerged along with telemedicine as a tool for drug allergy evaluations. E-consults are a clinician-to-clinician exchange in the electronic health record aimed at improving specialist access and reducing unnecessary in-person evaluations.[35] E-consults are more formal than the traditional "curbside consult" but do not involve a patient interaction. Phadke and colleagues[36] reported the Massachusetts General/Brigham experience of e-consults in allergy/immunology. The study looked at 306 completed e-consults, of which 201 were for ADRs, with penicillin allergy being the most common ADR in 60.6% of patients. One hundred forty-six of the initial ADR e-consults were subsequently referred for in-person evaluations for skin testing or challenges. However, 55 patients were fully evaluated via e-consult without the need for an in-person appointment. The study demonstrated that ADR e-consults were fast to complete, with an average of 10 minutes. The investigators also discussed that even in instances where the e-consult led to an in-person appointment, it allowed for testing materials and/or medication dilutions to be prepared in advance of the in-person appointment.[36]

Massachusetts General/Brigham colleagues also investigated e-consults for evaluating penicillin allergy in obstetric patients. In this study, there were 389 e-consults completed, and 363 (93%) of these recommended an in-person evaluation. However, 26 patients avoided an in-person visit because of either a recent severe recurrent reaction or an intolerance. The investigators concluded that the e-consult facilitated a high-volume triage process whereby patients who did present for in-person care after the e-consult had a significant reduction in second-line antibiotic use for group B *Streptococcus* prophylaxis and caesarean-section prophylaxis. This study demonstrated a degree of attrition in patients undergoing e-consults in that 39% of patients recommended for an in-person evaluation did not present for this evaluation.[37]

Mustafa and colleagues[38] reported their experience with e-consults for allergy/immunology inpatients. They received 109 consults during a 6-month period. Of these, 78 were completed through an e-consult, and 65 of these consults were for drug allergy. The potential recommendations for drug allergy included continued avoidance of the medication or an oral challenge in low-risk patients. The investigators demonstrated a shorter turnaround time to recommendations with the use of e-consults, along with saved allergy/immunology physician time. E-consults also allowed allergy/immunology physicians to complete the e-consult during the workday while seeing outpatients. The investigators also demonstrated that recommendations were followed similarly between patients evaluated via e-consults and patients evaluated in person. Furthermore, the investigators surveyed providers requesting the e-consults, and 97% of providers rated their impression of e-consults as "excellent" or "good." In-person consults were necessary in this analysis for evaluating SCARs or if penicillin skin testing was warranted.[38]

Telemedicine and Drug Allergy During the COVID-19 Pandemic

Despite encouraging studies with telemedicine, there was not widespread use of telemedicine in allergy/immunology before the COVID-19 pandemic.[39] The COVID-19 pandemic forced rapid transition to telemedicine in most outpatient offices owing to social distancing recommendations.[40] Thomas and colleagues[41] reported their experience with 637 synchronous telephone visits in the United Kingdom during the COVID-19 pandemic, of which 98 (18.3%) were for suspected ADRs. Ninety-seven of these evaluations were new patients, with 58% referred for beta-lactam allergy, 8.25% for non-beta-lactam allergy, 8.25% for local anesthetic allergy, and 7.2% for nonsteroidal anti-inflammatory drugs. Although 69 (71%) patients required a future in-person visit, 29% had a complete visit via telephone without need for further follow-up.

Tsao and colleagues[42] reported their experience with the rapid transition to telemedicine-based care during the COVID-19 shut down from March 10, 2020 until June 30, 2020. Their transition included the ability to schedule patients deemed appropriate for in-person testing for an office visit. This triaging of patients allowed for the office to maintain its 2019 level of drug allergy evaluations.

Interestingly, Mustafa and colleagues[43] also examined office encounters during New York State's reopening in May 2020 after the strict COVID-19 lockdown, specifically focusing on patient satisfaction with in-person, video, or telephone visits. In this analysis, there were 303 in-person visits, 98 video visits, and 46 telephone visits. Of these total visits, 21 in-person visits were for drug allergy, whereas no drug-allergy visits were conducted by video or telephone. This reflected the investigators' triaging of high-priority drug allergy appointments to be in person to conduct drug challenges where indicated.[43]

Similarly, the COVID-19 pandemic appears to have substantially expanded the adoption of telemedicine for dermatologic issues across multiple care settings.[44–46] Some practices scrambled to introduce telemedicine for the purpose of triaging alone at the outset of the pandemic, whereas others expanded to comprehensive telemedicine.[45–47] Parity of reimbursement with in-person visits has incentivized comprehensive telemedicine care for the time being, but its future is uncertain, and practices may capitalize variably on the telemedicine model. For example, academic institutions have more often offered telemedicine services, but are shown to lag behind private practices in publicizing them as an available format even during the pandemic.[44,48] Fortunately, the trend of quickly integrating telemedicine services brought on by the COVID-19 pandemic appears favorable overall. A review by Farr and colleagues[49] outlines the general successes of recently established telemedicine practices, with encouragingly high satisfaction rates despite accelerated rollouts and limitations that are often surmountable with improvements in technology and process flow.

The authors could not find any reports of telemedicine mobilized specifically for evaluation of acute drug or vaccine-related eruptions during the COVID-19 pandemic, but a new algorithm for high-acuity telemedicine provides a sound starting point in addition to the approaches reported by Wong and colleagues and Georgesen and colleagues. Rismiller and colleagues[50] described a telemedicine triaging system that they developed for inpatient consults that considers COVID-19 status and use of personal protective equipment using a store-and-forward approach with high-quality imaging

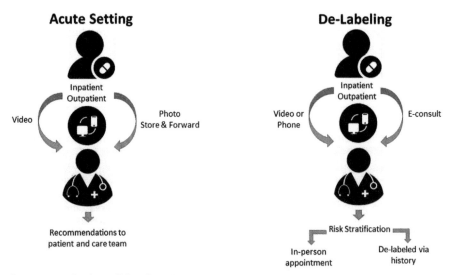

Fig. 1. Uses of telemedicine for ADRs.

capture. The algorithm begins with a request for photographs in response to *all* inpatient dermatology consults, after which the medical record is reviewed, and the case determined a good fit for telemedicine only versus need for in-person evaluation. COVID-19 status is assessed, and risk of transmission influences the number of dermatology team members present for in-person care.[50] The authors propose a similar algorithm whereby initial consultation and pertinent clinical information are presented to the consulting specialist in the most fitting telemedicine format (eg, store-and-forward for an acute rash), whose medical decision making would then include triaging and risk stratification before assessment and more comprehensive management recommendations (**Fig. 1**).

Despite its promise, practitioners using the telemedicine model may face numerous, sometimes shifting challenges. For example, state licensure boundaries, which had been relaxed by some states during the beginning of the COVID-19 pandemic, are being reinstated, prohibiting some providers from engaging in telemedicine care with patients living out of state. For those states that do allow care for out-of-state patients, malpractice coverage may nevertheless be restricted to providers' registered states of medical licensure. Many patient-driven modalities for capturing, storing, and sending images, such as smartphones, do not use a HIPAA-compliant level of encryption and pose the risk of unwitting privacy violations. Last, many patients may not possess the image and video-capturing computers or mobile devices necessary for telemedicine.[49] Fortunately, expansion of secure clinical interfaces and technological aids, such as superior camera hardware and mobile device "apps" designed to enhance image capture, may improve the quality of assessment in a medicolegally sound manner, and increasing demand for telemedicine may spur more providers to offer in-state options for their patients.

SUMMARY

Drug hypersensitivity reactions are relatively common and potentially life-threatening. Telemedicine has emerged as a useful tool for risk stratification, in particular, for assessment of common drug allergies, such as penicillin allergies and SCARs. Telemedicine can potentially overcome common issues, such as poor access to specialists, prohibitive geographic distance from a tertiary care center, or unavailability of in-person care owing to the COVID-19 pandemic, ensuring care when and where patients need it most.

CLINICS CARE POINTS

- Consider calling a telemedicine consult for drug hypersensitivity reactions.
- Evaluation of severe adverse cutaneous reactions and penicillin allergies hold particular promise by telemedicine.
- Drug hypersensitivity reactions are a subset of adverse drug reactions that most often entail type I or immunoglobulin E-mediated hypersensitivity reactions and type IV, T cell-mediated hypersensitivity reactions. Manifestations of type I hypersensitivity include urticaria, angioedema, and/or anaphylaxis, whereas type IV drug hypersensitivity reactions span benign, morbilliform, or exanthematous eruptions to severe cutaneous adverse reactions, such as Stevens-Johnson syndrome/toxic epidermal necrolysis and drug-induced hypersensitivity syndrome. Telemedicine has emerged as a potentially effective, safe, and time-saving tool to evaluate drug hypersensitivity reactions.
- Telemedicine may be useful for risk stratification when delabeling occurs in the outpatient setting. In one study based in a pediatric primary care setting, a risk-stratification approach was used in which pertinent historical information was gathered via video-visit telemedicine. Patients who were classified as low risk underwent an oral challenge in person, with the vast majority successfully being delabeled without need for additional in-person evaluation. Another study examined the use of telemedicine as the platform for risk stratification and its cost-effectiveness, noting a total cost of 56,456 USD to delabel 99 children compared with an estimated cost of 146,242 USD for the typical scenario of outpatient evaluation followed by a challenge in an acute care setting.
- Synchronous video has also been reported for delabeling in the acute care setting. One study used an advanced practice provider who performed skin prick and intradermal testing to penicillin on hospitalized patients undergoing evaluation for penicillin allergy, with the allergy/immunology physician then conducting a synchronous video visit for interpretation of results and counseling.
- Store-and-forward telemedicine has been shown to provide timely assessment and triaging of potential severe cutaneous adverse reactions, namely Stevens-Johnson syndrome/toxic epidermal necrolysis, and to guide decision making regarding transferring patients to a regional burn unit. At one institution, this triaging system was found to increase the positive predictive value of identifying Stevens-Johnson syndrome/toxic epidermal necrolysis and decrease the number of unnecessary transfers for uncomplicated drug rashes, resulting in substantial cost savings.
- Although there are limitations to basing clinical assessments on photographs, such as the quality and scope of images, there appears to be fair to good concordance between dermatologic assessments rendered through store-and-forward telemedicine and in-person clinical encounters.
- E-consults may be considered a category of telemedicine that specifically entails clinician-to-clinician communication. E-consults have been used to evaluate potential drug hypersensitivity reactions successfully and swiftly and with high satisfaction reported by the consulting providers, but e-consults have also faced high attrition rates when a subsequent in-person evaluation was recommended.
- There is new evidence on the rapid adoption of telemedicine practices brought about by the COVID-19 pandemic in allergy/immunology and dermatology. Despite accelerated rollouts and variable technological limitations, the incorporation of telemedicine has been met with overall high patient satisfaction and has played a vital role in both triaging and expanding access to care.

DISCLOSURE

D. Wells: No relevant disclosures. K. DeNiro: No relevant disclosures. A. Ramsey: Speakers Bureau for Sanofi/Regeneron and GlaxoSmithKline (not relevant for article).

REFERENCES

1. What is telehealth. NEJM Catalyst. February 1, 2018. Accessed March 10, 2022. https://catalyst.nejm.org/doi/full/10.1056/CAT.18.0268.
2. Rational pharmaceutical management plus center for pharmaceutical management. Management sciences for health. Drug and therapeutics committee training course. Geneva, Switzerland: Management Sciences for Health and World Health Organization; 2007. Available at: https://www.who.int/medicines/technical_briefing/tbs/Participant-s-Guide-All-Sessions.pdf.
3. Lazarou J, Pomeranz BH, Corey PN. Incidence of adverse drug reactions in hospitalized patients: a meta-analysis of prospective studies. JAMA 1998;279(15): 1200–5.
4. Impicciatore P, Choonara I, Clarkson A, et al. Incidence of adverse drug reactions in paediatric in/out-patients: a systematic review and meta-analysis of prospective studies. Br J Clin Pharmacol 2001;52(1):77–83.
5. Waibel KH. Synchronous telehealth for outpatient allergy consultations: a 2-year regional experience. Ann Allergy Asthma Immunol 2016;116(6):571–5.e1.
6. Allen HI, Vazquez-Ortiz M, Murphy AW, et al. De-labeling penicillin-allergic children in outpatients using telemedicine: potential to replicate in primary care. J Allergy Clin Immunol Pract 2020;8(5):1750–2.
7. Anstey KM, Choi L, Dawson D, et al. Enabling antibiotic allergy evaluations and reintroduction of first-line antibiotics for patients with cystic fibrosis. Ann Allergy Asthma Immunol 2021;127(4):456–61.
8. Allen HI, Gillespie P, Vazquez-Ortiz M, et al. A cost-analysis of outpatient paediatric penicillin allergy de-labelling using telemedicine. Clin Exp Allergy 2021; 51(3):495–8.
9. Wong CY, Colven RM, Gibran NS, et al. Accuracy and cost-effectiveness of a telemedicine triage initiative for patients with suspected Stevens-Johnson syndrome/toxic epidermal necrolysis. JAMA Dermatol 2021;157(1):114–5.
10. Georgesen C, Karim SA, Liu R, et al. Response: "distinguishing Stevens-Johnson syndrome/toxic epidermal necrolysis from clinical mimickers during inpatient dermatologic consultation-a retrospective chart review.". J Am Acad Dermatol 2020;82(3):e111–2.
11. Staicu ML, Holly AM, Conn KM, et al. The use of telemedicine for penicillin allergy skin testing. J Allergy Clin Immunol Pract 2018;6(6):2033–40.
12. Trubiano JA, Vogrin S, Copaescu A, et al. Direct oral penicillin challenge for penicillin allergy delabeling as a health services intervention: a multicenter cohort study. Allergy 2021. https://doi.org/10.1111/all.15169.
13. Steenvoorden L, Bjoernestad EO, Kvesetmoen TA, et al. De-labelling penicillin allergy in acutely hospitalized patients: a pilot study. BMC Infect Dis 2021;21(1): 1083.
14. Iammatteo M, Lezmi G, Confino-Cohen R, et al. Direct challenges for the evaluation of beta-lactam allergy: evidence and conditions for not performing skin testing. J Allergy Clin Immunol Pract 2021;9(8):2947–56.
15. Cooper L, Harbour J, Sneddon J, et al. Safety and efficacy of de-labelling penicillin allergy in adults using direct oral challenge: a systematic review. JAC Antimicrob Resist 2021;3(1):dlaa123.

16. Hoetzenecker W, Nägeli M, Mehra ET, et al. Adverse cutaneous drug eruptions: current understanding. Semin Immunopathol 2016;38(1):75–86.

17. Gerson D, Sriganeshan V, Alexis JB. Cutaneous drug eruptions: a 5-year experience. J Am Acad Dermatol 2008;59(6):995–9.

18. Zhang J, Lei Z, Xu C, et al. Current perspectives on severe drug eruption. Clin Rev Allergy Immunol 2021;1–17.

19. Schöpf E, Stühmer A, Rzany B, et al. Toxic epidermal necrolysis and Stevens-Johnson syndrome: an epidemiologic study from West Germany. Arch Dermatol 1991;127(6):839–42.

20. Roujeau JC, Stern RS. Severe adverse cutaneous reactions to drugs. New Engl J Med 1994;331(19):1272–85.

21. Duong TA, Valeyrie-Allanore L, Wolkenstein P, et al. Severe cutaneous adverse reactions to drugs. Lancet 2017;390(10106):1996–2011.

22. Stavropoulos PG, Soura E, Antoniou C. Drug-induced pemphigoid: a review of the literature. J Eur Acad Dermatol Venereol 2014;28(9):1133–40.

23. Bauer J, Maroon M. Dermatology inpatient consultations: a retrospective study. J Am Acad Dermatol 2010;62(3):518–9.

24. Hines AS, Zayas J, Wetter DA, et al. Retrospective analysis of 450 emergency department dermatology consultations: an analysis of in-person and teledermatology consultations from 2015 to 2019. J Telemed Telecare 2021. 1357633x211024844.

25. Prada-García C, Gonzalo-Orden JM, Benítez-Andrades JA, et al. Inpatient dermatology consultations in a tertiary care hospital in Spain: a retrospective study of 750 patients. Rev Clin Esp (Barc) 2020;220(7):426–31.

26. Phillips GS, Freites-Martinez A, Hsu M, et al. Inflammatory dermatoses, infections, and drug eruptions are the most common skin conditions in hospitalized cancer patients. J Am Acad Dermatol 2018;78(6):1102–9.

27. McMahon P, Goddard D, Frieden IJ. Pediatric dermatology inpatient consultations: a retrospective study of 427 cases. J Am Acad Dermatol 2013;68(6):926–31.

28. Charlston S, Siller G. Teledermatologist expert skin advice: a unique model of care for managing skin disorders and adverse drug reactions in hepatitis C patients. Australas J Dermatol 2018;59(4):315–7.

29. Phang KF, Santosa A, Low BPL, et al. A nurse-led, rheumatologist-assisted telemedicine intervention for dose escalation of urate-lowering therapy in gout. Int J Rheum Dis 2020;23(9):1136–44.

30. Gordon J. Dermatologic assessment from a distance: the use of teledermatology in an outpatient chemotherapy infusion center. Clin J Oncol Nurs 2012;16(4):418–20.

31. Dhaduk K, Miller D, Schliftman A, et al. Implementing and optimizing inpatient access to dermatology consultations via telemedicine: an experiential study. Telemed J E Health 2021;27(1):68–73.

32. Gabel CK, Nguyen E, Karmouta R, et al. Use of teledermatology by dermatology hospitalists is effective in the diagnosis and management of inpatient disease. J Am Acad Dermatol 2021;84(6):1547–53.

33. Keller JJ, Johnson JP, Latour E. Inpatient teledermatology: diagnostic and therapeutic concordance among a hospitalist, dermatologist, and teledermatologist using store-and-forward teledermatology. J Am Acad Dermatol 2020;82(5):1262–7.

34. Barbieri JS, Nelson CA, James WD, et al. The reliability of teledermatology to triage inpatient dermatology consultations. JAMA Dermatol 2014;150(4):419–24.

35. Vimalananda VG, Gupte G, Seraj SM, et al. Electronic consultations (e-consults) to improve access to specialty care: a systematic review and narrative synthesis. J Telemed Telecare 2015;21(6):323–30.

36. Phadke NA, Wolfson AR, Mancini C, et al. Electronic consultations in allergy/immunology. J Allergy Clin Immunol Pract 2019;7(8):2594–602.

37. Wolfson AR, Mancini CM, Banerji A, et al. Penicillin allergy assessment in pregnancy: safety and impact on antibiotic use. J Allergy Clin Immunol Pract 2021; 9(3):1338–46.

38. Mustafa SS, Staicu ML, Yang L, et al. Inpatient electronic consultations (E-consults) in allergy/immunology. J Allergy Clin Immunol Pract 2020;8(9):2968–73.

39. Kane CK, Gillis K. The use of telemedicine by physicians: still the exception rather than the rule. Health Aff (Millwood) 2018;37(12):1923–30.

40. Shaker MS, Oppenheimer J, Grayson M, et al. COVID-19: pandemic contingency planning for the allergy and immunology clinic. J Allergy Clin Immunol Pract 2020;8(5):1477–88.e5.

41. Thomas I, Siew LQC, Rutkowski K. Synchronous telemedicine in allergy: lessons learned and transformation of care during the COVID-19 pandemic. J Allergy Clin Immunol Pract 2020;9(1):170–6.e1.

42. Tsao LR, Villanueva SA, Pines DA, et al. Impact of rapid transition to telemedicine-based delivery on allergy/immunology care during COVID-19. J Allergy Clin Immunol Pract 2021;9(7):2672–9.e2.

43. Mustafa SS, Vadamalai K, Ramsey A. Patient satisfaction with in-person, video, and telephone allergy/immunology evaluations during the COVID-19 pandemic. J Allergy Clin Immunol Pract 2021;9(5):1858–63.

44. Yim KM, Florek AG, Oh DH, et al. Teledermatology in the United States: an update in a dynamic era. Telemed J E Health 2018;24(9):691–7.

45. Elsner P. Teledermatology in the times of COVID-19: a systematic review. J Dtsch Dermatol Ges 2020;18(8):841–5.

46. Moscarella E, Pasquali P, Cinotti E, et al. A survey on teledermatology use and doctors' perception in times of COVID-19. J Eur Acad Dermatol Venereol 2020; 34(12):e772–3.

47. Yeboah CB, Harvey N, Krishnan R, et al. The impact of COVID-19 on teledermatology: a review. Dermatol Clin 2021. https://doi.org/10.1016/j.det.2021.05.007.

48. Gorrepati PL, Smith GP. Analysis of availability, types, and implementation of teledermatology services during COVID-19. J Am Acad Dermatol 2020;83(3):958–9.

49. Farr MA, Duvic M, Joshi TP. Teledermatology during COVID-19: an updated review. Am J Clin Dermatol 2021;22(4):467–75.

50. Rismiller K, Cartron AM, Trinidad JCL. Inpatient teledermatology during the COVID-19 pandemic. J Dermatolog Treat 2020;31(5):441–3.

Pharmacogenomics of Drug Hypersensitivity

Technology and Translation

Rebecca Kuruvilla, MB ChB, MRCP, Kathryn Scott, PhD,
Sir Munir Pirmohamed, PhD, FRCP, FMedSci*

KEYWORDS

- Drug hypersensitivity • HLA • Pharmacogenetics • Implementation

KEY POINTS

- Drug hypersensitivity reactions are uncommon and genetically mediated adverse effects that contribute significantly to drug-related morbidity and mortality.
- Genetic variability in different HLA loci has been associated with different types of hypersensitivity reactions to several drugs, and the importance of particular HLA alleles has been validated by functional studies.
- Implementation of genetic testing as a precision medicine approach to prevent drug hypersensitivity reactions has been slow and challenging and further work is essential to maximize the impact of pharmacogenomic discoveries to improve translation to the clinic and patient outcomes.

INTRODUCTION

Pharmacogenomics aims to understand how genetic variation influences drug response. This understanding has the potential to support clinicians to deliver personalized therapy and to reduce the incidence of adverse drug reactions, including drug hypersensitivity reactions.[1]

Drug hypersensitivity reactions are an inappropriate response leading to tissue damage from an otherwise nontoxic agent.[2] They can affect multiple organs in isolation or in combination including the liver, skin, bone marrow, and muscle[3] **(Fig. 1)**. They vary in severity and can sometimes cause death. They usually affect a small percentage of the population and although they can be dose-dependent, unlike predictable pharmacologic adverse drug reactions, they do not show a typical dose-response relationship. Pharmacogenomic studies have shown associations between several human leukocyte antigen (HLA) markers and hypersensitivity to a wide range of

Department of Pharmacology and Therapeutics, Wolfson Centre for Personalised Medicine, The University of Liverpool, Liverpool, L69 3GL, UK
* Corresponding author: Institute of Systems, Molecular and Integrative Biology (ISMIB), University of Liverpool, Block A: Waterhouse Building 1-5, Brownlow Street, Liverpool L69 3GL
E-mail address: munirp@liverpool.ac.uk

Immunol Allergy Clin N Am 42 (2022) 335–355
https://doi.org/10.1016/j.iac.2022.01.006
0889-8561/22/© 2022 Elsevier Inc. All rights reserved.

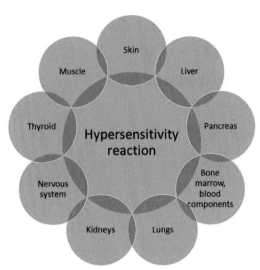

Fig. 1. Some of the many different organ systems which can be affected in hypersensitivity, either in isolation or in combination.

drugs.[3] As pharmacogenomics becomes part of mainstream medicine, it is important that researchers start to develop strategies, and the evidence base, to implement these HLA associations into clinical practice.

HLA AND IMMUNOGENOMIC CONTRIBUTORS TO DRUG HYPERSENSITIVITY

The HLA system is the human form of the vertebrate major histocompatibility complex. It plays a crucial role in allowing the immune system to discriminate between self and nonself. HLA proteins contain peptide-binding grooves which collectively present a repertoire of thousands of different peptides to T cells. Self-derived peptides are ignored because of exposure during thymic development and foreign peptides are recognized by the T cells, initiating an immune response under the control of regulatory pathways. The HLA locus, located on the short arm of chromosome 6, is highly polygenic, with HLA molecules classified according to function. Class I HLA molecules, HLA-A, -B, and -C, are found on the surface of all nucleated cells and present intracellularly derived peptides to CD8+-T cells. Class II HLA molecules, HLA-DRA, -DRB1, -DRB3, -DRB4, -DRB5, -DQA1, -DQB1, -DPA1, and -DPB1, are located on the surface of antigen-presenting cells and present a variety of extracellularly derived peptides to CD4+ T cells. The HLA class I loci, and in particular HLA-B, are highly polymorphic, giving rise to numerous variant HLA alleles; the IPD-IMGT/HLA database currently reports 7354, 8456, and 7307 HLA-A, -B, and -C alleles, respectively.[4] The HLA peptide-binding grooves show the highest sequence variation, maximizing the range of different peptides that can bind. The prevalence of specific HLA alleles can vary widely between ethnic groups, and as a result, the incidence of some HLA-associated hypersensitivity reactions also vary between groups.

The HLA system is essential for our response to disease. However, the same HLA alleles can predispose certain individuals to drug hypersensitivity reactions. In such reactions, the drug or drug metabolites interfere with the natural HLA-T-cell interaction leading to T-cell activation and an aberrant immune response.[5] Drug molecules are proposed to act on HLA molecules and activate T cells through 3 different mechanisms. In the hapten model, the drug forms a covalent bond with a protein, which is then processed, bound by an HLA molecule, and presented to the T-Cells. In the p-i model, the drug forms noncovalent interactions resulting in the formation of a complex comprising the drug, a peptide, HLA protein, and T-cell receptor. This complex seems to be stable enough to trigger an immune response. In the altered peptide repertoire model, the drug molecule forms a noncovalent interaction with the peptide-binding groove of the HLA molecule, altering the repertoire of bound peptides. It is important to note that these mechanisms are not mutually exclusive and there is good evidence for each of them occurring for different drugs, and sometimes for the same drug.[5]

Research over the last two decades has highlighted some important aspects of the associations between drugs, their propensity to cause hypersensitivity reactions, and specific HLA alleles, which are outlined in **Box 1** Box 2 provides some examples of other factors which may modulate the incidence of hypersensitivity, over and above the presence of risk HLA alleles.

EXAMPLES OF HLA ASSOCIATIONS

It is not the purpose of this article to provide a comprehensive overview of the many associations that have been reported with different drug-induced hypersensitivity reactions. Readers are referred to recent reviews.[5,20,21] Here we provide a description of some key examples.

Cutaneous Adverse Reactions

The skin is the organ most commonly affected in hypersensitivity reactions, either in isolation or as part of multisystem adverse reactions. The phenotypes vary greatly, from mild maculopapular exanthema to serious, often fatal reactions, such as toxic epidermal necrolysis.

Abacavir hypersensitivity is the poster child of HLA pharmacogenomics. The initial description of the association of abacavir hypersensitivity[9] with *HLA-B*57:01* in 2002

Box 1
Some caveats about HLA associations with drug hypersensitivity reactions

- Although strong associations have been identified with many drug hypersensitivity reactions and HLA alleles, the possession of an allele does not mean that the individual will develop the reaction (resulting in a low positive predictive value).[6] This is not fully understood (see **Box 2**).

- The same drug and the presence of the same HLA allele can lead to different clinical manifestations in different individuals. For example, *HLA-A*31:01* has been associated with different phenotypes of carbamazepine hypersensitivity (maculopapular exanthem, DRESS, and drug-induced liver injury).[7] The mechanism of this is unclear.

- For reasons which are unclear, the clinical severity of a reaction can vary between different individuals despite being exposed to the same drug, and carrying the same HLA allele.

- Different HLA alleles can predispose to hypersensitivity reactions to the same drug in different ethnic groups, which largely relates to the population frequency of that HLA allele. For example, *HLA-B*15:02* is associated with carbamazepine-induced Stevens-Johnson syndrome in South-East Asian populations but not in Northern European populations, where *HLA-A*31:01* is more important.[8]

- One HLA allele can be associated with different types of hypersensitivity reactions with many different drugs. For example, *HLA-B*57:01* is associated with abacavir hypersensitivity syndrome,[9] carbamazepine-associated Stevens-Johnson syndrome in European ancestry populations,[7] flucloxacillin-induced liver injury,[10] and pazopanib-induced liver injury.[11]

Box 2
Factors that modulate the frequency of occurrence of hypersensitivity reactions

- Underlying disease factors
  - Patients with HIV have an increased risk of hypersensitivity reactions with certain drugs such as sulfonamides but this can be ameliorated by controlling their disease using combination antiretroviral therapy.[12]
  - Patients with cystic fibrosis are at higher risk of hypersensitivity reactions with antibiotics received multiple times during the course of their illness.[13]
  - Patients with cancer being treated with immune checkpoint inhibitors have a higher risk of hypersensitivity reactions to concomitant drugs despite the fact that they may have been previously tolerant to these drugs.[14]
  - HLA-B*58:01 increases the risk of allopurinol-induced serious cutaneous adverse reactions, but this risk is further increased in patients with coexisting renal impairment.[15]
- Other genetic factors
  - Besides the presence of the predisposing HLA allele, other HLA alleles carried by the individual may either co-operate and increase the risk or may protect against the hypersensitivity reaction.[5]
  - Polymorphisms in drug-metabolizing genes may affect the pharmacokinetics of the drug and its metabolites, and thereby increase the risk of hypersensitivity. The best example of this is predisposition to phenytoin-induced serious cutaneous adverse reaction by the low-activity CYP2C9 variant, CYP2C9*3.[16]
  - Specific T-cell receptor clonotypes may interact with specific HLA alleles and increase the risk of a drug hypersensitivity reaction, as shown for carbamazepine.[17]
  - Genes encoding enzymes involved in peptide processing before HLA loading may modulate the risk as shown for nevirapine[18] and abacavir.[19]

---

has subsequently been replicated many times in different ethnic groups (**Table 1**). The utility of preprescription genotyping was shown in the PREDICT-1 trial.[22] Determination of whether a patient is positive for HLA-B*57:01 before prescribing abacavir is considered to be routine clinical practice in the developed world. Since 2008, it has been mandated in drug labels and in guidelines and has reduced the incidence of abacavir hypersensitivity.[23]

Carbamazepine hypersensitivity manifests in many different ways. Skin manifestations can vary in severity, and may be accompanied by internal organ involvement, in particular the liver. However, the liver can also be affected in isolation. In South-East Asian populations, a strong association has been shown between HLA-B*15:02 and carbamazepine-induced Stevens-Johnson syndrome and toxic epidermal necrolysis (SJS/TEN).[35] Carbamazepine-induced SJS/TEN can also be caused by the most common B75 serotype alleles in Southeast Asia,[36] HLA-B*15:08, HLA-B*15:11, and HLA-B*15:21. By contrast, in European ancestry populations, HLA-A*31:01 has been associated with various carbamazepine hypersensitivity phenotypes, ranging from maculopapular exanthem to SJS/TEN,[37] and more recently with liver injury.[7] These associations have been replicated in many different ethnic groups (**Table 2**). Although HLA-B*15:02 genotyping is recommended in many regulatory labels, HLA-A*31:01 is only mentioned for information. However, a Clinical Pharmacogenetics Implementation Consortium (CPIC) guideline suggests that genotyping for both alleles before carbamazepine prescription be considered.[36]

Allopurinol, a drug used for the treatment of gout, can cause serious cutaneous adverse reactions, including "drug reaction with eosinophilia and systemic symptoms" (DRESS) and SJS/TEN. Work from Taiwan showed a strong association between these hypersensitivity reactions and HLA-B*58:01[77]; this has now been replicated in many studies worldwide, but in particular in SE Asian populations, where the

Table 1
Associations of abacavir hypersensitivity with *HLA-B*57:01* in different ethnic groups

Drug	HLA Allele	Region/Ethnicity	Reference
Abacavir	*HLA B*57:01*	Western Australia (White)	Mallal et al,[9] 2002
		North America (majority White, also Black, American Hispanic and other)	Hetherington et al,[24] 2002
		North America (majority White, also Hispanic and other)	Stekler et al,[25] 2006
		Spanish (White)	Rodriguez-Novoa et al,[26] 2007
		French (majority White, black)	Zucman et al,[27] 2007
		White (majority), Arabic, Black, American Indian/Alaskan native, mixed other	Mallal et al,[22] 2008
		North America (White and Black)	Saag et al,[28] 2008
		North America (majority White, others including Blacks, aboriginals, Indo-Asians, Hispanics, Metis and Orientals and unknown)	Berka et al,[29] 2012
		European descent (majority White)	Martin et al,[30] 2004
		United Kingdom (White)	Hughes et al,[31] 2004
		Switzerland (White, Black, and other)	Rauch et al,[32] 2008
		White, African American, and other (American-Indian and Asian)	Young et al,[33] 2008
		White, African-American, and Hispanic	Mounze et al,[34] 2019

frequency of *HLA-B*58:01* is higher than in European Ancestry populations (**Table 3**). *HLA-B*58:01* has also recently been shown to be associated with allopurinol hepato-toxicity, where some of the cases also had manifest allopurinol DRESS.[78] Preprescrip-tion genotyping has shown to be cost-effective in some Asian countries.[79] In European and African populations, HLA-B*58:01 explains approximately 60% of allopurinol-associated DRESS and SJS/TEN.

Other important hypersensitivity reactions with predominantly cutaneous manifes-tations which have been reported recently include *HLA-B*13:01* and dapsone hyper-sensitivity[95], *HLA-A*32:01* and vancomycin DRESS,[96] and *HLA-DRB1*10:01* and β-lactam–induced immediate hypersensitivity reactions.[97]

Hepatic Adverse Reactions

Many different HLA and non-HLA alleles have been associated with drug-induced liver injury (DILI) caused by a variety of therapeutic substances—readers are referred to more comprehensive reviews of this subject.[21,98] Perhaps the most striking example is that of flucloxacillin-induced hepatic injury and its association with *HLA-B*57:01*. This was first described by Daly and colleagues[10] in 2009—a GWAS in 51 cases of flu-cloxacillin DILI showed a very strong association ($P = 10^{-33}$) with rs2395029, which was in linkage disequilibrium with *HLA-B*57:01*. Functional immunologic analysis showed the presence of drug-specific CD8+ HLA-restricted T-cell clones in patients with liver injury, with T-cell activation being processing-dependent.[99] A more recent evaluation of a larger number of patients has shown that *HLA-B*57:03* also predis-poses to flucloxacillin DILI, with valine at position 97 being common to both predispos-ing alleles. Flucloxacillin DILI is rare (incidence about 8.5 per 100,000), and over 13,500 people would need to be tested to prevent one case of DILI.[100] Therefore, prospective testing for *HLA-B*57:01* before flucloxacillin prescription would not be cost-effective. However, typing for *HLA-B*57:01* may still have diagnostic utility (see below).

Table 2
Studies reporting the association of different phenotypes of carbamazepine hypersensitivity with HLA alleles

Drug	HLA Allele	[a]Hypersensitivity Reaction	Ethnicity	Reference
Carbamazepine	HLA-B*15:02	SJS/TEN	Han Chinese	Chung et al,[38] 2004
		SJS/TEN, HSS, MPE	Han Chinese	Hung et al,[39] 2006
		SJS/TEN/HSS	Han Chinese	Man et al,[40] 2007
		SJS	Thai	Locharernkul et al,[41] 2008
		SJS	Indian	Mehta et al,[42] 2009
		SJS/TEN	Malay, Chinese, Indian	Chang et al,[43] 2011
		SJS/TEN	Han Chinese	Chen et al,[44] 2011
		SJS/TEN	Southern Han Chinese	Shi et al,[45] 2012
		SJS/TEN	Thai	Tassaneeyakul et al,[46] 2010
		SJS	Malay/Chinese	Then et al,[47] 2011
		SJS/TEN	Han Chinese	Wu et al,[48] 2010
		SJS/TEN	Han Chinese	Zhang et al,[49] 2011
		SJS/TEN	Indian	Aggarwal et al,[50] 2014
		SJS/TEN	Han Chinese	Genin et al,[51] 2014
		SJS/TEN	Javanese/Sudanese	Yuliwulandari et al,[52] 2017
		SJS/TEN and MPE	Thai	Sukasem et al,[53] 2018
		SJS/TEN	Han Chinese	Wang et al,[54] 2011
		SJS/TEN	Thai	Kulkantrakorn et al,[55] 2012
		SJS	European, Asian, African, Aboriginal, mixed and unknown	Amstutz et al,[56] 2013
		SJS	Han Chinese	Cheung et al,[57] 2013
		SJS/TEN	Han Chinese	Lin et al,[58] 2013
		SJS/TEN	Malay, Chinese	Chong et al,[59] 2014
		SJS/TEN	Southern Indian	Khor et al,[60] 2014
		SJS/TEN	Han Chinese	Kwan et al,[61] 2014
		SJS	Han Chinese	Sun et al,[62] 2014
		SJS/TEN	Han Chinese	Hsiao et al,[63] 2014
		SJS/TEN	Malay, Chinese	Toh et al,[64] 2014
		SJS/TEN	Han Chinese	Wang et al,[65] 2014
		SJS/TEN	Vietnamese	Nguyen et al,[66] 2015
		SJS/TEN	Han Chinese	Yang et al,[67] 2015
		SJS/TEN	Malay, Chinese, Indian	Teh et al,[68] 2016

Carbamazepine	HLA-A*31:01	MPE/HSS	Han Chinese	Hung et al,[39] 2006
		MPE, erythroderma, DIHS, and other drug eruptions.	Japanese	Kashiwagi et al,[69] 2008
		HSS, MPE	Northern European	McCormack et al,[70] 2011
		SJS/TEN/DIHS	Japanese	Ozeki et al,[71] 2011
		HSS	Koreans	Kim et al,[72] 2011
		SJS/TEN, DIHS, EEM, MPE	Japanese	Niihara et al,[73] 2013
		HSS, MPE	European, Asian, African, Aboriginal, mixed and unknown	Amstutz et al,[56] 2013
		DRESS	Europeans, Chinese	Genin et al,[51] 2014
		DRESS/MPE	Han Chinese	Hsiao et al,[63] 2014
		DRESS	Tunisian	Ksouda et al,[74] 2017
		SCAR	European	Nicoletti et al,[7] 2019
		MPE	North Indian	Ihtisham et al,[75] 2019
		DRESS	European	Mockenhaupt et al,[76] 2019

Abbreviations: DIHS, drug-induced hypersensitivity syndrome; DRESS, drug reaction with eosinophilia and systemic symptoms; EEM, erythema exudativum multiforme; HSS, hypersensitivity syndrome; MPE, maculopapular exanthem; SCAR, serious cutaneous adverse reaction; SJS, Stevens-Johnson syndrome; TEN, toxic epidermal necrolysis.

[a] Phenotype described as per the original study.

Table 3
Associations between allopurinol-induced cutaneous reactions and *HLA-B*58:01*

Drug	HLA Allele	[a]Hypersensitivity Reaction	Ethnicity/Region	Reference
Allopurinol	*HLA B*58: 01*	HSS, SJS, TEN.	Han Chinese	Hung et al,[77] 2005
		SJS/TEN	Japanese	Tohkin et al,[80] 2013
		DRESS/SJS/TEN	Han Chinese	Cheng et al,[81] 2015
		MPE/DRESS/SJS/TEN	Han Chinese	Ng et al,[15] 2016
		SJS/TEN	Koreans	Park et al,[82] 2016
		DRESS/SJS/TEN	Portuguese	Goncalo et al,[83] 2013
		MPE/DRESS/SJS/TEN	Han Chinese	Gao et al,[84] 2012
		EEM/SJS	Japanese	Niihara et al,[73] 2013
		EEM/DRESS/SJS/TEN	Han Chinese	Chiu et al,[85] 2012
		MPE/DRESS/SJS/TEN	Han Chinese	Cao et al,[86] 2012
		HSS/SJS/TEN	Koreans	Kang et al,[87] 2011
		HSS/SJS	Koreans	Jung et al,[88] 2011
		SJS/TEN	Italian (Caucasian)	Cristallo et al,[89] 2011
		SJS/TEN	Thai	Tassaneeyakul et al,[90] 2009
		SJS/TEN	Japanese	Kaniwa et al,[91] 2008
		SJS/TEN	European (majority), African, Asian, South American.	Lonjou et al,[92] 2008
		MPE/DRESS/SJS/TEN	Thai	Sukasem et al,[93] 2016
		DRESS/SJS/TEN	Thai	Nicoletti et al,[94] 2021

Abbreviations: DRESS, drug reaction with eosinophilia and systemic symptoms; HSS, hypersensitivity syndrome; SJS, Stevens-Johnson syndrome; TEN, toxic epidermal necrolysis.
[a] Phenotype described as per the original study.

Muscle Injury

Statins are a widely used group of drugs that have been associated with different forms of muscle injury.[101] In most instances, the muscle injury has been related to a genetic polymorphism in the influx transporter gene *SLCO1B1*.[102] However, statins can also cause necrotizing autoimmune myopathy, which is relatively rare, and is associated proximal myopathy with creatine kinase levels raised up to 50,000 IU/L.[102] This form of myopathy can present after years of use of statins, and may persist after stopping the statin, requiring treatment with immunosuppressants. Interestingly, patients with statin-induced necrotizing autoimmune myopathy often have circulating anti-HMG CoA-reductase (HMGCR) antibodies, and this adverse reaction has been associated with *HLA-DRB1*11:01*.[103]

Agranulocytosis

Agranulocytosis, a reduction in the absolute neutrophil count below 100 neutrophils per microliter, can be caused by nonimmune (usually due to cancer chemotherapy) or immune mechanisms. Antithyroid drugs (propylthiouracil, carbimazole, and methimazole) can cause immune-mediated agranulocytosis. The frequency is approximately 0.35%.[104] Patients are warned to seek medical attention if they experience symptoms that may be indicative of agranulocytosis, which is not ideal (as some patients can become seriously ill and warnings can also lead to patient anxiety).

An early case-control study in Japanese participants[105] (24 cases, 68 methimazole-treated controls, and 525 healthy controls) showed an association of methimazole-induced agranulocytosis with *HLA DRB1*08:03* (P = .007, odds ratio [OR] = 4.18). A study in a Taiwanese population[106] (42 cases and 1208 Graves' disease controls) confirmed the association with *HLA-DRB1*08:03* ($P = 1.83 \times 10^{-9}$, OR = 6.13). In addition, a significant association was also seen for *HLA-B*38:02* ($P = 7.75 \times 10^{-32}$, OR = 21.48). For those with both *HLA-B*38:02* and *HLA-DRB1*08:03,* the OR increased to 48.41. *HLA-B*38:02* and *HLA-DRB1*08:03* have been reported as markers for antithyroid drug-induced agranulocytosis in these other populations:

- Southern Chinese—20 cases, 775 controls, *HLA-B*38:02:01* was associated with carbimazole/methimazole-induced agranulocytosis ($P = 2.5 \times 10^{-14}$, OR = 265.5), but not associated with propylthiouracil.[107]
- Vietnamese—21 cases, 81 drug-tolerant controls, *HLA-B*38:02* was associated with carbimazole/methimazole-induced agranulocytosis ($P = 5.2 \times 10^{-7}$, OR = 28.6).[108]
- Han Chinese—29 cases, 140 drug-tolerant controls, associations with *HLA-B*38:02* ($P = 2.41 \times 10^{-4}$, OR = 7.525), *HLA-DRB1*08:03* ($P = 1.57 \times 10^{-3}$, OR = 4.316), and *HLA-B*27:05* ($P = 1.1 \times 10^{-4}$, OR = 66.24).[109]

Most recently, a study in a Japanese population[110] (87 cases and 384 antithyroid drug-treated controls) identified *HLA-B*39:01:01* ($P = 1.4 \times 10^{-3}$, OR = 3.35) as a novel risk factor for agranulocytosis. This association was replicated in Chinese ($P = 9.0 \times 10^{-3}$), Taiwanese ($P = 1.1 \times 10^{-3}$), and European populations ($P = 5.2 \times 10^{-4}$), with a meta-analysis of pooled results including cases from this and previous studies confirming the importance of this HLA allele ($P = 1.2 \times 10^{-9}$, OR = 3.66). In addition, analysis of the discovery cohort also replicated the association between *HLA-DRB1*08:03:02* and antithyroid drug-induced agranulocytosis ($P = 5.2 \times 10^{-7}$, OR = 2.80).

Implementing Genetic Testing into Clinical Practice

Strength of evidence: As highlighted in previous sections, there have been many discoveries of genetic factors predisposing to drug hypersensitivity reactions, but implementation into clinical practice has been much slower. Uptake into clinical practice depends on the strength of evidence of the association between a genetic marker and the drug hypersensitivity. In addition, it has become increasingly important to show that introduction of the genetic test will be cost-effective.

The highest level of evidence according to the evidence hierarchy is the randomized controlled trial (RCT). A recent systematic review showed that only one RCT has been undertaken in this area[111]—this was the PREDICT-1 trial,[22] which showed that *HLA-B*57:01* genotyping was clinically effective in preventing abacavir hypersensitivity reactions. Interestingly, implementation of *HLA-B*57:01* testing occurred before the completion of the PREDICT-1 trial in some countries such as the United Kingdom and Australia, countries that also participated in the study, largely because of the strength of the evidence (from observational studies), demonstration of cost-effectiveness, and a clinical and patient community that was willing to accept innovative change. It is also interesting to note that although testing for *HLA-B*57:01* was initially reactive (ie, testing just before prescription of abacavir), this has now become a pre-emptive test, that is, patients are tested for *HLA-B*57:01* at the time of HIV diagnosis as part of the initial clinical workup even if abacavir may not be used as first-line therapy, and the test result kept in the clinical records, for when (and if) abacavir is needed.

Instead of undertaking RCTs, some investigators have undertaken prospective studies where HLA genotyping is undertaken before drug prescription, and the culprit drug is avoided if the patient is positive for the HLA allele. This requires the use of historical controls, which has its limitations,[112] including the need to accurately determine the historical incidence of a rare adverse drug reaction. Such prospective studies have focused on carbamazepine (*HLA-B*15:02* and *HLA-A*31:01*), allopurinol (*HLA-B*58:01*), and dapsone (*HLA-B*13:01*)[113] — all have shown that preprescription testing for the specific HLA alleles reduced the incidence of hypersensitivity reactions compared with data derived from historical controls.

Most of the other drug hypersensitivity genetic studies which have been reported since 2000 have used a case-control design.[3] Various genotyping strategies have been used including genome-wide association studies, and some of these have found striking associations, with many of them being replicated in subsequent studies. Such observational studies may not be regarded as providing the strength of evidence needed to implement a genetic test into clinical practice. However, undertaking RCTs in this area is extremely difficult, if not impossible in many cases. This is due to the rarity of the reaction (which would therefore require a large sample size) and difficulty in raising funding because many of the compounds implicated in hypersensitivity reactions are generic drugs. It is our opinion that all types of evidence should be assessed, including observational data, rather than relying on the hierarchy of evidence,[114] which may have outlived its usefulness. All data should be interpreted in an intelligent fashion to determine whether the evidence is adequate to enable clinical implementation.

Predictive values: Studies of genetic testing often report various diagnostic parameters which indicate the predictive accuracy of the test. A recent systematic review has shown that most of the studies report sensitivity, specificity, positive and negative predictive values, while others also report values for number needed to test to prevent one reaction.[6] These parameters can vary for the same drug hypersensitivity reaction between different studies. In general, most of the studies have shown that the positive predictive values are low while the negative predictive values and specificity are high but not complete across different ethnicities in particular. This indicates the need to identify other factors (genetic and nongenetic) which increase the risk and therefore the predictive value of genetic testing.

Cost-effectiveness: Determination of the cost-effectiveness of a genetic test is an important piece of evidence that may be required by many health care systems before the test is taken up into clinical practice, and reimbursed.[79] As different health care systems have different models and costing structures, any cost-effectiveness analysis may only be relevant for the country where the data are derived from, and thus the same test may show different levels of cost-effectiveness in different countries. There are many reasons for this including health care costs, costs of genetic testing, and the population prevalence of the implicated genetic variant.[79] The latter can lead to policies which lead to recommending genetic testing in one ethnic group but not in another ethnic group within the same country. For example, in Singapore, a policy for genotyping of *HLA-B*15:02* before carbamazepine prescription was introduced for the Chinese and Malay populations based on cost-effectiveness analysis, but not for Indians.[115] This has the potential to introduce racial inequalities and inequity in access to care.

Drug labels and guidelines: Inclusion of a genetic test in the drug label will aid implementation. However, the information in the drug label can vary from a test that is mandated or recommended (which represents the minority) to a test that is included for information only. In most cases, the latter is ignored, and the evidence required for transitioning from an "information" label to a "recommended" label is not clear. Furthermore, there is a lack of harmonization in the wording used in drug labels from different regulatory agencies,[116] including when it comes to accurately identifying the at-risk populations based on self-reported ethnicity.

To aid implementation, several groups have started to develop guidelines, the 2 most well-known being the CPIC[117] and the Dutch Pharmacogenetics Working Group (DPWG).[118] This can lead to discordance between the guidance present in the drug label compared to the guideline. For instance, the CPIC guideline suggests that both *HLA-B*15:02* and *HLA-A*31:01* should be considered when prescribing carbamazepine,[36] whereas the FDA and EMA drug label recommend testing for *HLA-B*15:02* but include *HLA-A*31:01* for information only.

Behavior change: Changing the behavior of health care professionals is important in implementing a new test for drug hypersensitivity. This has been highlighted with respect to *HLA-B*15:02* testing to prevent carbamazepine hypersensitivity: physicians either did not undertake the testing as recommended or avoided the use of carbamazepine and prescribed alternative drugs, which also had a high risk of the hypersensitivity reactions (**Fig. 2**).[119–121]

Clearly, education and improving the knowledge of health care professionals is important in changing behavior, thereby increasing the uptake of pharmacogenetic testing. In the future, as more pharmacogenetic tests become implemented into clinical practice, developing decision support systems will be important to ensure that the relevant populations are tested, and test results are interpreted accurately.

Novel uses for genetic testing: Most genetic tests have been developed to predict susceptibility to an adverse drug reaction. However, it is possible to use genetic tests for other purposes as outlined in our framework for genetic testing[122]:

- Use in diagnosis: a genetic test that has a 100% negative predictive value could be used to improve the diagnosis of a drug hypersensitivity reaction and differentiate it from a non–drug-induced disease. For example, *HLA-B*57:01* has a 100% negative predictive value in relation to flucloxacillin-induced liver injury. Thus, it could be used to differentiate flucloxacillin-induced liver injury from another cause of abnormal liver function tests, for example, gallstones, to ensure that the patient not only receives appropriate treatment but also appropriate advice on whether to avoid flucloxacillin in the future.
- Stratification of monitoring: Many drug labels recommend blood test monitoring after starting a drug. This is inconvenient, costly, and unnecessary for most patients. Identification of a susceptible group using a genetic test may allow stratification of monitoring so that the susceptible group is monitored more frequently, whereas nonsusceptible individuals are monitored less frequently. This strategy only works in drugs where a genetic factor has a high negative predictive value.

Genetic testing technology: In the past, the lack and cost of genetic testing was often used as an excuse for not undertaking pharmacogenetic testing. However, with the advances in genotyping technologies, and the associated reduction in costs, this is no longer a viable excuse. The COVID-19 pandemic has shown that it is possible to implement genetic testing at scale in the community.[123] Currently, for most genetic tests, a reactive strategy is used, usually testing for a single locus before drug prescription. This requires waiting for the test result before prescribing the drug, which itself acts as a barrier to pharmacogenetic testing. We therefore need to move from a reactive to a pre-emptive strategy. This is starting to be implemented in some sentinel sites. For example, Boston Children's Hospital has been using a four-HLA (*HLA-A*31:01, HLA-B*15:02, HLA-B*57:01*, and *HLA-B*58:01*) panel-based test for years.[124] We have developed a globally relevant 23 HLA allele panel which has analytical validity equivalent to that of sequence-based typing, has a turnaround time of approximately 48 hours, has an accompanying decision support system, costs less than single locus testing, and is cost-effective.[125] The panel can be used when a

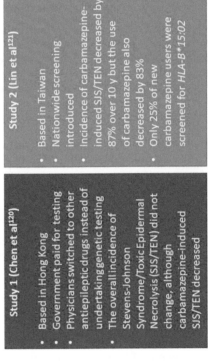

Study 1 (Chen et al[120])

- Based in Hong Kong
- Government paid for testing
- Physicians switched to other antiepileptic drugs instead of undertaking genetic testing
- The overall incidence of Stevens-Johnson Syndrome/Toxic Epidermal Necrolysis (SJS/TEN) did not change, although carbamazepine-induced SJS/TEN decreased

Study 2 (Lin et al[121])

- Based in Taiwan
- Nationwide screening introduced
- Incidence of carbamazepine–induced SJS/TEN decreased by 87% over 10 y but the use of carbamazepine also decreased by 83%
- Only 25% of new carbamazepine users were screened for HLA-B*15:02

Study 3 (Sung et al[122])

- Based in Singapore
- Genotyping introduced 2013 with a 75% subsidy
- Phenytoin not recommended as a substitute
- Led to a 92% reduction in carbamazepine-induced SJS/TEN
- Number of new carbamazepine users decreased by one-third

Fig. 2. Three studies[119–121] from SE Asia which have highlighted some of the difficulties in implementing genetic testing for HLA-B*15:02 in preventing carbamazepine-induced SJS and TEN at a country level.

particular HLA allele test is needed, with the other HLA allele results being stored in the patient's health record for use later if the patient is prescribed the relevant drugs, thus moving from a reactive to a pre-emptive approach.

SUMMARY

There is increasing evidence that genetic factors, and primarily HLA class I alleles, are important in predisposing to drug hypersensitivity reactions. Much of the research has focused on discovery, with many associations having been identified since the beginning of this century. This excellent work needs to continue and should be intensified by (a) using newer technologies such as whole human genome sequencing to identify novel genetic factors; (b) increasing international collaboration to increase the breadth and depth of patients and drugs evaluated; and (c) identifying genomic predisposing factors both within and outside the HLA region, including those which interact with HLA alleles to modulate the risk of hypersensitivity. By comparison to discovery, the application of genetic findings into clinical practice has lagged. Further work in this area is essential over the next few years to realize the promise of novel genetic discoveries and make a real impact on patient outcomes.

CLINICS CARE POINTS

- A patient who develops features of a hypersensitivity reaction should be carefully evaluated for both the clinical manifestations and drug causality. This will help to reach the correct diagnosis, identify the culprit drug, and recruit to studies on drug hypersensitivity.

- Before prescribing a drug, the clinician should be aware of the propensity of that drug to cause hypersensitivity, and whether there are any clinical, genetic, and other factors increasing susceptibility to that reaction. Risk mitigation should be undertaken by minimizing clinical risk factors and undertaking any genetic tests, as appropriate.

- Genetic tests may sometimes be helpful in a patient who has developed a hypersensitivity reaction when the etiology is unclear; for example, when the patient has been started on multiple drugs, and it is difficult to identify the culprit, and when there is an alternative coexisting non–drug-induced cause of the same clinical manifestations.

ACKNOWLEDGMENTS

M. Pirmohamed is funded by the MRC Centre for Drug Safety Science and NIHR global research group on oral anticoagulation.

DISCLOSURE

R. Kuruvilla and K. Scott have nothing to disclose. M. Pirmohamed has received partnership funding for the following: MRC Clinical Pharmacology Training Scheme (co-funded by MRC and Roche, UCB, Eli Lilly, and Novartis); a PhD studentship jointly funded by EPSRC and AstraZeneca; and grant funding from VistaGen Therapeutics. He has also unrestricted educational grant support for the UK Pharmacogenetics and Stratified Medicine Network from Bristol-Myers Squibb. He has developed an HLA genotyping panel with MC Diagnostics, but does not benefit financially from this (the HLA panel is mentioned in the article). He is part of the IMI Consortium ARDAT (www.ardat.org/). None of these funding sources have been used for the current article.

REFERENCES

1. Pirmohamed M. Pharmacogenetics: past, present and future. Drug Discov Today 2011;16(19–20):852–61.
2. Park BK, Pirmohamed M, Kitteringham NR. Role of drug disposition in drug hypersensitivity: a chemical, molecular, and clinical perspective. Chem Res Toxicol 1998;11(9):969–88.
3. Pirmohamed M, Ostrov DA, Park BK. New genetic findings lead the way to a better understanding of fundamental mechanisms of drug hypersensitivity. J Allergy Clin Immunol 2015;136(2):236–44.
4. Robinson J, Barker DJ, Georgiou X, et al. IPD-IMGT/HLA database. Nucleic Acids Res 2019;48(D1):D948–55.
5. Jaruthamsophon K, Thomson PJ, Sukasem C, et al. HLA allele-restricted immune-mediated adverse drug reactions: framework for genetic prediction. Annu Rev Pharmacol Toxicol 2022;62:509–29. https://doi.org/10.1146/annurev-pharmtox-052120-014115.
6. Manson LEN, Swen JJ, Guchelaar H-J. Diagnostic test criteria for HLA genotyping to prevent drug hypersensitivity reactions: a systematic review of actionable HLA recommendations in CPIC and DPWG guidelines. Front Pharmacol 2020; 11:567048.
7. Nicoletti P, Barrett S, McEvoy L, et al. Shared genetic risk factors across carbamazepine-induced hypersensitivity reactions. Clin Pharmacol Ther 2019; 106(5):1028–36.
8. Alfirevic A, Jorgensen AL, Williamson PR, et al. HLA-B locus in Caucasian patients with carbamazepine hypersensitivity. Pharmacogenomics 2006;7(6): 813–8.
9. Mallal S, Nolan D, Witt C, et al. Association between presence of HLA-B*5701, HLA-DR7, and HLA-DQ3 and hypersensitivity to HIV-1 reverse-transcriptase inhibitor abacavir. Lancet 2002;359(9308):727–32.
10. Daly AK, Donaldson PT, Bhatnagar P, et al. HLA-B*5701 genotype is a major determinant of drug-induced liver injury due to flucloxacillin. Nat Genet 2009; 41(7):816–9.
11. Xu CF, Johnson T, Wang X, et al. HLA-B*57:01 confers susceptibility to pazopanib-associated liver injury in patients with cancer. Clin Cancer Res 2016;22(6):1371–7.
12. Chaponda M, Pirmohamed M. Hypersensitivity reactions to HIV therapy. Br J Clin Pharmacol 2011;71(5):659–71.
13. Roehmel JF, Schwarz C, Mehl A, et al. Hypersensitivity to antibiotics in patients with cystic fibrosis. J Cyst Fibros 2014;13(2):205–11.
14. Hammond S, Olsson-Brown A, Grice S, et al. Checkpoint inhibition reduces the threshold for drug-specific T-Cell priming and increases the incidence of sulfasalazine hypersensitivity. Toxicol Sci 2021;kfab144. https://doi.org/10.1093/toxsci/kfab144.
15. Ng CY, Yeh YT, Wang CW, et al. Impact of the HLA-B(*)58:01 allele and renal impairment on allopurinol-induced cutaneous adverse reactions. J Invest Dermatol 2016;136(7):1373–81.
16. Chung WH, Chang WC, Lee YS, et al. Genetic variants associated with phenytoin-related severe cutaneous adverse reactions. JAMA 2014;312(5): 525–34.
17. Pan RY, Chu MT, Wang CW, et al. Identification of drug-specific public TCR driving severe cutaneous adverse reactions. Nat Commun 2019;10(1):3569.

18. Carr DF, Bourgeois S, Chaponda M, et al. Genome-wide association study of nevirapine hypersensitivity in a sub-Saharan African HIV-infected population. J Antimicrob Chemother 2017;72(4):1152–62.

19. Pavlos R, Deshpande P, Chopra A, et al. New genetic predictors for abacavir tolerance in HLA-B*57:01 positive individuals. Hum Immunol 2020;81(6):300–4.

20. Li Y, Deshpande P, Hertzman RJ, et al. Genomic risk factors driving immune-mediated delayed drug hypersensitivity reactions. Front Genet 2021;12:641905.

21. Stephens C, Lucena MI, Andrade RJ. Genetic risk factors in the development of idiosyncratic drug-induced liver injury. Expert Opin Drug Metab Toxicol 2021; 17(2):153–69.

22. Mallal S, Phillips E, Carosi G, et al. HLA-B*5701 screening for hypersensitivity to abacavir. New Engl J Med 2008;358(6):568–79.

23. Rauch A, Nolan D, Martin A, et al. Prospective genetic screening decreases the incidence of abacavir hypersensitivity reactions in the Western Australian HIV cohort study. Clin Infect Dis 2006;43(1):99–102.

24. Hetherington S, Hughes AR, Mosteller M, et al. Genetic variations in HLA-B region and hypersensitivity reactions to abacavir. Lancet 2002;359(9312):1121–2.

25. Stekler J, Maenza J, Stevens C, et al. Abacavir hypersensitivity reaction in primary HIV infection. AIDS 2006;20(9):1269–74.

26. Rodriguez-Novoa S, Garcia-Gasco P, Blanco F, et al. Value of the HLA-B*5701 allele to predict abacavir hypersensitivity in Spaniards. AIDS Res Hum Retroviruses 2007;23(11):1374–6.

27. Zucman D, Truchis P, Majerholc C, et al. Prospective screening for human leukocyte antigen-B*5701 avoids abacavir hypersensitivity reaction in the ethnically mixed French HIV population. J Acquir Immune Defici Syndr 2007;45(1):1–3.

28. Saag M, Balu R, Phillips E, et al. High sensitivity of human leukocyte antigen-b*5701 as a marker for immunologically confirmed abacavir hypersensitivity in white and black patients. Clin Infect Dis 2008;46(7):1111–8.

29. Berka N, Gill JM, Liacini A, et al. Human leukocyte antigen (HLA) and pharmacogenetics: screening for HLA-B*57:01 among human immunodeficiency virus-positive patients from southern Alberta. Hum Immunol 2012;73(2):164–7.

30. Martin AM, Nolan D, Gaudieri S, et al. Predisposition to abacavir hypersensitivity conferred by HLA-B*5701 and a haplotypic Hsp70-Hom variant. Proc Natl Acad Sci U S A 2004;101(12):4180–5.

31. Hughes DA, Vilar FJ, Ward CC, et al. Cost-effectiveness analysis of HLA B*5701 genotyping in preventing abacavir hypersensitivity. Pharmacogenetics 2004; 14(6):335–42.

32. Rauch A, Nolan D, Thurnheer C, et al. Refining abacavir hypersensitivity diagnoses using a structured clinical assessment and genetic testing in the Swiss HIV Cohort Study. Antivir Ther 2008;13(8):1019–28.

33. Young B, Squires K, Patel P, et al. First large, multicenter, open-label study utilizing HLA-B*5701 screening for abacavir hypersensitivity in North America. AIDS 2008;22(13):1673–5.

34. Mounzer K, Hsu R, Fusco JS, et al. HLA-B*57:01 screening and hypersensitivity reaction to abacavir between 1999 and 2016 in the OPERA(®) observational database: a cohort study. AIDS Res Ther 2019;16(1):1.

35. Yip VL, Marson AG, Jorgensen AL, et al. HLA genotype and carbamazepine-induced cutaneous adverse drug reactions: a systematic review. Clin Pharmacol Ther 2012;92(6):757–65.

36. Phillips EJ, Sukasem C, Whirl-Carrillo M, et al. Clinical Pharmacogenetics Implementation Consortium Guideline for HLA Genotype and Use of Carbamazepine and Oxcarbazepine: 2017 Update. Clin Pharmacol Ther 2018;103(4):574–81.

37. Yip VL, Pirmohamed M. The HLA-A*31:01 allele: influence on carbamazepine treatment. Pharmgenomics Pers Med 2017;10:29–38.

38. Chung WH, Hung SI, Hong HS, et al. Medical genetics: a marker for Stevens-Johnson syndrome. Nature 2004;428(6982):486.

39. Hung SI, Chung WH, Jee SH, et al. Genetic susceptibility to carbamazepine-induced cutaneous adverse drug reactions. Pharmacogenetics and Genomics 2006;16(4):297–306.

40. Man CB, Kwan P, Baum L, et al. Association between HLA-B*1502 allele and antiepileptic drug-induced cutaneous reactions in Han Chinese. Epilepsia 2007;48(5):1015–8.

41. Locharernkul C, Loplumlert J, Limotai C, et al. Carbamazepine and phenytoin induced Stevens-Johnson syndrome is associated with HLA-B*1502 allele in Thai population. Epilepsia 2008;49(12):2087–91.

42. Mehta TY, Prajapati LM, Mittal B, et al. Association of HLA-B*1502 allele and carbamazepine-induced Stevens-Johnson syndrome among Indians. Indian J Dermatol Venereol Leprol 2009;75(6):579–82.

43. Chang CC, Too CL, Murad S, et al. Association of HLA-B*1502 allele with carbamazepine-induced toxic epidermal necrolysis and Stevens-Johnson syndrome in the multi-ethnic Malaysian population. Int J Dermatol 2011;50(2):221–4.

44. Chen P, Lin JJ, Lu CS, et al. Carbamazepine-induced toxic effects and HLA-B*1502 screening in Taiwan. New Engl J Med 2011;364(12):1126–33.

45. Shi YW, Min FL, Qin B, et al. Association between HLA and Stevens-Johnson syndrome induced by carbamazepine in Southern Han Chinese: genetic markers besides B*1502? Basic Clin Pharmacol Toxicol 2012;111(1):58–64.

46. Tassaneeyakul W, Tiamkao S, Jantararoungtong T, et al. Association between HLA-B*1502 and carbamazepine-induced severe cutaneous adverse drug reactions in a Thai population. Epilepsia 2010;51(5):926–30.

47. Then SM, Rani ZZ, Raymond AA, et al. Frequency of the HLA-B*1502 allele contributing to carbamazepine-induced hypersensitivity reactions in a cohort of Malaysian epilepsy patients. Asian Pac J Allergy Immunol 2011;29(3):290–3.

48. Wu XT, Hu FY, An DM, et al. Association between carbamazepine-induced cutaneous adverse drug reactions and the HLA-B*1502 allele among patients in central China. Epilepsy Behav 2010;19(3):405–8.

49. Zhang Y, Wang J, Zhao LM, et al. Strong association between HLA-B*1502 and carbamazepine-induced Stevens-Johnson syndrome and toxic epidermal necrolysis in mainland Han Chinese patients. Eur J Clin Pharmacol 2011;67(9):885–7.

50. Aggarwal R, Sharma M, Modi M, et al. HLA-B * 1502 is associated with carbamazepine induced Stevens-Johnson syndrome in North Indian population. Hum Immunol 2014;75(11):1120–2.

51. Genin E, Chen DP, Hung SI, et al. HLA-A*31:01 and different types of carbamazepine-induced severe cutaneous adverse reactions: an international study and meta-analysis. Pharmacogenomics J 2014;14(3):281–8.

52. Yuliwulandari R, Kristin E, Prayuni K, et al. Association of the HLA-B alleles with carbamazepine-induced Stevens-Johnson syndrome/toxic epidermal necrolysis in the Javanese and Sundanese population of Indonesia: the important role of the HLA-B75 serotype. Pharmacogenomics 2017;18(18):1643–8.

53. Sukasem C, Chaichan C, Nakkrut T, et al. Association between HLA-B alleles and carbamazepine-induced maculopapular exanthema and severe cutaneous reactions in Thai patients. J Immunol Res 2018;2018:2780272.

54. Wang Q, Zhou JQ, Zhou LM, et al. Association between HLA-B*1502 allele and carbamazepine-induced severe cutaneous adverse reactions in Han people of southern China mainland. Seizure 2011;20(6):446–8.

55. Kulkantrakorn K, Tassaneeyakul W, Tiamkao S, et al. HLA-B*1502 strongly predicts carbamazepine-induced Stevens-Johnson syndrome and toxic epidermal necrolysis in Thai patients with neuropathic pain. Pain Pract 2012;12(3):202–8.

56. Amstutz U, Ross CJ, Castro-Pastrana LI, et al. HLA-A 31:01 and HLA-B 15:02 as genetic markers for carbamazepine hypersensitivity in children. Clin Pharmacol Ther 2013;94(1):142–9.

57. Cheung YK, Cheng SH, Chan EJ, et al. HLA-B alleles associated with severe cutaneous reactions to antiepileptic drugs in Han Chinese. Epilepsia 2013; 54(7):1307–14.

58. Lin YT, Chang YC, Hui RC, et al. A patch testing and cross-sensitivity study of carbamazepine-induced severe cutaneous adverse drug reactions. J Eur Acad Dermatol Venereol 2013;27(3):356–64.

59. Chong KW, Chan DW, Cheung YB, et al. Association of carbamazepine-induced severe cutaneous drug reactions and HLA-B*1502 allele status, and dose and treatment duration in paediatric neurology patients in Singapore. Arch Dis Child 2014;99(6):581–4.

60. Khor AH, Lim KS, Tan CT, et al. HLA-B*15:02 association with carbamazepine-induced Stevens-Johnson syndrome and toxic epidermal necrolysis in an Indian population: a pooled-data analysis and meta-analysis. Epilepsia 2014;55(11): e120–4.

61. Kwan PK, Ng MH, Lo SV. Association between HLA-B*15:02 allele and antiepileptic drug-induced severe cutaneous reactions in Hong Kong Chinese: a population-based study. Hong Kong Med J 2014;20(Suppl 7):16–8.

62. Sun D, Yu CH, Liu ZS, et al. Association of HLA-B*1502 and *1511 allele with antiepileptic drug-induced Stevens-Johnson syndrome in central China. J Huazhong Univ Sci Technolog Med Sci 2014;34(1):146–50.

63. Hsiao YH, Hui RC, Wu T, et al. Genotype-phenotype association between HLA and carbamazepine-induced hypersensitivity reactions: strength and clinical correlations. J Dermatol Sci 2014;73(2):101–9.

64. Toh DS, Tan LL, Aw DC, et al. Building pharmacogenetics into a pharmacovigilance program in Singapore: using serious skin rash as a pilot study. Pharmacogenomics J 2014;14(4):316–21.

65. Wang W, Hu FY, Wu XT, et al. Genetic predictors of Stevens-Johnson syndrome and toxic epidermal necrolysis induced by aromatic antiepileptic drugs among the Chinese Han population. Epilepsy Behav 2014;37:16–9.

66. Nguyen DV, Chu HC, Nguyen DV, et al. HLA-B*1502 and carbamazepine-induced severe cutaneous adverse drug reactions in Vietnamese. Asia Pac Allergy 2015;5(2):68–77.

67. Yang F, Yang Y, Zhu Q, et al. Research on susceptible genes and immunological pathogenesis of cutaneous adverse drug reactions in Chinese hans. J Investig Dermatol Symp Proc 2015;17(1):29–31.

68. Teh LK, Selvaraj M, Bannur Z, et al. Coupling genotyping and computational modeling in prediction of anti-epileptic drugs that cause stevens johnson syndrome and toxic epidermal necrolysis for carrier of HLA-B*15:02. J Pharm Pharm Sci 2016;19(1):147–60.

69. Kashiwagi M, Aihara M, Takahashi Y, et al. Human leukocyte antigen genotypes in carbamazepine-induced severe cutaneous adverse drug response in Japanese patients. J Dermatol 2008;35(10):683–5.

70. McCormack M, Alfirevic A, Bourgeois S, et al. HLA-A*3101 and carbamazepine-induced hypersensitivity reactions in Europeans. New Engl J Med 2011;364(12):1134–43.

71. Ozeki T, Mushiroda T, Yowang A, et al. Genome-wide association study identifies HLA-A*3101 allele as a genetic risk factor for carbamazepine-induced cutaneous adverse drug reactions in Japanese population. Hum Mol Genet 2011;20(5):1034–41.

72. Kim SH, Lee KW, Song WJ, et al. Carbamazepine-induced severe cutaneous adverse reactions and HLA genotypes in Koreans. Epilepsy Res 2011;97(1–2):190–7.

73. Niihara H, Kaneko S, Ito T, et al. HLA-B*58:01 strongly associates with allopurinol-induced adverse drug reactions in a Japanese sample population. J Dermatol Sci 2013;71(2):150–2.

74. Ksouda K, Affes H, Mahfoudh N, et al. HLA-A*31:01 and carbamazepine-induced DRESS syndrom in a sample of North African population. Seizure 2017;53:42–6.

75. Ihtisham K, Ramanujam B, Srivastava S, et al. Association of cutaneous adverse drug reactions due to antiepileptic drugs with HLA alleles in a North Indian population. Seizure 2019;66:99–103.

76. Mockenhaupt M, Wang CW, Hung SI, et al. HLA-B*57:01 confers genetic susceptibility to carbamazepine-induced SJS/TEN in Europeans. Allergy 2019;74(11):2227–30.

77. Hung SI, Chung WH, Liou LB, et al. HLA-B*5801 allele as a genetic marker for severe cutaneous adverse reactions caused by allopurinol. Proc Natl Acad Sci U S A 2005;102(11):4134–9.

78. Fontana RJ, Li YJ, Phillips E, et al. Allopurinol hepatotoxicity is associated with human leukocyte antigen Class I alleles. Liver Int 2021;41(8):1884–93.

79. Plumpton CO, Roberts D, Pirmohamed M, et al. A systematic review of economic evaluations of pharmacogenetic testing for prevention of adverse drug reactions. PharmacoEconomics 2016;34(8):771–93.

80. Tohkin M, Kaniwa N, Saito Y, et al. A whole-genome association study of major determinants for allopurinol-related Stevens-Johnson syndrome and toxic epidermal necrolysis in Japanese patients. Pharmacogenomics J 2013;13(1):60–9.

81. Cheng L, Xiong Y, Qin CZ, et al. HLA-B*58:01 is strongly associated with allopurinol-induced severe cutaneous adverse reactions in Han Chinese patients: a multicentre retrospective case-control clinical study. Br J Dermatol 2015;173(2):555–8.

82. Park HJ, Kim YJ, Kim DH, et al. HLA allele frequencies in 5802 Koreans: varied allele types associated with SJS/TEN according to culprit drugs. Yonsei Med J 2016;57(1):118–26.

83. Goncalo M, Coutinho I, Teixeira V, et al. HLA-B*58:01 is a risk factor for allopurinol-induced DRESS and Stevens-Johnson syndrome/toxic epidermal necrolysis in a Portuguese population. Br J Dermatol 2013;169(3):660–5.

84. Gao S, Gui XE, Liang K, et al. HLA-dependent hypersensitivity reaction to nevirapine in Chinese Han HIV-infected patients. AIDS Res Hum Retroviruses 2012;28(6):540–3.

85. Chiu ML, Hu M, Ng MH, et al. Association between HLA-B*58:01 allele and severe cutaneous adverse reactions with allopurinol in Han Chinese in Hong Kong. Br J Dermatol 2012;167(1):44–9.

86. Cao ZH, Wei ZY, Zhu QY, et al. HLA-B*58:01 allele is associated with augmented risk for both mild and severe cutaneous adverse reactions induced by allopurinol in Han Chinese. Pharmacogenomics 2012;13(10):1193–201.

87. Kang HR, Jee YK, Kim YS, et al. Positive and negative associations of HLA class I alleles with allopurinol-induced SCARs in Koreans. Pharmacogenetics and Genomics 2011;21(5):303–7.

88. Jung JW, Song WJ, Kim YS, et al. HLA-B58 can help the clinical decision on starting allopurinol in patients with chronic renal insufficiency. Nephrol Dial Transpl 2011;26(11):3567–72.

89. Cristallo AF, Schroeder J, Citterio A, et al. A study of HLA class I and class II 4-digit allele level in Stevens-Johnson syndrome and toxic epidermal necrolysis. Int J Immunogenet 2011;38(4):303–9.

90. Tassaneeyakul W, Jantararoungtong T, Chen P, et al. Strong association between HLA-B*5801 and allopurinol-induced Stevens-Johnson syndrome and toxic epidermal necrolysis in a Thai population. Pharmacogenetics and Genomics 2009;19(9):704–9.

91. Kaniwa N, Saito Y, Aihara M, et al. HLA-B locus in Japanese patients with antiepileptics and allopurinol-related Stevens-Johnson syndrome and toxic epidermal necrolysis. Pharmacogenomics 2008;9(11):1617–22.

92. Lonjou C, Borot N, Sekula P, et al. A European study of HLA-B in Stevens-Johnson syndrome and toxic epidermal necrolysis related to five high-risk drugs. Pharmacogenetics and Genomics 2008;18(2):99–107.

93. Sukasem C, Jantararoungtong T, Kuntawong P, et al. HLA-B (*) 58:01 for allopurinol-induced cutaneous adverse drug reactions: implication for clinical interpretation in Thailand. Front Pharmacol 2016;7:186.

94. Saksit N, Tassaneeyakul W, Nakkam N, et al. Risk factors of allopurinol-induced severe cutaneous adverse reactions in a Thai population. Pharmacogenetics and Genomics 2017;27(7):255–63.

95. Zhang FR, Liu H, Irwanto A, et al. HLA-B*13:01 and the dapsone hypersensitivity syndrome. N Engl J Med 2013;369(17):1620–8.

96. Konvinse KC, Trubiano JA, Pavlos R, et al. HLA-A*32:01 is strongly associated with vancomycin-induced drug reaction with eosinophilia and systemic symptoms. J Allergy Clin Immunol 2019;144(1):183–92.

97. Nicoletti P, Carr DF, Barrett S, et al. Beta-lactam-induced immediate hypersensitivity reactions: A genome-wide association study of a deeply phenotyped cohort. J Allergy Clin Immunol 2021;147(5):1830–1837 e1815.

98. Kaliyaperumal K, Grove JI, Delahay RM, et al. Pharmacogenomics of drug-induced liver injury (DILI): molecular biology to clinical applications. J Hepatol 2018;69(4):948–57.

99. Monshi MM, Faulkner L, Gibson A, et al. Human leukocyte antigen (HLA)-B*57:01-restricted activation of drug-specific T cells provides the immunological basis for flucloxacillin-induced liver injury. Hepatology 2013;57(2):727–39.

100. Alfirevic A, Pirmohamed M. Predictive genetic testing for drug-induced liver injury: considerations of clinical utility. Clin Pharmacol Ther 2012;92(3):376–80.

101. Alfirevic A, Neely D, Armitage J, et al. Phenotype standardization for statin-induced myotoxicity. Clin Pharmacol Ther 2014;96(4):470–6.

102. Carr DF, Francis B, Jorgensen AL, et al. Genomewide association study of statin-induced myopathy in patients recruited Using the UK clinical practice research datalink. Clin Pharmacol Ther 2019;106(6):1353–61.

103. Mammen AL, Gaudet D, Brisson D, et al. Increased frequency of DRB1*11:01 in anti-hydroxymethylglutaryl-coenzyme a reductase-associated autoimmune myopathy. Arthritis Care Res (Hoboken) 2012;64(8):1233–7.

104. Abraham P, Acharya S. Current and emerging treatment options for Graves' hyperthyroidism. Ther Clin Risk Manag 2010;6:29–40.

105. Tamai H, Sudo T, Kimura A, et al. Association between the DRB1*08032 histocompatibility antigen and methimazole-induced agranulocytosis in Japanese patients with Graves disease. Ann Intern Med 1996;124(5):490–4.

106. Chen P-L, Shih S-R, Wang P-W, et al. Genetic determinants of antithyroid drug-induced agranulocytosis by human leukocyte antigen genotyping and genome-wide association study. Nat Commun 2015;6:7633.

107. Cheung CL, Sing CW, Tang CS, et al. HLA-B*38:02:01 predicts carbimazole/methimazole-induced agranulocytosis. Clin Pharmacol Ther 2016;99(5):555–61.

108. Thao MP, Tuan PVA, Linh LGH, et al. Association of HLA-B(*)38:02 with Antithyroid Drug-Induced Agranulocytosis in Kinh Vietnamese Patients. Int J Endocrinol 2018;2018:7965346.

109. He Y, Zheng J, Zhang Q, et al. Association of HLA-B and HLA-DRB1 polymorphisms with antithyroid drug-induced agranulocytosis in a Han population from northern China. Sci Rep 2017;7(1):11950.

110. Nakakura S, Hosomichi K, Uchino S, et al. HLA-B*39:01:01 is a novel risk factor for antithyroid drug-induced agranulocytosis in Japanese population. Pharmacogenomics J 2021;21(1):94–101.

111. Alfirevic A, Pirmohamed M, Marinovic B, et al. Genetic testing for prevention of severe drug-induced skin rash. Cochrane Database Syst Rev 2019;7: CD010891.

112. Viele K, Berry S, Neuenschwander B, et al. Use of historical control data for assessing treatment effects in clinical trials. Pharm Stat 2014;13(1):41–54.

113. Oussalah A, Yip V, Mayorga C, et al. Genetic variants associated with T cell-mediated cutaneous adverse drug reactions: A PRISMA-compliant systematic review-An EAACI position paper. Allergy 2020;75(5):1069–98.

114. Rosner AL. Evidence-based medicine: Revisiting the pyramid of priorities. J Bodywork Movement Therapies 2012;16(1):42–9.

115. Dong D, Sung C, Finkelstein EA. Cost-effectiveness of HLA-B*1502 genotyping in adult patients with newly diagnosed epilepsy in Singapore. Neurology 2012; 79(12):1259–67.

116. Yamazaki S. A retrospective analysis of actionable pharmacogenetic/genomic biomarker language in FDA labels. Clin Transl Sci 2021;14(4):1412–22.

117. Relling MV, Klein TE, Gammal RS, et al. The Clinical Pharmacogenetics Implementation Consortium: 10 Years Later. Clin Pharmacol Ther 2020;107(1):171–5.

118. Swen JJ, Nijenhuis M, van Rhenen M, et al. Pharmacogenetic Information in Clinical Guidelines: The European Perspective. Clin Pharmacol Ther 2018; 103(5):795–801.

119. Chen Z, Liew D, Kwan P. Effects of a HLA-B*15:02 screening policy on antiepileptic drug use and severe skin reactions. Neurology 2014;83(22):2077–84.

120. Lin C-W, Huang W-I, Chao P-H, et al. Temporal trends and patterns in carbamazepine use, related severe cutaneous adverse reactions, and HLA-B*15:02 screening: A nationwide study. Epilepsia 2018;59(12):2325–39.

121. Sung C, Tan L, Limenta M, et al. Usage Pattern of Carbamazepine and Associated Severe Cutaneous Adverse Reactions in Singapore Following Implementation of HLA-B*15:02 Genotyping as Standard-of-Care. Front Pharmacol 2020; 11:527.
122. Alfirevic A, Pirmohamed M. Genomics of Adverse Drug Reactions. Trends Pharmacol Sci 2017;38(1):100–9.
123. Mercer TR, Salit M. Testing at scale during the COVID-19 pandemic. Nat Rev Genet 2021;22(7):415–26.
124. Manzi SF, Fusaro VA, Chadwick L, et al. Creating a scalable clinical pharmacogenomics service with automated interpretation and medical record result integration - experience from a pediatric tertiary care facility. J Am Med Inform Assoc 2017;24(1):74–80.
125. Plumpton CO, Pirmohamed M, Hughes DA. Cost-Effectiveness of panel tests for multiple pharmacogenes associated with adverse drug reactions: an evaluation framework. Clin Pharmacol Ther 2019;105(6):1429–38.

Advances in the Pathomechanisms of Delayed Drug Hypersensitivity

Chuang-Wei Wang, PhD[a,b,c], Sherrie Jill Divito, MD, PhD[d],
Wen-Hung Chung, MD, PhD[a,b,c,e,f,*], Shuen-Iu Hung, PhD[a,b,g,*]

KEYWORDS

- Delayed drug hypersensitivity • Human leukocyte antigens
- Immune checkpoint blockade • Severe cutaneous adverse reactions
- T cell receptor • Cytotoxic proteins

KEY POINTS

- Delayed drug hypersensitivity mainly involves a T-cell-mediated immune response against different pharmaceutical substances.
- Delayed drug hypersensitivity has strong genetic associations with human leukocyte antigens (HLA), which may present the drugs, and/or reactive metabolites to T-cell receptors (TCR), resulting in T cell activation.
- In addition to HLA, TCR, drug metabolism, the pathogenesis of delayed drug hypersensitivity also involves the reactivation of virus, and activation of many immune mediators, cytotoxicity proteins, cytokines, and chemokines.

[a] Cancer Vaccine & Immune Cell Therapy Core Lab, Department of Medical Research, Chang Gung Memorial Hospital, Linkou Branch, No. 5, Fuxing St., Guishan Dist., Taoyuan 333, Taiwan; [b] Department of Dermatology, Drug Hypersensitivity Clinical and Research Center, Chang Gung Memorial Hospital, Linkou Branch, No. 5, Fuxing St., Guishan Dist., Taoyuan 333, Taiwan; [c] Department of Dermatology, Xiamen Chang Gung Hospital, No. 123, Xiafei Road, Haicang District, Xiamen, China; [d] Department of Dermatology, Brigham & Women's Hospital, Harvard Medical School, 221 Longwood Avenue, EBRC Room 513, Boston, MA 02115, USA; [e] Whole-Genome Research Core Laboratory of Human Diseases, Chang Gung Memorial Hospital, Keelung Branch, No. 222, Maijin Rd., Anle Dist., Keelung 204, Taiwan; [f] College of Medicine, Chang Gung University, No.259, Wenhua 1st Rd., Guishan Dist., Taoyuan 333, Taiwan; [g] Department and Institute of Pharmacology, National Yang Ming Chiao Tung University, No. 155, Sec.2, Linong Street, Taipei, 112 Taiwan
* Corresponding author. Department of Medical Research, Cancer Vaccine & Immune Cell Therapy Core Lab, Chang Gung Memorial Hospital, Linkou Branch, Taoyuan 333, Taiwan
E-mail addresses: chung1@cgmh.org.tw; wenhungchung@yahoo.com (W.-H.C.); sihung@cgmh.org.tw; hungshueniu@gmail.com (S.-I.H.)

Immunol Allergy Clin N Am 42 (2022) 357–373
https://doi.org/10.1016/j.iac.2022.01.002
0889-8561/22/© 2022 Elsevier Inc. All rights reserved.

Abbreviations	
HLA	human leukocyte antigens
TCR	T cell receptor
MPE	maculopapular exanthema
FDE	fixed drug eruption
SCAR	severe cutaneous adverse reactions
AGEP	acute generalized exanthematous pustulosis
DRESS	drug reaction with eosinophilia and systemic symptoms
SJS	Stevens–Johnson syndrome
TEN	toxic epidermal necrolysis
CBZ	carbamazepine
CDR3	third complementarity-determining region
CTL	cytotoxic T lymphocytes
TCM	central memory T cells
TEM	effector memory T cells
TRM	tissue-resident memory T cells
TEMRA	terminally differentiated effector memory Tcells
GVHD	graft versus host disease
NK	natural killer
IL	interleukin
HHV	human herpesvirus
EBV	Epstein–Barr virus
CMV	cytomegalovirus
irAEs	immune-related adverse events
CYP	cytochrome P450
IVIg	intravenous immunoglobulins

INTRODUCTION
Drug Hypersensitivity Reactions

Delayed drug hypersensitivity is off-target reactions, traditionally classified as type B or unpredictable reactions that are rare and occur in individuals with an underlying genetic predisposition.[1–3]

Clinical Phenotypes and Epidemiology of Delayed Drug Hypersensitivity

Delayed drug hypersensitivity typically develops from 3 to 7 days to weeks following drug exposure, with variable clinical presentations that can range from mild symptoms, such as maculopapular exanthema (MPE), or fixed drug eruption (FDE), to life-threatening severe cutaneous adverse reactions (SCARs), including acute generalized exanthematous pustulosis (AGEP), drug reaction with eosinophilia and systemic symptoms (DRESS), Stevens–Johnson syndrome (SJS), and toxic epidermal necrolysis (TEN).[4]

Maculopapular exanthema (MPE) presents as a mild, generalized, widespread skin rash without evidence of blistering or internal organ involvement. FDE is characterized as well-demarcated, dusky red patches involving the skin or mucosa, which tends to appear on the same sites during recurrence.

Acute generalized exanthematous pustulosis (AGEP) is characterized by the rapid development of many numerous spongiform subcorneal pustules that are nonfollicular and sterile located in the epidermis, and marked papillary edema under histopathology.[5] DRESS is defined by a suspected drug reaction involving skin rash, dysregulation of at least one internal organ, one blood abnormality (eosinophilia or atypical lymphocytes), lymphadenopathy, and fever greater than 38.5°C.[6] DRESS typically presents with little to no skin detachment or mucocutaneous involvement but includes internal organ involvement and hematological abnormalities (eg, liver damage, eosinophilia, atypical lymphocytes, high fever, and so forth). The characteristic histopathologic changes in DRESS include epidermal spongiosis, dyskeratosis, and interface vacuolization.[7,8]

SJS, SJS–TEN overlap, and TEN are known as disorders along a continuous disease spectrum, according to the disease severity and the extent of epidermal detachment.[9–11] SJS/TEN is characterized by mucocutaneous involvement, which more commonly occurs with the oral mucosa than the ocular, genital, or anal mucosa. SJS, SJS–TEN overlap, and TEN are defined by the degree of skin detachment, affecting 10%, 10%–30%, and more than 30% of the BSA, respectively. Epidermal necrosis is one of the important pathologic features of SJS/TEN.[10]

MOLECULAR MECHANISMS OF DELAYED DRUG HYPERSENSITIVITY
Human Leukocyte Antigens

Delayed drug hypersensitivity is thought to be elicited by the excessive activation of CD4[+] and CD8[+] T-lymphocytes, leading to the dysregulation of the immune system.[12] Drugs or pharmaceutical substances could become foreign antigens when they directly or indirectly bind to receptors and then activate the immune reactions. Human leukocyte antigens (HLA) are the primary immune anchors for presenting foreign antigens and are responsible for the initiation of immune response.[13] The highly polymorphic properties of HLA molecules among individuals provide diverse opportunities for interactions with various drugs and pharmaceutical substances. The pathogenetic interactions between HLAs and drug antigens have been supported by the discovery of strong genetic associations, for example, HLA-B*15:02 and carbamazepine (CBZ)-induced SJS/TEN,[14] HLA-B*58:01 and allopurinol-induced SCAR,[15] HLA-B*57:01 and abacavir hypersensitivity,[16] and HLA-B*13:01 and dapsone/co-trimoxazole-induced DRESS.[17–19] These data support the essential role of HLA in the initiation of immune recognition and the induction of downstream inflammation of delayed drug hypersensitivity.

T-Cell Receptors

In addition to HLA alleles, several studies have shown that specific T-cell receptors (TCRs) play important roles in the pathogenesis of delayed drug hypersensitivity.[20,21] Chung and colleagues found that oxypurinol stimulation resulted in T-cell activation, associated with a significant increase in granulysin. TCR sequencing revealed that blister cells and oxypurinol-expanded T cells possessed preferential TCR-Vβ usage and the clonal expansion of specific CDR3 (third complementarity-determining region).[21] Pan and colleagues identified a public TCR composed of a TCRα CDR3 "VFDNTDKLI" paired with a TCRβ CDR3 "ASSLAGELF" in clonotypes derived from patients from Asia and Europe with CBZ-induced SJS/TEN, which may explain how patients with different HLA alleles associated with different ethnicities can develop similar hypersensitivity reactions. This public TCR shows drug-specificity and phenotype-specificity in an HLA-B*15:02-favored manner. Functional assays, cocultures, and adoptive transfers of TCR-T cells into animal models suggest that drug-specific TCRs expressed by cytotoxic T lymphocytes (CTL) may be essential for the immune synapse that mediates CBZ-induced SJS/TEN.[20,22]

In addition, Zhao and colleagues analyzed the immune response associated with HLA Class-II–restricted T cells in patients with dapsone-induced DRESS.[23] However, the detailed interactions and mechanisms that underlie HLA-B*13:01/dapsone-restricted CTL responses remain poorly understood.

Taken together, the recent discovery of HLA genetic predispositions and clonotype-specific TCR usages[21,24] support the concept that an immune synapse involving an HLA–drug–TCR interaction is essential for inducing delayed drug hypersensitivity.

When an offending drug binds with an HLA molecule or TCR, the HLA–drug/peptide–TCR complex may trigger a series of activations, resulting in the expansion of T lymphocytes.[25] The detailed pathomechanisms underlying the development of delayed drug hypersensitivity reactions are outlined in **Fig. 1.**

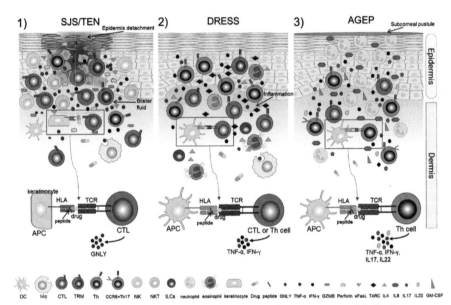

Fig. 1. Pathogenic mechanisms of severe delayed drug hypersensitivity.(1) The immune responses of SJS/TEN can be triggered by the binding of an antigenic drug with a specific HLA allele on antigen-presenting cells (APC)/keratinocyte, resulting in CTL activations. A specific TCR expressed by T cells recognizes the drug/HLA complex. Upon activation, CTL can produce large quantities of immune mediators (eg, GNLY, perforin/GZMB, sFasL, and cytokines/chemokines). In particular, secretory GNLY (15 kDa), which is expressed at a very high level in skin lesions associated with SJS/TEN, is a primary mediator for epidermal necrosis and blister formation. By comparison, GZMB/perforin and Fas/FasL are produced by granule exocytosis on cell–cell contact and present at lower concentrations than granulysin in inflammatory skin lesions. After being attacked by cytotoxic proteins, keratinocytes become damaged, and skin rash or extensive epidermal detachment occurred. (2) DRESS-affected skin reactions are primarily infiltrated with drug-induced CTL or CD4+T cells into the dermis and the release of TNF-α and IFN-γ as well as the recruitment of eosinophil, Dermal macrophages produce TARC/CCL17, which attracts memory CD4+T cells. The CD4+T cells are thought to release IL-4, which work together with chemokines/cytokines to promote systemic inflammation with eosinophilia. In addition, ILC2s, which can secret cytokines to stimulate eosinophils, also play roles in the pathogenesis of skin inflammation. (3) Regarding the pathogenesis of AGEP, drug-specific T cells can produce large amounts of GM-CSF, and in addition to IFN-γ, TNF-α, IL-17, and IL-22. Subcorneal pustules are filled with neutrophils recruited through IL-8, which is produced by keratinocytes and infiltrating CCR6+CD4+ Th17 cells. AGEP, Acute generalized exanthematous pustulosis; APC, antigen-presenting cell; CTL, cytotoxic CD8+T cells; DC, dendritic cell; DRESS, drug reaction with eosinophilia and systemic symptoms; GM-CSF; granulocyte-macrophage colony-stimulating factor; GNLY, granulysin; GZMB, Granzyme B; HLA, human leukocyte antigen; IFN-γ, Interferon-γ; IL-4, Interleukin-4; ILCs, innate lymphoid cells; Mφ, macrophage; NK, natural killer cell; NKT, natural killer T cell; sFasL, soluble Fas ligand; SJS, Stevens–Johnson syndrome; TARC, thymus- and activation-regulated chemokine; TCR, T cell receptor; TEN, toxic epidermal necrolysis; TNF-α, tumor necrosis factor-a; TRM, tissue-resident T cells.

T-Cell Subsets Mediating Delayed Drug Hypersensitivity Reactions

There exist multiple types of T cells that are classified largely on their phenotype and function (**Fig. 2**). Classification is increasingly complex and populations are not always clearly defined; however, simplistically, conventional T cells express the $\alpha\beta$ type T cell receptor and either the CD4$^+$ or CD8$^+$ coreceptor. They are then further classified as naïve, effector, or memory, and within the memory group they are subdivided into central memory T cells (TCM), effector memory T cells (TEM), or tissue-resident memory T cells (TRM). A final population in humans is increasingly appreciated termed terminally differentiated effector memory T cells (TEMRA). While evidence directly supports T cells as primary mediators of delayed drug hypersensitivity reactions, the T cell subset(s) mediating the different forms of delayed drug hypersensitivity reactions remains unknown. Illuminating the T cell subset(s) involved in disease is critically important to understanding disease pathogenesis, and moreover has direct implications for clinical care as it could potentially impact prediction, treatment, and testing to identify culprit drugs.

1) T cell inhibition

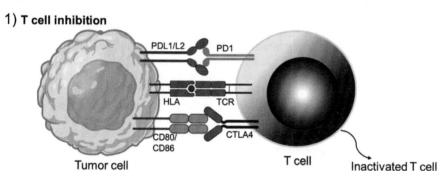

2) ICB-mediated T cell activation

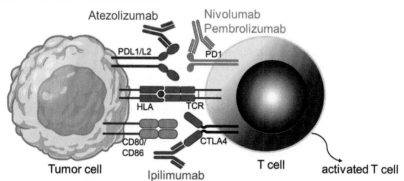

Fig. 2. Delayed drug hypersensitivity induced by immune checkpoint blockades. (1) The expression of CTLA4 and PD1 on T cells serves as an immune checkpoint through tumor cells which can bind to their coreceptors to inactivate T cells. (2) Immune checkpoint blockades, including anti-CTLA4 (ipilimumab), anti-PDL1 (Atezolizumab), and anti-PD1 (nivolumab and pembrolizumab) antibodies, can activate T cells by blocking the CTLA-4-CD80/CD86 and PD-1-PDL1/L2-mediated immunoinhibitory signaling, resulting in dysregulated T-cell activation and trigger hypersensitivity reactions. CTLA-4, cytotoxic T-lymphocyte-associated antigen 4; HLA, human leukocyte antigen; PD-1, programmed cell death protein 1; PDL1/L2, Programmed cell death 1 ligand 1/ligand 2; TCR, T cell receptor.

Human skin at steady-state contains a large population of TRM[26,27] that has been shown to play significant roles in other inflammatory skin conditions such as contact dermatitis, graft versus host disease (GVHD), psoriasis, and atopic dermatitis.[28–35] Skin TRM have been speculated to be causal or contributory to delayed drug hypersensitivity reactions; however, data are currently circumstantial. Trubiano and colleagues demonstrated that skin TRM are generated as a result of DRESS and MPE, and that skin tissue-resident (TRM) cells could likely mediate localized response to intradermal challenge with culprit drug.[36] Similarly, in some cases patients with resolved disease react to a drug applied in a skin patch test, further supporting the presence of drug-specific TRM in skin after disease resolution.[37] Whether skin TRM are present and functional during active disease has not been directly studied, but Villani and colleagues, recently identified CD8[+] CD45RA[−]CCR7[−]CD57[−] cytotoxic T cells, consistent with either an effector (TEM) or tissue-resident (TRM) phenotype, as the main T cell subset present in blister fluid of patients with SJS/TEN.[38] Further work is necessary to distinguish these 2 populations. Skin TRM have also been incriminated in the pathogenesis of FDE through demonstration that CD69[+] T cells residing in skin at steady-state became functional on exposure to drug.[39]

The presence of drug-reactive tissue resident (TRM) in skin before the development of a delayed drug hypersensitivity reaction has interesting implications for disease pathogenesis and raises the possibility of antigen cross-reactivity. In this scenario, tissue resident (TRM) specific for another antigen, most likely a virus, are present in skin from prior infection, but cross-react to drug presented in the context of a specific HLA. This heterologous immune hypothesis could explain why some patients react to a drug upon first exposure, and potentially why only a low percentage of patients expressing an at-risk HLA allele react to drug (they must also have been previously exposed to a particular virus and generated skin TRM).[40,41] Mechanistic interrogation in this field is currently underway.

Cytotoxic Signals, Cytokines, and Potential Apoptosis Pathways Involved in Stevens–Johnson Syndrome/Toxic Epidermal Necrolysis

Chung and colleagues reported that 15-kDa granulysin, known as a cytotoxic protein produced by CTL, natural killer (NK)/NK T cells, was strongly expressed by blister cells found in skin lesions and served as a key mediator for widespread keratinocyte apoptosis in SJS/TEN.[42,43] Granulysin protein levels show a larger increase than the levels of other cytotoxic proteins, such as perforin, granzyme B, and sFasL, in the blister fluids of patients with SJS/TEN.[42] In addition, the granulysin has been known to stimulate C-C motif chemokine ligand 20 (CCL20) expression in monocytes,[44] is capable of promoting leukocyte or dendritic cells recruitment, and acts as an immune alarm that activates specific immune responses.[45] Studies have also demonstrated high amounts of granulysin in patients with drug-induced DRESS, and FDE, but not in MPE.[46–48]

High levels of tumor necrosis factor-α (TNF-α) have also been observed in SJS/TEN, and TNF-α has been suggested to be involved in the extensive necrosis of TEN skin lesions.[49,50] In addition, interferon (IFN)-γ was identified as being upregulated in patients with SJS/TEN.[51,52] Furthermore, interleukin (IL)-6, IL-8, IL-15, TNF-α, and granulysin showed increased plasma levels in patients with SJS/TEN.[53] Other cytokines, such as IL-2, IL-5, IL-6, IL-12, IL-17, and IL-18, have also been identified as exacerbating the extensive collateral damage associated with SJS/TEN pathogenesis.[42,46,54–57]

Regarding the cell populations, higher proportions of NK and NK T cells have been reported in the blister fluids of patients with SJS/TEN.[42] The high amounts of granulysin released by NK/NK T cells, together with the expression of other cytotoxic proteins in the blister environment, is regulated by the balance between NK receptor activation and inhibition.[58] The activating receptor CD94/NKG2C is expressed in NK cells and CTL that infiltrate the skin of patients with SJS/TEN.[59] Moreover, the nonclassical HLA molecule, soluble HLA-E (sHLA-E), is a CD94/NKG2C ligand, and sHLA-E expression increases in the keratinocytes identified in the skin lesions of patients with SJS/TEN.[59]

Fas–FasL interaction has previously been reported to be involved in keratinocyte apoptosis in SJS/TEN.[60] However, no differences in the expression of membrane-bound FasL were found between keratinocytes obtained from patients with TEN and those from healthy individuals.[61]

A recent study indicated that Annexin A1 was involved in keratinocyte apoptosis in an SJS/TEN-like response generated in a murine model.[62] Annexin A1 was upregulated in the culture supernatant of drug-stimulated PBMCs from patients who recovered from SJS/TEN.[62] The anti–intrinsic apoptosis protein B-cell lymphoma/leukemia-2-like protein 10 (BCL2L10), which is silenced by miR-18a-5p, was reported to be abnormally low in patients with TEN, resulting in the induction of intrinsic keratinocyte apoptosis.[63]

Immunopathogenesis of Drug Reaction with Eosinophilia and Systemic Symptoms

The immunopathogenesis of DRESS has been proposed to involve both the activation of T lymphocytes and virus reactivation.[64] The symptoms of DRESS were demonstrated to be a result of activated T cells directed at the human virus antigens, which involves the reactivated virus home to the skin and visceral organs[64–66] The activated T lymphocytes release IL-4, IL-5, and IL-13, which work together with chemokines, and pro-inflammatory cytokines, such as TNF-α, IFN-γ, IL-6, and IL-15, to promote systemic inflammation with eosinophilia, resulting in the development of DRESS.[53,67,68]

DRESS has been reported to involve the reactivation of the different virus, for example, human herpesvirus (HHV)-6, HHV-7, Epstein–Barr virus (EBV), or cytomegalovirus (CMV).[65,67–69] Particularly, HHV-6 is suggested to play an essential role in the immunopathogenesis of DRESS.[70,71] Hashizume and colleagues found that mono-myeloid precursor cells harboring HHV-6 are activated by high-mobility group box 1 (HMGB-1), which is critical for the reactivation of HHV-6 in the skin lesions of patients with DRESS.[72]

Innate lymphoid cell type 2 cells (ILC2s) also play important roles in the pathogenesis of skin inflammation in patients with DRESS.[73] ILC2s secrete IL-5 to stimulate eosinophils. In addition, thymic stromal lymphopoietin (TSLP) elicits IL-33 expression, which binds to its receptor, ST2 (a member of the IL 1 receptor family), and activates Th2 cells, ILC2s, eosinophils, and mast cells.[74,75] Tsai and colleagues observed that the levels of ST2$^+$ILC2s, IL-5, and TSLP in blood and serum were significantly elevated in patients with DRESS.[73]

Recently, Kim and colleagues performed the single-cell RNA-sequencing (scRNA-seq) analysis of both skin and blood samples obtained from a patient with refractory DRESS.[76] The study showed that DRESS-associated lymphocytes had the upregulated expression of C-C chemokine receptor 10 (CCR10), Janus kinase 3 (JAK3), and signal transducer and activator of transcription 1 (STAT1). They further identified the CCR4$^+$CCR10$^+$CD4$^+$ memory T cell in the blood of the examined patient with DRESS.[76]

Immunopathogenesis of Acute Generalized Exanthematous Pustulosis

AGEP has been characterized by increased neutrophilic inflammatory processes, which are triggered by T lymphocytes and contribute to AGEP pathogenesis. High levels of IL-

8 (also known as CXCL8) have been identified in patients with AGEP, and the recruitment of neutrophils has also been observed in the skin lesions of patients during the late phase of disease development.[77,78] Drug-specific T cells isolated from patients with AGEP produce large amounts of granulocyte-macrophage colony-stimulating factor (GM-CSF), and IFN-γ and TNF-α.[78] In addition, IL-17 and IL-22 have been shown to cooperate with IFN-γ and TNF-α in stimulating the production of IL-8 by keratinocytes and further activate CCR6+CD4+Th17 cells in patients with AGEP.[78,79]

Co-inhibitory Signaling of Delayed Drug Hypersensitivity

The co-inhibitory receptors that mediate interactions between the T cells and antigen-presenting cells involved in hypersensitivity-associated immune responses have recently been identified. The most well-known co-inhibitory receptors are cytotoxic T-lymphocyte-associated protein 4 (CTLA-4) and programmed cell death protein 1 (PD-1), which are targeted by immune checkpoint blockade (ICB) immunotherapy in cancer.[80] ICB immunotherapy may lead to disequilibrium in the immune system, which manifests as an upregulated T-cell response, resulting in induced hypersensitivity reactions (shown in **Fig. 2**). CTLA-4 and CD28 are homologous receptors that are expressed on both CD4$^+$ and CD8$^+$ T cells and bind to CD80/CD86 on antigen-presenting cells. CTLA-4 serves to ultimately inhibit T-cell responses.[81] PD-1 is a checkpoint receptor that is primarily expressed on activated CD4$^+$ T cells and CD8$^+$ CTLs in the peripheral blood. PD-1 transmits an immunosuppressive signal during ligation, inhibiting T-cell proliferation, cytokine release, and cytotoxicity.[82,83] The ligands of PD-1, including programmed death-ligand 1 (PD-L1) and PD-L2, expressed primarily on antigen-presenting cells.[84] The blockade of the PD-1/PD-L1 axis plays a role in drug hypersensitivity. The *in vitro* PD-1 blockade assay shows to increase the reactivity of epidermal CD8$^+$ memory T cells.[35] Another study in human subjects revealed that priming drug-naive CD4$^+$ and CD8$^+$ T cells against drug antigens may be more effective when the PD-L1-mediated pathway was blocked.[85]

The detailed immune pathomechanism that underlies immune-checkpoint blockade (ICB)-induced delayed drug hypersensitivity is not yet fully understood. Although ICB is successful for treating various cancer types, ICB usage is associated with immune-related adverse events (irAEs).[86] Immune checkpoint blockade-induced irAEs could affect different organs and tissues. Pruritus and MPE are commonly reported, whereas severe cutaneous manifestations, such as SJS/TEN, DRESS, and Sweet's Syndrome, are uncommon.[87–90] In addition to irAE, ICB usage has been suggested to increase the risk of delayed hypersensitivity to other drugs.[91] Watanabe and colleagues reported that a patient developed TEN 1 month after discontinuing nivolumab.[92] Vivar and colleagues reported on a melanoma patient who was treated with ipilimumab and nivolumab, in whom MPE progressed to TEN over a 3-month period. An increase of CD8$^+$ T cells and upregulated PD-L1 expression in both T cells and keratinocytes were observed.[93] Goldinger and colleagues reported a case series in which 22% of 68 patients on pembrolizumab or nivolumab developed inflammatory skin lesions, ranging from a mild maculopapular rash to SJS-like lesions with upregulated PD-1.[94] These studies suggest that ICB therapy may render patients more vulnerable to have a hypersensitivity reaction to other drugs and autoimmunity, or it may directly activate T cells to trigger immune responses in skin lesions, contributing to the occurrence of irAEs.[95]

Other Risk Factors Associated with Delayed Drug Hypersensitivity

In addition to HLA alleles and TCR, genetic variants in drug-metabolizing enzymes, such as the cytochrome P450 (CYP) system, have also been associated with the development of delayed drug hypersensitivity.[70,96] Toxic intermediates produced during drug metabolism can accumulate and cause cell death or bind to T cells, provoking immune responses. Chung and colleagues[97] identified that *CYP2C* variants, including *CYP2C9*3*, are strongly associated with phenytoin-related SCARs. Phenytoin-induced SCAR patients who carried *CYP2C9*3* showed delayed clearance of plasma phenytoin, resulting in an increased risk of phenytoin-induced SCAR.[98]

Renal impairment or chronic kidney disease (CKD) can significantly delay drug clearance and metabolism, which has been associated with an increase in the plasma concentration of oxypurinol,[99] resulting in an increased risk of allopurinol-SCAR development and poor prognosis. Increased risk of allopurinol hypersensitivity, including SJS/TEN and DRESS, have been significantly associated with female sex, CKD, CVD, allopurinol use starting after 60 years of age, and an initial dosage greater than 100 mg/d. Allopurinol-associated mortality was also significantly higher in patients with CKD, CVD, and older age.[100] Allopurinol prescribed for patients with asymptomatic hyperuricemia with underlying CKD or CVD significantly increases the risk of hypersensitivity reactions and mortality.[100,101]

Genetic Testing Before Drug Use

Genetic HLA alleles associated with different drugs-induced delayed hypersensitivity reactions have been identified, and several important pharmacogenetic markers have been successfully applied in clinical practice. Cost-effectiveness studies have examined the application of genetic testing before drug treatment to prevent SCAR development,[102–104] indicating that genetic screening is an important SCAR prevention strategy.

According to accumulated evidence, the prescreening for *HLA-B*15:02* among patients of Asian descent before CBZ administration has been recommended by the US Food and Drug Administration (FDA) since 2007, and the drug-regulatory agencies in Asia countries.[105] So far, a preventive genetic test for *HLA-B*15:02* gene among potential new users of CBZ is supported by the national health insurance programs in Taiwan, Hong Kong, Singapore, Thailand, and mainland China.[106,107] Furthermore, and the US FDA now recommends genetic *HLA-B*15:02* screening before oxcarbazepine treatment.

Genetic *HLA-B*57:01* testing before abacavir treatment of HIV treatment is strongly evidence-based and widely used in clinical practice[37] and is recommended by the US FDA, and European Medicines Agency (EMA), Canada Health Canada. *HLA-B*58:01* screening is commonly used to protect patients from the risk of allopurinol-induced SCAR.[108] Several medical centers in Taiwan, Hong Kong, Thailand, Korea, and mainland China provide such prescreening.[109] To prevent dapsone-induced hypersensitivity reaction, *HLA-B*13:01* testing is recommended for new patients with leprosy being initiated on dapsone therapy in China.[110] For the prevention of phenytoin-induced SCAR, an ongoing clinical trial is examining the presence of *CYP2C9*3* and *HLA-B*15:02* alleles screening in Taiwan and China.[111]

TREATMENT STRATEGIES FOR DELAYED DRUG HYPERSENSITIVITY

Corticosteroids remain the most common immunosuppressant treatment of various phenotypes of delayed drug hypersensitivity. Although a tendency toward improved survival, recent systemic reviews have shown that systemic corticosteroid monotherapy does not significantly improve mortality relative to supportive care among patients with SJS/TEN.[112,113]

Anti-TNF-α biologic agents can block the TNF-α secretion, which is the pro-inflammatory cytokine most strongly associated with SCAR pathogenesis.[114,115]

Wang and colleagues performed a randomized controlled study comparing anti-TNF-α agents-etanercept with systemic corticosteroids and found that etanercept can improve SJS/TEN outcomes compared with corticosteroids.[116] Several case reports have also revealed that beneficial treatments with anti-TNF-α biologic agents in patients with TEN and TEN-like acute cutaneous lupus erythematosus.[117–122] Combination therapy, such as the add-on use of a biologic anti-TNF-α agent, may represent a well-tolerated and effective strategy for reducing the -related adverse events and to inhibiting disease progression in patients with severe and fulminant clinical courses. Other common treatments for SJS/TEN contain intravenous immunoglobulins (IVIg) and cyclosporine. However, the clinical benefits for IVIg and cyclosporine remain controversial.[123,124]

Although systemic corticosteroids remain the standard treatment of DRESS, their abilities to improve clinical outcomes and decrease sequelae production remain unclear.[125] Few case–control studies have been reported to support the efficacy or benefits of systemic corticosteroids for the treatment of DRESS.[126,127] Other therapies, such as IVIg, plasmapheresis, acetylcysteine, or combinations of these therapies, have also been tested in patients with DRESS,[125,127] with varying results.[127,128] Recently, Kim and colleagues[76] identified a population of memory T cells in the skin of a refractory DRESS patient with enhanced JAK–STAT signaling. The JAK1 and JAK3 inhibitor tofacitinib were able to successfully control the DRESS.

SUMMARY

There are increasing evidence revealing that the immune receptors and mediators play crucial roles in delayed drug hypersensitivity development. The immunopathogenic mechanisms underlying delayed drug hypersensitivity are complex, involving the presentation of drug antigens to initiate the immune recognition responses, resulting in cell death due to the upregulation of cytotoxic proteins and enhanced inflammatory reactions due to the dysregulation of cytokines/chemokines. We also discussed the proposed mechanisms through which delayed drug hypersensitivity is induced by ICB. In addition, genetic factors that predispose individuals to the development of delayed drug hypersensitivity have been identified and translated into clinical practice. Understanding the underlying pathomechanisms will facilitate the development of new approaches for the prevention and management of delayed drug hypersensitivity.

CLINICS CARE POINTS

- Pharmacogenomic screening of variants of *HLAs* and *CYP* metabolizing enzymes prior to prescribing some medicines is an important strategy for preventing severe delayed drug hypersensitivity with genetic predispositions.
- Corticosteroids remain the most commonly used immunosuppressant treatment of delayed drug hypersensitivity.
- Anti-TNF-α biologic agents (eg, etanercept) have been reported to improve SJS/TEN outcomes, and the add-on use with corticosteroids may represent a well-tolerated and effective strategy for delayed drug hypersensitivity.

ACKNOLEDGEMENTS

We thank the support of members of Drug Hypersensitivity Clinical and Research Center, and Cancer Vaccine and Immune Cell Therapy core lab, Chang Gung Memorial Hospital, Linkou branch. This work was supported by grants from Chang Gung

Memorial Hospital (CIRPG3I0041 ~ 43), and the Ministry of Science and Technology of Taiwan (MOST 108-2320-B-010 -021 -MY3, MOST 109-2320-B-182A-008 -MY3).

DISCLOSURE

The authors have declared that they have no conflicts of interest.

REFERENCES

1. Knowles SR, Uetrecht J, Shear NH. Idiosyncratic drug reactions: the reactive metabolite syndromes. Lancet 2000;356(9241):1587–91.
2. Hausmann O, Schnyder B, Pichler WJ. Drug hypersensitivity reactions involving skin. Handbook Exp Pharmacol 2010;196:29–55.
3. Harp JL, Kinnebrew MA, Shinkai K. Severe cutaneous adverse reactions: impact of immunology, genetics, and pharmacology. Semin Cutan Med Surg 2014; 33(1):17–27.
4. Mockenhaupt M. Epidemiology of cutaneous adverse drug reactions. Chem Immunol Allergy 2012;97:1–17.
5. Sidoroff A, Halevy S, Bavinck JN, et al. Acute generalized exanthematous pustulosis (AGEP)–a clinical reaction pattern. J Cutan Pathol 2001;28(3):113–9.
6. Kardaun SH, Sekula P, Valeyrie-Allanore L, et al. Drug reaction with eosinophilia and systemic symptoms (DRESS): an original multisystem adverse drug reaction. Results from the prospective RegiSCAR study. Br J Dermatol 2013; 169(5):1071–80.
7. Bocquet H, Bagot M, Roujeau JC. Drug-induced pseudolymphoma and drug hypersensitivity syndrome (Drug Rash with Eosinophilia and Systemic Symptoms: DRESS). Semin Cutan Med Surg 1996;15(4):250–7.
8. Chi MH, Hui RC, Yang CH, et al. Histopathological analysis and clinical correlation of drug reaction with eosinophilia and systemic symptoms (DRESS). Br J Dermatol 2014;170(4):866–73.
9. Roujeau JC. The spectrum of Stevens-Johnson syndrome and toxic epidermal necrolysis: a clinical classification. J Invest Dermatol 1994;102(6):28S–30S.
10. Roujeau JC, Stern RS. Severe adverse cutaneous reactions to drugs. N Engl J Med 1994;331(19):1272–85.
11. Assier H, Bastuji-Garin S, Revuz J, et al. Erythema multiforme with mucous membrane involvement and Stevens-Johnson syndrome are clinically different disorders with distinct causes. Arch Dermatol 1995;131(5):539–43.
12. Lerch M, Pichler WJ. The immunological and clinical spectrum of delayed drug-induced exanthems. Curr Opin Allergy Clin Immunol 2004;4(5):411–9.
13. Chung WH, Hung SI, Chen YT. Human leukocyte antigens and drug hypersensitivity. Curr Opin Allergy Clin Immunol 2007;7(4):317–23.
14. Chung WH, Hung SI, Hong HS, et al. Medical genetics: a marker for Stevens-Johnson syndrome. Nature 2004;428(6982):486.
15. Hung SI, Chung WH, Liou LB, et al. HLA-B*5801 allele as a genetic marker for severe cutaneous adverse reactions caused by allopurinol. Proc Natl Acad Sci U S A 2005;102(11):4134–9.
16. Mallal S, Nolan D, Witt C, et al. Association between presence of HLA-B*5701, HLA-DR7, and HLA-DQ3 and hypersensitivity to HIV-1 reverse-transcriptase inhibitor abacavir. Lancet 2002;359(9308):727–32.
17. Zhang FR, Liu H, Irwanto A, et al. HLA-B*13:01 and the dapsone hypersensitivity syndrome. N Engl J Med 2013;369(17):1620–8.

18. Wang CW, Tassaneeyakul W, Chen CB, et al. Whole genome sequencing identifies genetic variants associated with co-trimoxazole hypersensitivity in Asians. J Allergy Clin Immunol 2021;147(4):1402–12.
19. Wang H, Yan L, Zhang G, et al. Association between HLA-B*1301 and dapsone-induced hypersensitivity reactions among leprosy patients in China. J Invest Dermatol 2013;133(11):2642–4.
20. Pan RY, Chu MT, Wang CW, et al. Identification of drug-specific public TCR driving severe cutaneous adverse reactions. Nat Commun 2019;10(1):3569.
21. Chung WH, Pan RY, Chu MT, et al. Oxypurinol-specific T cells possess preferential TCR clonotypes and express granulysin in allopurinol-induced severe cutaneous adverse reactions. J Invest Dermatol 2015;135(9):2237–48.
22. Chu MT, Wang CW, Chang WC, Chen CB, Chung WH, Hung SI. Granulysin-based lymphocyte activation test for evaluating drug causality in antiepileptics-induced severe cutaneous adverse reactions. J Invest Dermatol 2021;141(6):1461–72.e10.
23. Zhao Q, Almutairi M, Tailor A, et al. HLA Class-IIRestricted CD8(+) T cells contribute to the promiscuous immune response in dapsone-hypersensitive patients. J Invest Dermatol 2021;141(10):2412–25.e2.
24. Ko TM, Chung WH, Wei CY, et al. Shared and restricted T-cell receptor use is crucial for carbamazepine-induced Stevens-Johnson syndrome. J Allergy Clin Immunol 2011;128(6):1266–76.e11.
25. Naisbitt DJ, Britschgi M, Wong G, et al. Hypersensitivity reactions to carbamazepine: characterization of the specificity, phenotype, and cytokine profile of drug-specific T cell clones. Mol Pharmacol 2003;63(3):732–41.
26. Clark RA, Chong B, Mirchandani N, et al. The vast majority of CLA+ T cells are resident in normal skin. J Immunol 2006;176(7):4431–9.
27. Clark RA, Chong BF, Mirchandani N, et al. A novel method for the isolation of skin resident T cells from normal and diseased human skin. J Invest Dermatol 2006;126(5):1059–70.
28. Gaide O, Emerson RO, Jiang X, et al. Common clonal origin of central and resident memory T cells following skin immunization. Nat Med 2015;21(6):647–53.
29. Divito SJ, Aasebo AT, Matos TR, et al. Peripheral host T cells survive hematopoietic stem cell transplantation and promote graft-versus-host disease. J Clin Invest 2020;130(9):4624–36.
30. Brunner PM, Emerson RO, Tipton C, et al. Nonlesional atopic dermatitis skin shares similar T-cell clones with lesional tissues. Allergy 2017;72(12):2017–25.
31. Matos TR, O'Malley JT, Lowry EL, et al. Clinically resolved psoriatic lesions contain psoriasis-specific IL-17-producing alphabeta T cell clones. J Clin Invest 2017;127(11):4031–41.
32. Gallais Serezal I, Classon C, Cheuk S, et al. Resident T Cells in resolved psoriasis steer tissue responses that stratify clinical outcome. J Invest Dermatol 2018;138(8):1754–63.
33. Gallais Serezal I, Hoffer E, Ignatov B, et al. A skewed pool of resident T cells triggers psoriasis-associated tissue responses in never-lesional skin from patients with psoriasis. J Allergy Clin Immunol 2019;143(4):1444–54.
34. Gadsboll AO, Jee MH, Funch AB, et al. Pathogenic CD8(+) epidermis-resident memory T cells displace dendritic epidermal T cells in allergic dermatitis. J Invest Dermatol 2020;140(4):806–15. e5.
35. Gamradt P, Laoubi L, Nosbaum A, et al. Inhibitory checkpoint receptors control CD8(+) resident memory T cells to prevent skin allergy. J Allergy Clin Immunol 2019;143(6):2147–57.e9.

36. Trubiano JA, Gordon CL, Castellucci C, et al. Analysis of skin-resident memory T cells following drug hypersensitivity reactions. J Invest Dermatol 2020;140(7): 1442–5.e4.

37. Mallal S, Phillips E, Carosi G, et al. HLA-B*5701 screening for hypersensitivity to abacavir. N Engl J Med 2008;358(6):568–79.

38. Villani AP, Rozieres A, Bensaid B, et al. Massive clonal expansion of polycyto-toxic skin and blood CD8(+) T cells in patients with toxic epidermal necrolysis. Sci Adv 2021;7(12). https://doi.org/10.1126/sciadv.abe0013.

39. Mizukawa Y, Yamazaki Y, Teraki Y, et al. Direct evidence for interferon-gamma production by effector-memory-type intraepidermal T cells residing at an effector site of immunopathology in fixed drug eruption. Am J Pathol 2002; 161(4):1337–47.

40. White KD, Chung WH, Hung SI, et al. Evolving models of the immunopathogen-esis of T cell-mediated drug allergy: The role of host, pathogens, and drug response. J Allergy Clin Immunol Aug 2015;136(2):219–34 [quiz: 235].

41. White KD, Abe R, Ardern-Jones M, et al. SJS/TEN 2017: building multidisci-plinary networks to drive science and translation. J Allergy Clin Immunol Pract 2018;6(1):38–69.

42. Chung WH, Hung SI, Yang JY, et al. Granulysin is a key mediator for dissemi-nated keratinocyte death in Stevens-Johnson syndrome and toxic epidermal necrolysis. Nat Med 2008;14(12):1343–50.

43. Wang CW, Chung WH, Cheng YF, et al. A new nucleic acid-based agent inhibits cytotoxic T lymphocyte-mediated immune disorders. J Allergy Clin Immunol 2013;132(3):713–22.e11.

44. Hogg AE, Bowick GC, Herzog NK, et al. Induction of granulysin in CD8+ T cells by IL-21 and IL-15 is suppressed by human immunodeficiency virus-1. J Leukoc Biol 2009;86(5):1191–203.

45. Tewary P, Yang D, de la Rosa G, et al. Granulysin activates antigen-presenting cells through TLR4 and acts as an immune alarmin. Blood 2010;116(18): 3465–74.

46. Abe R, Yoshioka N, Murata J, et al. Granulysin as a marker for early diagnosis of the Stevens-Johnson syndrome. Ann Intern Med 2009;151(7):514–5.

47. Weinborn M, Barbaud A, Truchetet F, et al. Histopathological study of six types of adverse cutaneous drug reactions using granulysin expression. Int J Derma-tol 2016;55(11):1225–33.

48. Hsu HC, Thiam TK, Lu YJ, et al. Mutations of KRAS/NRAS/BRAF predict cetux-imab resistance in metastatic colorectal cancer patients. Oncotarget 2016; 7(16):22257–70.

49. Paquet P, Nikkels A, Arrese JE, et al. Macrophages and tumor necrosis factor alpha in toxic epidermal necrolysis. Arch Dermatol 1994;130(5):605–8.

50. Paul C, Wolkenstein P, Adle H, et al. Apoptosis as a mechanism of keratinocyte death in toxic epidermal necrolysis. Br J Dermatol 1996;134(4):710–4.

51. Nassif A, Moslehi H, Le Gouvello S, et al. Evaluation of the potential role of cy-tokines in toxic epidermal necrolysis. J Invest Dermatol 2004;123(5):850–5.

52. Viard-Leveugle I, Gaide O, Jankovic D, et al. TNF-alpha and IFN-gamma are po-tential inducers of Fas-mediated keratinocyte apoptosis through activation of inducible nitric oxide synthase in toxic epidermal necrolysis. J Invest Dermatol 2013;133(2):489–98.

53. Su SC, Mockenhaupt M, Wolkenstein P, et al. Interleukin-15 Is Associated with severity and mortality in Stevens-Johnson syndrome/toxic epidermal necrolysis. J Invest Dermatol 2017;137(5):1065–73.

54. Chen C-B, Abe R, Pan R-Y, et al. An updated review of the molecular mechanisms in drug hypersensitivity. J Immunol Res 2018;2018:6431694.

55. Hashizume H, Fujiyama T, Tokura Y. Reciprocal contribution of Th17 and regulatory T cells in severe drug allergy. J Dermatol Sci 2016;81(2):131.

56. Posadas SJ, Padial A, Torres MJ, et al. Delayed reactions to drugs show levels of perforin, granzyme B, and Fas-L to be related to disease severity. J Allergy Clin Immunol 2002;109(1):155–61.

57. Caproni M, Torchia D, Schincaglia E, et al. Expression of cytokines and chemokine receptors in the cutaneous lesions of erythema multiforme and Stevens–Johnson syndrome/toxic epidermal necrolysis. Br J Dermatol 2006;155(4):722–8.

58. Lanier LL. NK cell recognition. Annu Rev Immunol 2005;23:225–74.

59. Morel E, Escamochero S, Cabanas R, et al. CD94/NKG2C is a killer effector molecule in patients with Stevens-Johnson syndrome and toxic epidermal necrolysis. J Allergy Clin Immunol 2010;125(3):703–10, 710 e1-710 e8.

60. Viard I, Wehrli P, Bullani R, et al. Inhibition of toxic epidermal necrolysis by blockade of CD95 with human intravenous immunoglobulin. Science 1998;282(5388):490–3.

61. Abe R, Shimizu T, Shibaki A, et al. Toxic epidermal necrolysis and Stevens-Johnson syndrome are induced by soluble Fas ligand. Am J Pathol 2003;162(5):1515–20.

62. Saito N, Qiao H, Yanagi T, et al. An annexin A1-FPR1 interaction contributes to necroptosis of keratinocytes in severe cutaneous adverse drug reactions. Sci Transl Med 2014;6(245):245ra95.

63. Ichihara A, Wang Z, Jinnin M, et al. Upregulation of miR-18a-5p contributes to epidermal necrolysis in severe drug eruptions. J Allergy Clin Immunol 2014;133(4):1065–74.

64. Picard D, Janela B, Descamps V, et al. Drug reaction with eosinophilia and systemic symptoms (DRESS): a multiorgan antiviral T cell response. Sci Transl Med 2010;2(46):46ra62.

65. Yoshikawa T, Fujita A, Yagami A, et al. Human herpesvirus 6 reactivation and inflammatory cytokine production in patients with drug-induced hypersensitivity syndrome. J Clin Virol 2006;37(Suppl 1):S92–6.

66. Shiohara T, Mizukawa Y. Drug-induced hypersensitivity syndrome (DiHS)/drug reaction with eosinophilia and systemic symptoms (DRESS): An update in 2019. Allergol Int 2019;68(3):301–8.

67. Bellon T. Mechanisms of severe cutaneous adverse reactions: recent advances. Drug Saf Aug 2019;42(8):973–92.

68. Shiohara T, Mizukawa Y, Aoyama Y. Monitoring the acute response in severe hypersensitivity reactions to drugs. Curr Opin Allergy Clin Immunol 2015;15(4):294–9.

69. Shiohara T, Kano Y. A complex interaction between drug allergy and viral infection. Clin Rev Allergy Immunol 2007;33(1–2):124–33.

70. Chung WH, Wang CW, Dao RL. Severe cutaneous adverse drug reactions. J Dermatol 2016;43(7):758–66.

71. Descamps V, Valance A, Edlinger C, et al. Association of human herpesvirus 6 infection with drug reaction with eosinophilia and systemic symptoms. Arch Dermatol 2001;137(3):301–4.

72. Hashizume H, Fujiyama T, Kanebayashi J, et al. Skin recruitment of monomyeloid precursors involves human herpesvirus-6 reactivation in drug allergy. Allergy 2013;68(5):681–9.

73. Tsai YG, Liou JH, Hung SI, et al. Increased Type 2 innate lymphoid cells in patients with drug reaction with eosinophilia and systemic symptoms syndrome. J Invest Dermatol 2019;139(8):1722–31.

74. Cayrol C, Girard JP. IL-33: an alarmin cytokine with crucial roles in innate immunity, inflammation and allergy. Curr Opin Immunol 2014;31:31–7.

75. Lott JM, Sumpter TL, Turnquist HR. New dog and new tricks: evolving roles for IL-33 in type 2 immunity. J Leukoc Biol 2015;97(6):1037–48.

76. Mack MR, Kim BS. A precision medicine-based strategy for a severe adverse drug reaction. Nat Med 2020;26(2):167–8.

77. Halevy S. Acute generalized exanthematous pustulosis. Curr Opin Allergy Clin Immunol 2009;9(4):322–8.

78. Schaerli P, Britschgi M, Keller M, et al. Characterization of human T cells that regulate neutrophilic skin inflammation. J Immunol 2004;173(3):2151–8.

79. Kabashima R, Sugita K, Sawada Y, et al. Increased circulating Th17 frequencies and serum IL-22 levels in patients with acute generalized exanthematous pustulosis. J Eur Acad Dermatol Venereol 2011;25(4):485–8.

80. Wei SC, Duffy CR, Allison JP. Fundamental mechanisms of immune checkpoint blockade therapy. Cancer Discov 2018;8(9):1069.

81. Stamper CC, Zhang Y, Tobin JF, et al. Crystal structure of the B7-1/CTLA-4 complex that inhibits human immune responses. Nature 2001;410(6828):608–11.

82. Wu Y, Chen W, Xu ZP, et al. PD-L1 distribution and perspective for cancer immunotherapy—blockade, knockdown, or inhibition. review. Front Immunol 2019;10:2022.

83. Zhao H, Liao X, Kang Y. Tregs: Where We Are and What Comes Next? Review. Front Immunol 2017;8:1578.

84. Keir ME, Butte MJ, Freeman GJ, et al. PD-1 and Its Ligands in Tolerance and Immunity. Annu Rev Immunol 2008;26(1):677–704.

85. Gibson A, Ogese M, Sullivan A, et al. Negative Regulation by PD-L1 during Drug-Specific Priming of IL-22–Secreting T Cells and the Influence of PD-1 on Effector T Cell Function. J Immunol 2014;192(6):2611.

86. Sibaud V. Dermatologic Reactions to Immune Checkpoint Inhibitors. Am J Clin Dermatol 2018;19(3):345–61.

87. Phillips GS, Wu J, Hellmann MD, et al. Treatment Outcomes of Immune-Related Cutaneous Adverse Events. J Clin Oncol 2019;37(30):2746–58.

88. Pintova S, Sidhu H, Friedlander PA, et al. Sweet's syndrome in a patient with metastatic melanoma after ipilimumab therapy. Melanoma Res 2013;23(6):498–501.

89. Lu J, Thuraisingam T, Chergui M, et al. Nivolumab-associated DRESS syndrome: A case report. JAAD case Rep 2019;5(3):216–8.

90. Maloney NJ, Ravi V, Cheng K, et al. Stevens-Johnson syndrome and toxic epidermal necrolysis-like reactions to checkpoint inhibitors: a systematic review. Int J Dermatol 2020;59(6):183–8.

91. Ford M, Sahbudin I, Filer A, et al. High proportion of drug hypersensitivity reactions to sulfasalazine following its use in anti-PD-1-associated inflammatory arthritis. Rheumatology 2018;57(12):2244–6.

92. Watanabe Y, Yamaguchi Y, Takamura N, et al. Toxic epidermal necrolysis accompanied by several immune-related adverse events developed after discontinuation of nivolumab. Eur J Cancer 2020;131:1–4.

93. Vivar KL, Deschaine M, Messina J, et al. Epidermal programmed cell death-ligand 1 expression in TEN associated with nivolumab therapy. J Cutan Pathol 2017;44(4):381–4.

94. Goldinger SM, Stieger P, Meier B, et al. Cytotoxic Cutaneous Adverse Drug Reactions during Anti-PD-1 Therapy. Clin Cancer Res 2016;22(16):4023.

95. Postow MA, Sidlow R, Hellmann MD. Immune-related adverse events associated with immune checkpoint blockade. New Engl J Med 2018;378(2):158–68.

96. Pirmohamed M, Park BK. Adverse drug reactions: back to the future. Br J Clin Pharmacol 2003;55(5):486–92.

97. Chung WH, Chang WC, Lee YS, et al. Genetic variants associated with phenytoin-related severe cutaneous adverse reactions. JAMA 2014;312(5):525–34.

98. Su SC, Chen CB, Chang WC, et al. HLA Alleles and CYP2C9*3 as Predictors of Phenytoin Hypersensitivity in East Asians. Clin Pharmacol Ther 2019;105(2):476–85.

99. Chung WH, Chang WC, Stocker SL, et al. Insights into the poor prognosis of allopurinol-induced severe cutaneous adverse reactions: the impact of renal insufficiency, high plasma levels of oxypurinol and granulysin. Ann Rheum Dis 2015;74(12):2157–64.

100. Yang CY, Chen CH, Deng ST, et al. Allopurinol Use and Risk of Fatal Hypersensitivity Reactions: A Nationwide Population-Based Study in Taiwan. JAMA Intern Med 2015;175(9):1550–7.

101. Ng CY, Yeh YT, Wang CW, et al. Impact of the HLA-B(*)58:01 Allele and Renal Impairment on Allopurinol-Induced Cutaneous Adverse Reactions. J Invest Dermatol 2016;136(7):1373–81.

102. Hughes DA, Vilar FJ, Ward CC, et al. Cost-effectiveness analysis of HLA B*5701 genotyping in preventing abacavir hypersensitivity. Pharmacogenetics 2004;14(6):335–42.

103. Plumpton CO, Alfirevic A, Pirmohamed M, et al. Cost effectiveness analysis of HLA-B*58:01 genotyping prior to initiation of allopurinol for gout. Rheumatology (Oxford) 2017;56(10):1729–39.

104. Ke CH, Chung WH, Wen YH, et al. Cost-effectiveness analysis for genotyping before allopurinol treatment to prevent severe cutaneous adverse drug reactions. J Rheumatol 2017;44(6):835–43.

105. Chen P, Lin JJ, Lu CS, et al. Carbamazepine-induced toxic effects and HLA-B*1502 screening in Taiwan. N Engl J Med 2011;364(12):1126–33.

106. Chen Z, Liew D, Kwan P. Effects of a HLA-B*15:02 screening policy on antiepileptic drug use and severe skin reactions. Neurology 2014;83(22):2077–84.

107. Tiamkao S, Jitpimolmard J, Sawanyawisuth K, et al. Cost minimization of HLA-B*1502 screening before prescribing carbamazepine in Thailand. Int J Clin Pharm 2013;35(4):608–12.

108. Khanna D, Fitzgerald JD, Khanna PP, et al. 2012 American College of Rheumatology guidelines for management of gout. Part 1: systematic nonpharmacologic and pharmacologic therapeutic approaches to hyperuricemia. Arthritis Care Res (Hoboken) 2012;64(10):1431–46.

109. Ke CH, Chung WH, Tain YL, et al. Utility of human leukocyte antigen-B*58: 01 genotyping and patient outcomes. Pharmacogenet Genomics 2019;29(1):1–8.

110. Liu H, Wang Z, Bao F, et al. Evaluation of prospective HLA-B*13:01 screening to prevent dapsone hypersensitivity syndrome in patients with leprosy. JAMA Dermatol 2019;155(6):666–72.

111. Chang CJ, Chen CB, Hung SI, et al. Pharmacogenetic testing for prevention of severe cutaneous adverse drug reactions. Front Pharmacol 2020;11:969.

112. Zimmermann S, Sekula P, Venhoff M, et al. Systemic immunomodulating therapies for Stevens-Johnson syndrome and toxic epidermal necrolysis: a systematic review and meta-analysis. JAMA Dermatol 2017;153(6):514–22.

113. Tsai TY, Huang IH, Chao YC, et al. Treating toxic epidermal necrolysis with systemic immunomodulating therapies: a systematic review and network meta-analysis. J Am Acad Dermatol 2021;84(2):390–7.

114. Scott LJ. Etanercept: a review of its use in autoimmune inflammatory diseases. Drugs 2014;74(12):1379–410.

115. Hunger RE, Hunziker T, Buettiker U, et al. Rapid resolution of toxic epidermal necrolysis with anti-TNF-alpha treatment. J Allergy Clin Immunol 2005;116(4):923–4.

116. Wang CW, Yang LY, Chen CB, et al. Randomized, controlled trial of TNF-α antagonist in CTL-mediated severe cutaneous adverse reactions 2018;128(3).

117. Famularo G, Di Dona B, Canzona F, et al. Etanercept for toxic epidermal necrolysis. Ann Pharmacother 2007;41(6):1083–4.

118. Gunawardane ND, Menon K, Guitart J, et al. Purpura fulminans from meningococcemia mimicking Stevens-Johnson syndrome in an adult patient taking etanercept. Arch Dermatol 2012;148(12):1429–31.

119. Paradisi A, Abeni D, Bergamo F, et al. Etanercept therapy for toxic epidermal necrolysis. J Am Acad Dermatol 2014;71(2):278–83.

120. Fischer M, Fiedler E, Marsch WC, et al. Antitumour necrosis factor-alpha antibodies (infliximab) in the treatment of a patient with toxic epidermal necrolysis. Br J Dermatol 2002;146(4):707–9.

121. Kreft B, Wohlrab J, Bramsiepe I, et al. Etoricoxib-induced toxic epidermal necrolysis: successful treatment with infliximab. J Dermatol 2010;37(10):904–6.

122. Zarate-Correa LC, Carrillo-Gomez DC, Ramirez-Escobar AF, et al. Toxic epidermal necrolysis successfully treated with infliximab. J Investig Allergol Clin Immunol 2013;23(1):61–3.

123. Schneck J, Fagot JP, Sekula P, et al. Effects of treatments on the mortality of Stevens-Johnson syndrome and toxic epidermal necrolysis: A retrospective study on patients included in the prospective EuroSCAR Study. J Am Acad Dermatol 2008;58(1):33–40. https://doi.org/10.1016/j.jaad.2007.08.039.

124. Walsh SA, Creamer D. Drug reaction with eosinophilia and systemic symptoms (DRESS): a clinical update and review of current thinking. Clin Exp Dermatol Jan 2011;36(1):6–11.

125. Shiohara T, Kano Y, Takahashi R, et al. Drug-induced hypersensitivity syndrome: recent advances in the diagnosis, pathogenesis and management. Chem Immunol Allergy 2012;97:122–38.

126. Tas S, Simonart T. Management of drug rash with eosinophilia and systemic symptoms (DRESS syndrome): an update. Dermatology 2003;206(4):353–6.

127. Criado PR, Criado RF, Avancini JM, et al. Drug reaction with Eosinophilia and Systemic Symptoms (DRESS)/Drug-induced Hypersensitivity Syndrome (DIHS): a review of current concepts. An Bras Dermatol 2012;87(3):435–49.

128. Moling O, Tappeiner L, Piccin A, et al. Treatment of DIHS/DRESS syndrome with combined N-acetylcysteine, prednisone and valganciclovir–a hypothesis. Med Sci Monit 2012;18(7):CS57–62.

A Risk-Based Approach to Penicillin Allergy

Jason A. Trubiano, BBiomedSci, MBBS, PhD[a,b,*]

KEYWORDS

- Antibiotic allergy • Oral provocation • Oral challenge • Antimicrobial stewardship
- Drug challenge • Allergy assessment • Allergy risk assessment

KEY POINTS

- Penicillin allergy is associated with antimicrobial resistance, inappropriate and restricted prescribing, and poor patient and health care outcomes.
- Readily available tools and clinician rules are available to enable risk assessment of reported penicillin allergies by allergists and nonallergists.
- Low-risk penicillin allergies once assessed are amenable to direct oral penicillin challenge, with an increased literature base to support safety and efficacy.
- Risk assessment should be incorporated into health care to assign testing and antibiotic prescribing directions to clinicians for patients reporting a penicillin allergy.

INTRODUCTION

Penicillin allergy remains highly prevalent and a major public health issue.[1,2] The known association of penicillin allergy with appropriate antibiotic prescribing and antimicrobial resistance has increased the spotlight on penicillin allergy as a target for antimicrobial stewardship program (ASP) intervention.[3] Penicillin allergy is associated with increased methicillin-resistant *Staphylococcus aureus* and *Clostridium Difficile* infection,[4,5] surgical site infection,[6] delayed time to antibiotic therapy,[7] inappropriate antibiotic utilization,[8] increased length of stay,[9] intensive care unit admission, and outpatient mortality.[10] In response, penicillin allergy delabeling has been proposed as an active intervention to prevent or arrest the public health implications of such a "label."

Delabeling is defined as the removal of a patient's penicillin allergy through a formal allergy testing procedure or medical reconciliation.[3] Although the term delabeling was first introduced in 2013, penicillin allergy testing in the inpatient setting as a tool to improve antibiotic utilization was first reported over 40 years ago.[11,12] Since then

[a] Department of Infectious Diseases, Centre for Antibiotic Allergy and Research, Austin Health, 145 Studley Road, Heidelberg, Victoria 3084, Australia; [b] Department of Medicine, Austin Health, University of Melbourne, Heidelberg 3084, Australia
* Department of Infectious Diseases, Centre for Antibiotic Allergy and Research, Austin Health, 145 Studley Road, Heidelberg, Victoria 3084, Australia.
E-mail address: Jason.TRUBIANO@austin.org.au

Immunol Allergy Clin N Am 42 (2022) 375–389
https://doi.org/10.1016/j.iac.2021.12.002
0889-8561/22/© 2021 Elsevier Inc. All rights reserved.
immunology.theclinics.com

penicillin allergy testing has been incorporated primarily into inpatient ASP programs, with examples of successful whole-of-hospital programs implemented that include risk stratification deployed to improve antibiotic usage.[13,14] The same or similar programs have also been found to reduce inappropriate antibiotic usage,[14,15] restricted antibiotic usage,[14] length of stay, and hospital costs.[16] A body of evidence now exists that enable the allergist and nonallergist to perform penicillin allergy risk assessment to appropriately match the resultant phenotype with a management plan.

DISCUSSION
Evaluation

The assessment of risk regarding a patient-reported penicillin allergy is essential to assigning the correct management—(1) direct delabeling or oral challenge (low risk), (2) skin testing ± oral challenge (moderate risk), or (3) specialist review (high risk). This assessment historically has been performed by allergists as routine clinical practice, however, to enable nonallergists to deploy a range of assessment tools that have been developed. The essential components of all antibiotic allergy assessment tools need to center on ascertaining the correct phenotype.[17,18]

On review of the literature 8 assessment tools or algorithms were identified, all derived from expert opinion with the predominance of adult applications and either a testing (direct oral challenge or skin testing) and/or beta-lactam utilization output (**Table 1**). Devchand and colleagues produced an assessment tool that can be used by the nonallergist to enable an allergy history and subsequent risk stratification, with a resultant sensitivity of 91.8% and specificity of 97.5% (see **Table 1**).[19,20] This tool has been adapted for pediatric use,[21] implemented in whole-of-hospital programs,[14] and implemented into AMS programs in Australia.[22] In addition, Shenoy and colleagues presented an expert opinion algorithm for extrapolating antibiotic allergy assessment into risk stratification (see **Table 1**),[17] which has subsequently been referenced and adapted for widespread clinical use.

Clinical decision rules have also been of increased interest to enable prompt risk stratification of patients at the point-of-care, moving beyond assessment algorithms to key variables. There are 4 published clinical decision rules for penicillin or beta-lactam allergy, from across Europe, United States, and Australia (**Table 2**). The negative predictive values (NPV) range from 80.6% to 96.3%, with 3 of the 4 tools providing a validated low-risk criteria (see **Table 2**). On review of the literature the only clinical decision rule derived from prospective data with subsequent international validation is PEN-FAST.[23] PEN-FAST is a 3-point clinical criterion derived from prospective data of 622 patients that underwent penicillin allergy testing in Melbourne (Australia). Following derivation, external validation was performed in penicillin allergy cohorts from Sydney (Australia), Perth (Australia), and Vanderbilt University Medical Center (Nashville, USA) (n = 945 patients).[23] The variables associated with a positive penicillin allergy test result on multivariable analysis were subsequently summarized in the mnemonic PEN-FAST: *PEN*icillin allergy, *F*ive or fewer years ago, *A*naphylaxis/angioedema, *S*evere cutaneous adverse reaction (SCAR), and *T*reatment required for allergy episode (or unknown). The major criteria included an allergy event occurring 5 or fewer years ago (2 points) and anaphylaxis/angioedema or SCAR (2 points); the minor criterion (1 point) included treatment required for an allergy episode (or unknown). A score of less than 3 points for PEN-FAST is considered low risk for penicillin allergy—17 of 460 patients (3.7%) positive on testing (area under the curve [AUC], 0.805; NPV 96.3% [95% confidence interval, 94.1%–97.8%]). There are also other successfully derived clinical decision rules, including that from Stevenson and

Table 1
Penicillin allergy risk assessment and clinical decision rules

Author/Region	Primary Derivation	User Group	Population	Assessment Outcomes	Outputs	Sensitivity	Specificity	External Validation or Usage	Special Population Adaption
Assessment tools									
Staicu et al,[39] 2016 (USA)	Expert opinion	Hospital clinicians	Adult inpatients	Mild-moderate/severe	Beta-lactam utilization[b]	—	—	USA[40]	—
Devchand et al,[19] 2019 (AUS)	Expert opinion	Pharmacists Doctors Nurses	Adult inpatients/outpatients[a]	No risk/low/moderate/high; *Low-risk criteria:* childhood rash, MPE >10 y, unknown > 10 y	Testing[b]	91.8%	97.5%–97.9%	AUS[14,20,41,42]	Pediatric adapation[21]
Blumenthal et al,[43] 2019 (USA)	Expert opinion	Allergists	Outpatients (n = 426)	Low/intermediate/high; *Low risk criteria:* Mild cutaneous or unknown > 5 y	Testing & beta-lactam utilisation[b]	95.1%	—	USA[44]	Perioperative assessment[44]
Shenoy et al,[17] 2019 (USA)	Expert opinion[c]	Clinicians	Not specified	Low/medium/high; *Low-risk criteria:* type A, pruritis without rash, unknown reactions > 10 y without IgE features, family history	Testing[b]	—	—	USA[45,46] Canada[46]	General practice[47]
Ramsey et al,[48] 2018 (USA)	Expert opinion	Pharmacists	Adult inpatients (n = 50)	No specific grading; *Low-risk criteria:* type A, family history	Testing[a] & penicillin utilization	94%	NA	USA[45]	—
Roberts et al,[49] 2020 (UK)	Expert opinion	Pharmacists	Pediatric out patients (n = 104)	Low/possible IgE/allergic/severe	DOC	91%	—	—	—
Reichel et al,[50] 2020 (Germany)	Expert opinion	Allergists	Outpatients (n = 200)	Low/moderate/high; Low risk—isolated urticaria, type A, childhood rash	Testing[b]	—	—	—	—

(continued on next page)

Table 1
(continued)

Author/Region	Primary Derivation	User Group	Population	Assessment Outcomes	Outputs	Sensitivity	Specificity	External Validation or Usage	Special Population Adaption
Manning et al,[46] 2021 (Canada)	Expert opinion[d]	Pharmacists	Inpatients (n = 48)	Low/medium/high. Low: unknown reaction or side effect; poorly described nonanaphylactic symptoms, delayed (>72 h) rash without IgE features	Allergy documentation	—	—	—	—
Clinical decision rules									
Chiriac et al,[16,26] 2019 (France)	Retrospective data—multivariable logistic regression	Allergists	(n = 1991 retrospective, 200 prospective)	5-point criteria. No validated low-risk criteria identified	Testing[b]	51% 83% NPV	75% 40% PPV	—	—
Siew et al,[25] 2019 (UK)	Retrospective data—multivariable logistic regression	Allergists	(n = 1092)	Low-risk criteria—no anaphylaxis, reaction > 1 y previous, inability to recall index drug	Testing[b]	80.6% NPV (98.4% low risk only)	—	—	—
Stevenson et al,[24] 2020 (AUS)	Retrospective—multivariable logistic regression	Allergists	(n = 447)	Low-risk criteria: non-SCAR rash OR rash without angioedema and > 1 y previous	Testing[b]	80.6% (NPV 97.1%)	60.8%	—	—
Trubiano et al,[23] 2020 (AUS/USA)	Prospective data—multivariable logistic regression	Clinicians	(n = 622 primary validation; 945 external validation)	3 point clinical criteria (max score 5). Low/moderate/high. Low-risk criteria: PEN-FAST score < 3	Testing[b]	70.7% (NPV 96.3%)	78.5%	Europe[51]	—

Low risk was defined as an assessment outcome that led to or recommended direct oral penicillin challenge.

Abbreviations: DOC, direct oral challenge; IDT, penicillin intradermal testing; IgE, immunoglobulin E; MPE, maculopapular exanthema; NPV, negative predictive value; PPV, positive predictive value; SPT, penicillin skin prick testing.

[a] Expert opinion derived and applied to real case scenarios (n = 8) from a prospective inpatient and outpatient testing database by 40 end users.

[b] An output of allergy testing could be direct oral penicillin challenge and/or skin testing.

[c] Approved and endorsed by IDSA, AAAAI, and SHEA ‡

[d] Adapted from References[17,52].

Table 2
Direct oral challenge in the inpatient and outpatient adult population

Author	Setting	N	Risk Assessed	ICH	Low-Risk Definition	Follow-up	Oral Challenge (Full Dose)	Immediate Positive	Delayed Positive	Total Positive
Tucker et al,[53] 2017 (USA)	Retrospective adult outpatients	328	A/I	No	All reactions EXCLUDING SCAR/hepatitis/hemolytic anemia/nephritis	—	1-step amoxicillin (250 mg)	1.5%[a] (5/328)	N/A	1.5%
Trubiano et al,[41] 2018 (AUS)	Prospective multicenter— adult inpatient/ outpatients	46	ID	Yes	ANY OF type A ADR/ unknown reaction >10 y/ benign childhood rash/ nonurticarial rash/ MPE >10 y prior EXCLUDING History of drug associated anaphylaxis/ hemodynamically unstable	5 d	1-step penicillin/ amoxicillin (250 mg)—2 h observation	0%	0%	0%
Banks et al,[27,e] 2019 (USA)	Retrospective single center— adult outpatients	708	A/I	U	ANY OF benign rash/GI Symptoms/headache/ benign somatic symptoms/unknown AND >1 y EXCLUDING Blistering rash, nephritis, hepatitis, hemolytic anemia	-	1-step amoxicillin (250 mg)	1.1% (8/708) [a,b]	—	1.1%
	Retrospective adult outpatients	806	A/I			-	1-step amoxicillin (250 mg)	1.2% (15/806) [a]	0.8% (10/806) [a]	2%
Iammatteo et al,[54] 2019 (USA)	Prospective single center— adult and	155	A/I	U	All reactions EXCLUDING Bronchospasm or laryngeal edema requiring intubation/anaphylactic shock/SCAR, AIN,	1 mo	2-step amoxicillin (500 mg)—2 h	2.6% (4/155) [a]	—	2.6%

(continued on next page)

Table 2
(continued)

Author	Setting	N	Risk Assessed	ICH	Low-Risk Definition	Follow-up	Oral Challenge (Full Dose)	Immediate Positive	Delayed Positive	Total Positive
	pediatric outpatients				hepatitis, hemolytic anemia, cutaneous/ mucosal blisters, hypersensitivity vasculitis, pneumonitis, pulmonary fibrosis and serum sickness)/ antihistamine use/ pregnancy					
Kuruvilla et al,[55] 2019 (USA)	Retrospective single center— adult outpatients	20	A/I	U	ANY OF nonspecific benign rash/Remote unknown reaction/benign somatic symptoms AND >1 y EXCLUDING Blistering rash/hemolytic anemia/organ involvement/steroids/ antihistamines	-	1-step amoxicillin (500 mg) – 1 h observation	0%	0%	0%
Stevenson et al. 2019 (AUS)[24]	Retrospective multicentre— adult outpatients	167	A/I	U	"Low-risk" defined by centre-specific protocols EXCLUDING Pregnancy/significant cardiorespiratory disease	3–7 d	1- or 2-step amoxicillin or implicated penicillin	3.6%	0%	3.6%[b] (6/167)[d]
Mustafa et al,[56] 2019 (USA)	Prospective single center RCT—adult/ pediatric outpatients	79	A/I	U	ANY OF skin rash/hives/ itching/unknown AND >10 y AND nil emergency medical attention EXCLUDING Age < 5 y/pregnancy/SCAR	-	2-step amoxicillin (400 mg)—1 h observation	3.8% (3/79) [a]	N/A	3.8%

Savic et al,[57] 2019 (UK)	Prospective single center—adult preoperative outpatients	56	Nurse	U	ANY OF GI/nonitchy rash/no hospital admission/ thrush/unknown AND >15 y EXCLUDING Unstable asthma/ pregnancy/breastfeeding	5–7 d	3-step amoxicillin then 3 d (500 mg)	2% (1/56)[a]	0%	2%
Devchand et al,[20] 2019 (AUS)	Prospective single center—adult inpatients	20	Nurse/ pharmacist	Yes	childhood exanthema Rash > 10 y Unknown > 10 y EXCLUDING History of drug-associated anaphylaxis/ hemodynamically unstable	24 h	1-step penicillin VK or amoxicillin (250 mg)—2 h observation	Nil	5%	5% (1/20)[a]
Blumenthal et al,[13] 2019 (USA)	Retrospective multicentre—adult inpatients	76 (6)[a]	AI/internal medicine/ nurse	U	ANY OF minor rash (not hives)/MPE/recorded allergy that patient denies	-	1-step or 2-step amoxicillin	—	–	3.9%[b] (3/76)
Du Plessis et al,[58] 2019 (NZ)	Prospective single center—adult inpatients	34	Pharmacist	U	Delayed onset rash AND > 5 y EXCLUDING COPD/asthma/significant cardiovascular disease/ β-blockers, ACE inhibitors/ hemodynamically unstable/> 70 y	1 mo + 1 y	5-step amoxicillin (500 mg)	—	8.8%	8.8% (3/34)[a]

(continued on next page)

Table 2
(continued)

Author	Setting	N	Risk Assessed	ICH	Low-Risk Definition	Follow-up	Oral Challenge (Full Dose)	Immediate Positive	Delayed Positive	Total Positive
Li et al,[59] 2019 (AUS)	Prospective single center—adult inpatients	56	A/I	Yes	Type A reaction (nonimmune mediated) OR immune-mediated reaction EXCLUDING Anaphylaxis (<10 y)/IgE mediated <1 y/hemolytic anemia/serum sickness/SCAR/pregnancy/hemodynamically unstable	3 d	3-step amoxicillin (500 mg)—3 h observation (then 3 days)	0%	3.6% (2/56)[a]	3.6%
Ramsey et al,[60] 2020 (USA)	Prospective single center—adult inpatients	48	A/I/Pharm	U	ANY OF rash/hives/itching/ unknown AND >20 y AND nil emergency medical attention EXCLUDING Pregnancy	2 wk	3-step amoxicillin (500 mg)— 1.5 h observation	2% (1/48)[a]	4% (2/48)[a]	6.25%
Stone et al,[61] 2020 (USA)	Prospective single center—adult critical care inpatients	54	A/I	U	ANY OF urticaria only >5 y/ self-limited rash/GI only/ remote childhood reaction with limited details/family history of alone/avoidant due to fear of allergy/known tolerance of penicillin postreaction/other symptoms: nonallergy	Chart review at 7 mo	1-step amoxicillin (250 mg)	0% (0)	0% (0)	0%

Chua et al,[14] 2020 (AUS)	Prospective multicentre adult general inpatients	200	ID	Yes	ANY OF type A ADR where direct delabeling not accepted by patient/ unknown reaction >10 y/ benign childhood rash/ injection site reaction/ MPE >10 y EXCLUDING History of drug-associated anaphylaxis/ hemodynamically unstable	90 d	1-step penicillin/ amoxicillin (250 mg)—2 h observation	1.5% (3/200c)	1.5% (3/200)	3%
Lin et al. 2020 (Netherlands)[62]	Prospective single center—adult inpatients	42	Internal medicine/ pharm	U	Mild rash, rhinitis or GI > 1 y - OR 1–2 immediate symptoms of any severity > 10 y EXCLUDING Day treatment patients		1-step amoxicillin 500 mg— 1 h observation	0	2/42	5% (2/42)a,b
Steenvoorden et al,[63] 2021 (Norway)	Prospective single center—adult inpatients	54	Internal medicine	U	ANY OF benign rash OR symptoms unlikely to be allergic cause OR no recollection of reaction EXCLUDING Penicillin: IgE mediated, SCAR, critical illness, recent anaphylaxis (any)	-	2-step amoxicillin (75 mg/250 mg) — 1 h observation	1.9% (1/54)	3.7% (2/54)	5.5% (3/54)a

Abbreviations: A/I, allergy/immunology; ACE, angiotensin-converting enzyme; ADR, adverse drug reaction; GI, gastrointestinal; ICH, immunocompromised host; ID, infectious diseases; mg, milligrams; MPE, maculopapular exanthema; Pharm, pharmacist; RCT, randomized controlled trial; SCAR, severe cutaneous adverse reactions; U, unknown.

a No serious adverse events (SAE)—as defined by not requiring intensive care support, adrenaline therapy, SCAR, or readmission to hospital.
b Unspecified if onset of reaction postchallenge was immediate or delayed.
c Nonimmune-mediated ADR.
d Unknown descriptions of positive challenges.
e Nonpeer-reviewed data, 708 patients from Walter Reed National Military Cent and Marine Corps Recruit Depot.
Adapted from Rose MT, Slavin M, Trubiano J. The democratization of de-labeling: a review of direct oral challenge in adults with low-risk penicillin allergy. Expert Rev Anti Infect Ther. 2020 Nov;18(11):1143-1153.

colleagues—derived from a multicenter Australian retrospective cohort 447 patients.[24] These investigators identified a reported penicillin allergy of benign rash more than 1 year previous as a low-risk criterion (97.1% NPV, sensitivity 80.6%; specificity 60.8%). Siew and colleagues used a retrospective cohort from the United Kingdom (n = 1092) to generate a low-risk criteria consisting of (1) no anaphylaxis, (2) reaction more than 1 year ago, and (3) no recall of index drug (NPV 98.4%).[25] Chiriac and colleagues from a French retrospective beta-lactam allergy cohort generated a clinical decision rule that in the authors' recommendations was unable to predict allergy (AUC, 0.67; sensitivity, 51%; NPV, 83%).[26] It is evident that a range of clinical decision rules are available; however, replication and external validation in the region of proposed use is still recommended before implementation.

RISK-BASED APPROACHES TO PENICILLIN ALLERGY TESTING

A risk-based approach has been increasingly applied to penicillin allergy testing, with most of the modern evidence for the use of direct oral penicillin challenge, without skin testing, in the low-risk clinical phenotypes.[27] The data for moderate to severe allergy testing supports skin prick and intradermal testing as the standard of care, evident in recent international consensus guidelines.[28–30] The use of in vivo skin testing (intradermal and/or patch testing) for the most severe end of the spectrum for delayed hypersensitivity reactions remains controversial, with recent recommendations made by an expert group detailing these should only be performed in specialist centers.[31] The role of in vitro and ex vivo testing in both severe immediate and delayed penicillin hypersensitivity also remains predominately in a research-only capacity,[30,31] and if used in practice they are to complement in vivo testing.[32]

Regarding risk-stratified approaches to penicillin allergy in adult-treated populations, the greatest evidence is available for low-risk penicillin allergy. A recent review of the available literature by Rose and colleagues examined data from 1912 accumulative low-risk direct oral penicillin allergy patients, with positive oral challenge rates of 0% to 4.2% and 0% to 8.8% for outpatient and inpatients noted, respectively. Heterogeneity was noted in selected phenotypes, challenge steps, and drug dosing.[33] Provided in **Table 2** is a current list of 17 cohort studies (12, 70.5% prospective; 1, 5.8% randomized controlled trial; 9, 52% single-step only protocols; 11, 64.7% allergist-led assessment) where direct oral penicillin challenge was performed in a risk-stratified low-risk population. The consistent finding among a heterogenous study population was the utilization of a "historical benign rash" or "childhood rash" as universally accepted definition for low-risk. Chua and colleagues[14] in the most recent multicenter prospective study integrated direct oral penicillin challenge following risk assessment into a whole-of-hospital ASP program, with demonstratable impacts on appropriateness of prescribing (2-fold increase) and narrow spectrum penicillin (10-fold increase) usage. The data provided enable clinicians to risk stratify patients into low risk using available tools and apply either a single-step or multistep direct oral penicillin challenge with an observation period of 1 to 2 hours posttesting.

Although a complete review was not performed, similar evidence of risk-stratified oral penicillin challenge in pediatric setting is evident.[34] In the outpatient arena direct amoxicillin challenge without skin testing has been successfully deployed in children.[35] Mill and colleagues demonstrated in 818 pediatric outpatients, the largest cohort, that graded direct oral amoxicillin challenge was tolerated in 94.1%, even when including potentially moderate- and high-risk allergies (eg, anaphylaxis).[36] The pediatric literature has recently been reviewed[37] and in conjunction with international

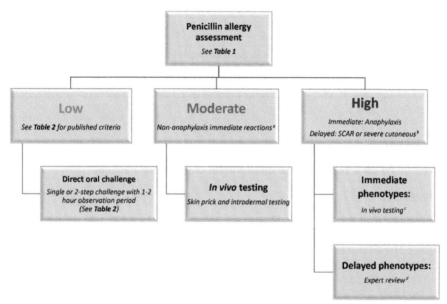

Fig. 1. Risk-based approach to penicillin allergy. [a] Urticaria has been considered as low risk in some oral challenge cohorts (see **Table 2**). [b] Delayed rashes with blistering, mucosal or desquamating components often have same testing approaches applied as SCAR. [c] In vitro testing, such as basophil activation test (BAT), if available can be applied for implicated drugs as outlined in recent consensus guidelines and position papers; however, this testing is not available in most centers outside of the research setting.[28,64] [d] In vitro testing, such as lymphocyte transformation test (LTT) or enzyme linked immunospot assay (ELISpot), has only been used in research setting and should be used with caution. In vivo testing (delayed intradermal testing or patch testing) may be performed in specialist centers, at a minimum of 6 weeks yet routinely 6 months postreaction.[28,31]

recommendations, direct oral challenge in children is suggested for nonimmediate, and potentially immediate but not severe, reactions to amoxicillin.[30,38]

SUMMARY

There is increased evidence that low-risk patients carefully assessed by expert-derived assessment tools or validated clinical decision rule can undergo direct oral penicillin challenge in both pediatrics and adults. A schematic approach to penicillin allergy testing, stratified for risk, is provided in **Fig. 1**. Future studies are required to externally validate clinical decision/assessment tools and standardize testing. International consensus is required regarding several challenge components, including number of challenge steps (1-step vs multistep), observation period, inclusion of some phenotypes as low risk (eg, urticaria), and stakeholder delivery.

CLINICS CARE POINTS

- When performing a penicillin allergy assessment ascertain the phenotype (eg, rash, anaphylaxis), timing (eg, childhood) to enable risk stratification into low, moderate, and high risk, irrespective of tool utilized.

- When undertaking direct oral penicillin challenge the greatest evidence remains for childhood exanthema or delayed reactions more than 5 to 10 years previous.
- Avoid direct oral penicillin challenge for severe reactions (eg, anaphylaxis, severe cutaneous adverse reactions) and only with caution in moderate phenotypes (ie, urticaria) where evidence is less.

DISCLOSURE

There are no commercial or financial conflicts of interest to declare.

REFERENCES

1. (CDC) CfDC. Evaluation and Diagnosis of Penicillin Allergy for Healthcare Professionals. 2017. Available at: https://www.cdc.gov/antibiotic-use/community/for-hcp/Penicillin-Allergy.html. October 23, 2019.
2. Blumenthal KG, Peter JG, Trubiano JA, et al. Antibiotic allergy. Lancet 2019; 393(10167):183–98.
3. Trubiano J, Phillips E. Antimicrobial stewardship's new weapon? A review of antibiotic allergy and pathways to 'de-labeling'. Curr Opin Infect Dis 2013;26(6): 526–37.
4. Blumenthal KG, Lu N, Zhang Y, et al. Risk of meticillin resistant Staphylococcus aureus and Clostridium difficile in patients with a documented penicillin allergy: population based matched cohort study. Bmj 2018;361:k2400.
5. Macy E, Contreras R. Health care use and serious infection prevalence associated with penicillin "allergy" in hospitalized patients: A cohort study. J Allergy Clin Immunol 2014;133(3):790–6.
6. Blumenthal KG, Ryan EE, Li Y, et al. The impact of a reported penicillin allergy on surgical site infection risk. Clin Infect Dis 2018;66(3):329–36.
7. Conway EL, Lin K, Sellick JA, et al. Impact of penicillin allergy on time to first dose of antimicrobial therapy and clinical outcomes. Clin Ther 2017;39(11):2276–83.
8. Trubiano JA, Chen C, Cheng AC, et al. Antimicrobial allergy 'labels' drive inappropriate antimicrobial prescribing: lessons for stewardship. J Antimicrob Chemother 2016;71(6):1715–22.
9. Charneski L, Deshpande G, Smith SW. Impact of an antimicrobial allergy label in the medical record on clinical outcomes in hospitalized patients. Pharmacotherapy 2011;31(8):742–7.
10. Blumenthal KG, Lu N, Zhang Y, et al. Recorded penicillin allergy and risk of mortality: a population-based matched cohort study. J Gen Intern Med 2019;34(9): 1685–7.
11. Adkinson NF Jr, Thompson WL, Maddrey WC, et al. Routine use of penicillin skin testing on an inpatient service. N Engl J Med 1971;285(1):22–4.
12. Levine BB, Redmond AP, Voss HE, et al. Prediction of penicillin allergy by immunological tests. Ann N Y Acad Sci 1967;145(2):298–309.
13. Blumenthal KG, Li Y, Hsu JT, et al. Outcomes from an inpatient beta-lactam allergy guideline across a large US health system. Infect Control Hosp Epidemiol 2019;40(5):528–35.
14. Chua KYL, Vogrin S, Bury S, et al. The penicillin allergy delabeling program: a multicenter whole-of-hospital health services intervention and comparative effectiveness study. Clin Infect Dis 2021;73(3):487–96.

15. Trubiano JA, Thursky KA, Stewardson AJ, et al. Impact of an integrated antibiotic allergy testing program on antimicrobial stewardship: a multicenter evaluation. Clin Infect Dis 2017;65(1):166–74.
16. Brusco NK, Bury S, Chua KYL, et al. Penicillin Allergy Delabeling Program: an exploratory economic evaluation in the Australian context. Intern Med J 2021. https://doi.org/10.1111/imj.15532.
17. Shenoy ES, Macy E, Rowe T, et al. Evaluation and management of penicillin allergy: a review. JAMA 2019;321(2):188–99.
18. Devchand M, Trubiano JA. Penicillin allergy: a practical approach to assessment and prescribing. Aust Prescr 2019;42(6):192–9.
19. Devchand M, Urbancic KF, Khumra S, et al. Pathways to improved antibiotic allergy and antimicrobial stewardship practice: The validation of a beta-lactam antibiotic allergy assessment tool. J Allergy Clin Immunol Pract 2019;7(3):1063–5.e5.
20. Devchand M, Kirckpatrick C, Stevenson W, et al. Evaluation of a pharmacist-led penicillin allergy de-labelling ward-round – A novel antimicrobial stewardship intervention. J Antimicrob Chemother 2019;74(6):1725–30.
21. Rischin KJ, Mostaghim M, Rao A, et al. ESCAPE-Allergy: Evaluating screening for children and adolescents with penicillin allergy. J Paediatr Child Health 2021. https://doi.org/10.1111/jpc.15657.
22. Clarke J, Graham N. Paediatric antibiotic allergy assessment, testing and de-labelling. 2020. Available at: https://www.childrens.health.qld.gov.au/wp-content/uploads/PDF/guidelines/gdl-01076.pdf. Accessed January 6, 2021.
23. Trubiano JA, Vogrin S, Chua KYL, et al. Development and validation of a penicillin allergy clinical decision rule. JAMA Intern Med 2020;180(5):745–52.
24. Stevenson B, Trevenen M, Klinken E, et al. Multicenter australian study to determine criteria for low- and high-risk penicillin testing in outpatients. J Allergy Clin Immunol Pract 2020;8(2):681–9.e3.
25. Siew LQC, Li PH, Watts TJ, et al. Identifying Low-Risk Beta-Lactam Allergy Patients in a UK Tertiary Centre. J Allergy Clin Immunol Pract 2019;7(7):2173–81.e1.
26. Chiriac AM, Wang Y, Schrijvers R, et al. Designing predictive models for beta-lactam allergy using the drug allergy and hypersensitivity database. J Allergy Clin Immunol Pract 2018;6(1):139–48.e2.
27. Banks TA, Tucker M, Macy E. Evaluating penicillin allergies without skin testing. Curr Allergy asthma Rep 2019;19(5):27.
28. Romano A, Atanaskovic-Markovic M, Barbaud A, et al. Towards a more precise diagnosis of hypersensitivity to beta-lactams - an EAACI position paper. Allergy 2020;75(6):1300–15.
29. Khan DA, Solensky R. Drug allergy. J Allergy Clin Immunol 2010;125(2 Suppl 2):S126–37.
30. Torres MJ, Adkinson NF Jr, Caubet JC, et al. Controversies in drug allergy: beta-lactam hypersensitivity testing. J Allergy Clin Immunol Pract 2019;7(1):40–5.
31. Phillips EJ, Bigliardi P, Bircher AJ, et al. Controversies in drug allergy: Testing for delayed reactions. J Allergy Clin Immunol 2019;143(1):66–73.
32. Mayorga C, Ebo DG, Lang DM, et al. Controversies in drug allergy: In vitro testing. J Allergy Clin Immunol 2019;143(1):56–65.
33. Rose MT, Slavin M, Trubiano J. The democratization of de-labeling: a review of direct oral challenge in adults with low-risk penicillin allergy. Expert Rev Anti Infect Ther 2020;18(11):1143–53.
34. Vyles D, Antoon JW, Norton A, et al. Children with reported penicillin allergy: Public health impact and safety of delabeling. Ann Allergy Asthma Immunol 2020;124(6):558–65.

35. Wang LA, Patel K, Kuruvilla ME, et al. Direct amoxicillin challenge without preliminary skin testing for pediatric patients with penicillin allergy labels. Ann Allergy Asthma Immunol 2020;125(2):226–8.

36. Mill C, Primeau MN, Medoff E, et al. Assessing the diagnostic properties of a graded oral provocation challenge for the diagnosis of immediate and nonimmediate reactions to amoxicillin in children. JAMA Pediatr 2016;170(6):e160033.

37. Abrams EM, Ben-Shoshan M. Should testing be initiated prior to amoxicillin challenge in children? Clin Exp Allergy 2019;49(8):1060–6.

38. Mirakian R, Leech SC, Krishna MT, et al. Management of allergy to penicillins and other beta-lactams. Clin Exp Allergy 2015;45(2):300–27.

39. Staicu ML, Brundige ML, Ramsey A, et al. Implementation of a penicillin allergy screening tool to optimize aztreonam use. Am J Health System Pharm 2016; 73(5):298–306.

40. Turner NA, Wrenn R, Sarubbi C, et al. Evaluation of a pharmacist-led penicillin allergy assessment program and allergy delabeling in a tertiary care hospital. JAMA Netw Open 2021;4(5):e219820.

41. Trubiano JA, Smibert O, Douglas A, et al. The safety and efficacy of an oral penicillin challenge program in cancer patients: a multicenter pilot study. Open Forum Infect Dis 2018;5(12):ofy306.

42. Caughey GE, Shakib S, Inglis JM, et al. External validation of beta-lactam antibiotic allergy assessment tools: implications for clinical practice and workforce capacity. J Allergy Clin Immunol Pract 2019;7(6):2094–5.

43. Blumenthal KG, Huebner EM, Fu X, et al. Risk-based pathway for outpatient penicillin allergy evaluations. J Allergy Clin Immunol Pract 2019;7(7):2411–4.e1.

44. Plager JH, Mancini CM, Fu X, et al. Preoperative penicillin allergy testing in patients undergoing cardiac surgery. Ann Allergy Asthma Immunol 2020;124(6): 583–8.

45. Song YC, Nelson ZJ, Wankum MA, et al. Effectiveness and feasibility of pharmacist-driven penicillin allergy de-labeling pilot program without skin testing or oral challenges. Pharmacy (Basel) 2021;9(3):127.

46. Manning J, Pammett RT, Hamour AO, et al. Assessing use of a standardized allergy history questionnaire for patients with reported allergy to penicillin. Can J Hosp Pharm 2021;74(2):104–9.

47. Gateman DP, Rumble JE, Protudjer JLP, et al. Amoxicillin oral provocation challenge in a primary care clinic: a descriptive analysis. CMAJ Open 2021;9(2): E394–9.

48. Ramsey A, Staicu ML. Use of a penicillin allergy screening algorithm and penicillin skin testing for transitioning hospitalized patients to first-line antibiotic therapy. J Allergy Clin Immunol Pract 2018;6(4):1349–55.

49. Roberts H, Soller L, Ng K, et al. First pediatric electronic algorithm to stratify risk of penicillin allergy. Allergy Asthma Clin Immunol 2020;16(1):103.

50. Reichel A, Roding K, Stoevesandt J, et al. De-labelling antibiotic allergy through five key questions. Clin Exp Allergy 2020;50(4):532–5.

51. Piotin A, Godet J, Trubiano JA, et al. Predictive factors of amoxicillin immediate hypersensitivity and validation of PEN-FAST clinical decision rule. Ann Allergy Asthma Immunol 2021;128(1):27–32.

52. Ontario. PH. Antimicrobial Stewardship Strategy: Systematic antibiotic allergy verification. Available at: https://www.publichealthontario.ca/apps/asp-strategies/data/pdf/ASP_Strategy_Systematic_Antibiotic_Allergy_Verification. pdf. 2021. Accessed January 6, 2021.

53. Tucker MH, Lomas CM, Ramchandar N, et al. Amoxicillin challenge without penicillin skin testing in evaluation of penicillin allergy in a cohort of Marine recruits. J Allergy Clin Immunol Pract 2017;5(3):813–5.

54. Iammatteo M, Alvarez Arango S, Ferastraoaru D, et al. Safety and outcomes of oral graded challenges to amoxicillin without prior skin testing. J Allergy Clin Immunol Pract 2019;7(1):236–43.

55. Kuruvilla M, Shih J, Patel K, et al. Direct oral amoxicillin challenge without preliminary skin testing in adult patients with allergy and at low risk with reported penicillin allergy. Allergy Asthma Proc 2019;40(1):57–61.

56. Mustafa SS, Conn K, Ramsey A. Comparing direct challenge to penicillin skin testing for the outpatient evaluation of penicillin allergy: a randomized controlled trial. J Allergy Clin Immunol Pract 2019;7(7):2163–70.

57. Savic L, Gurr L, Kaura V, et al. Penicillin allergy de-labelling ahead of elective surgery: feasibility and barriers. Br J Anaesth 2019;123(1):e110–6.

58. du Plessis T, Walls G, Jordan A, et al. Implementation of a pharmacist-led penicillin allergy de-labelling service in a public hospital. J Antimicrob Chemother 2019;74(5):1438–46.

59. Li J, Shahabi-Sirjani A, Figtree M, et al. Safety of direct drug provocation testing in adults with penicillin allergy and association with health and economic benefits. Ann Allergy Asthma Immunol 2019;123(5):468–75.

60. Ramsey A, Mustafa SS, Holly AM, et al. Direct challenges to penicillin-based antibiotics in the inpatient setting. J Allergy Clin Immunol Pract 2020;8(7):2294–301.

61. Stone CA Jr, Stollings JL, Lindsell CJ, et al. Risk-stratified management to remove low-risk penicillin allergy labels in the ICU. Am J Respir Crit Care Med 2020; 201(12):1572–5.

62. Lin L, Nagtegaal JE, Buijtels P, et al. Antimicrobial stewardship intervention: optimizing antibiotic treatment in hospitalized patients with reported antibiotic allergy. J Hosp Infect 2020;104(2):137–43.

63. Steenvoorden L, Bjoernestad EO, Kvesetmoen TA, et al. De-labelling penicillin allergy in acutely hospitalized patients: a pilot study. BMC Infect Dis 2021;21(1): 1083.

64. Mayorga C, Sanz ML, Gamboa P, et al. In vitro methods for diagnosing nonimmediate hypersensitivity reactions to drugs. J Investig Allergol Clin Immunol 2013;23(4):213–25 [quiz: preceding 225].

Allergy to Radiocontrast Dye

Knut Brockow, MD

KEYWORDS

- Radiocontrast media • Hypersensitivity • Anaphylaxis • Exanthem • Diagnosis
- Allergy test • Provocation test • Premedication

KEY POINTS

- Hypersensitivity to radiocontrast media (RCM) is common and is classified into immediate (IHR) and nonimmediate hypersensitivity reactions (NIHR).
- In IHR to RCM, an immediate-type allergy is demonstrated by skin test and basophil activation test predominantly in patients with severe reactions.
- Changing the RCM and selecting a skin test–negative RCM in these patients is effective in the prevention of future reactions and superior to premedication.
- Drug provocation test is an option to confirm tolerability of skin test–negative alternatives.
- NIHR to RCM presents with exanthemas, which are often skin test–positive and caused by T cell–mediated hypersensitivity.

INTRODUCTION: PREVALENCE, DEFINITIONS, AND RISK FACTORS

More than 70 million applications of iodinated radiocontrast media (RCM) are administered worldwide per year.[1] Adverse reactions are commonly encountered. Some reported reactions may causally be unrelated to RCM, such as spontaneous urticaria, exanthems of other causes, or anxiety-associated subjective symptoms. Most adverse reactions to RCM are predictable by their known toxicity (eg, nephrotoxicity or neurotoxicity, such as vasovagal reactions, transient warmth/flushing, pallor, weakness, nausea and vomiting, or bradycardia). However, hypersensitivity reactions (HR) to RCM do occur.[2] RCM HR are classified in either immediate HR (IHR) occurring typically within 1 hour but up to 6 hours after RCM administration presenting with cutaneous reactions (urticaria, erythema, pruritus, angioedema) with or without systemic manifestations including anaphylaxis[3,4]; or nonimmediate HR (NIHR) developing more than 6 hours, mostly 1 to 3 days and up to 10 days after RCM application[3,5,6] manifesting with exanthems, mostly benign maculopapular exanthems without systemic symptoms.[7] Among 196,081 Korean patients, an overall

Department of Dermatology and Allergy Biederstein, School of Medicine, Technical University of Munich, Biedersteiner Strasse 29, Munich 80802, Germany
E-mail address: knut.brockow@tum.de

Immunol Allergy Clin N Am 42 (2022) 391–401
https://doi.org/10.1016/j.iac.2021.12.001
0889-8561/22/© 2021 Elsevier Inc. All rights reserved.

immunology.theclinics.com

prevalence of 0.73% has been described, with severe reactions in 0.01%.[8] The major risk factor for these reactions was re-exposure after previous reaction to RCM (adjusted odds ratio, 199). Minor risk factors in this study were hyperthyroidism, drug allergy, other allergic diseases, and family history of RCM reactions (odds ratio, 3.6; 3.5; 6.8; 14.0). IHRs to RCM are substantially less often reported for intra-arterial than for extravascular (eg, gastrointestinal, genitourinary) administrations.[9,10] In a study assessing the risk of cardiac catheterization in 71,782 patients, there was no significant increased risk in patients exposed to β-blockers or angiotensin-converting enzyme inhibitors.[11]

CLINICAL RELEVANCE

IHR to RCM manifest as urticaria and symptoms of anaphylaxis.[12–14] Fatal anaphylaxis is rare with an estimated rate of 1 to 2/100,000 procedures.[15–17] Most IHR present with urticaria and/or angioedema and pruritus.[12] A transient angioedema of the small bowel has been reported.[18] Anaphylaxis commonly affects the skin and involves other organ systems (eg, with bronchospasm and wheezing, nausea or vomiting, and tachycardia and hypotension). An acute coronary syndrome caused by reduced blood flow to the heart may develop.[19,20] Maculopapular exanthem of mild or moderate severity is common after RCM exposure.[14] In addition, other NIHRs are often exanthems, and severe cutaneous adverse reactions (eg, drug reaction with eosinophilia and systemic symptoms, Stevens-Johnson syndrome, toxic epidermal necrolysis, or acute generalized exanthematous pustulosis) have been described.[21–25] RCM-induced sialoadenitis with neck swelling is another well-recognized NIHR.[26] Further exceptional NIHR reactions have been reported in individual cases.[27] It has, however, to be considered that the causal relationship between RCM exposure and reaction remains unconfirmed by allergy tests or re-exposition in most of these cases.

CURRENT EVIDENCE ON MECHANISMS

For IHR, the mechanism of most cases has been considered nonallergic. In mouse models, the RCMs iopamidol and iohexol activated the mast cell–specific receptor MRGPR X2.[28,29] However, a mechanism for nonallergic RCM reactions demonstrable selectively in reacting patients, but not in tolerant control subjects, has been demonstrated.[30]

During the last years, evidence for a possible IgE-mediated allergic mechanism for IHR to RCM is accumulating.[31] An increasing number of studies report positive skin tests in patients with IHR, particularly those with severe reactions.[4,32,33] Tryptase and histamine release during the reaction, and positive basophil activation tests have been demonstrated.[30] Whereas in most patients with IHR of mild to moderate severity no sensitization is demonstrated, positive skin tests are more common in those with severe and more recent reactions.[4,32,33] Genetic susceptibility genes have been sought for IHR to RCM; however, results from different studies found only weak associations that were not reproducible.[34,35]

The mechanism of NIHRs to RCM is believed to be T cell–mediated, although skin tests are not unequivocally positive. Nevertheless, the typical time of onset of delayed allergic reactions, clinical picture, duration of the exanthema, positive delayed intradermal skin and patch tests, ex vivo activated T cells, and positive lymphocyte transformation tests closely resemble T cell–mediated drug allergy.

TESTING APPROACH
Indication for Testing

Not all patients with reported adverse reactions after receiving RCM should be offered allergy testing.[36] Those with subjective or other nonspecific symptoms, such as feeling of warmth or erythema at injection side, nausea, paresthesia, headache, or dizziness, most likely suffer from a nonsevere toxic reaction or causally unrelated reaction. Because of the low pretest probability, prescreening unselected patients by skin testing cannot predict future HR.[37] However, patients reporting typical manifestations of IHR or NIHR have a much higher pretest probability and should be allergy tested (**Box 1**).[36]

Skin Tests

Sensitivity of skin testing in patients with RCM HS is higher when less time has elapsed from the date of reaction.[12,38] In Europe skin testing has been recommended in RCM hypersensitivity for some time and this recently has become more prevalent practice in the United States.[39,40] Skin tests may differentiate allergy from nonallergic reactions and identify safe skin test–negative alternatives, which has been confirmed by intravenous provocation or re-exposure.[32,33,38,41,42]

Skin test procedures are selected according to the suspected mechanism.[43] For IHR, skin prick tests (SPT) and intradermal tests (IDT) with immediate readings are done and for NIHR, patch test and late readings for SPT and IDT. In NIHR, IDT are more sensitive than patch tests.[41] Skin tests are done with the culprit RCM and, if possible, with a panel of alternative RCMs.[36,43] In IHR, most centers test RCM for SPT undiluted at 300 to 320 mg/mL and diluted at 1:10 for IDT for better specificity. In NIHR, patch test is done undiluted, IDT mostly 1:10 diluted, and both are read after 24 to 48 and 72 hours. Validity of different reading times for skin tests has not yet been formally compared and patients should be instructed to return for additional readings in case of any test site reaction.[36]

A higher rate of positive skin tests has been seen in more severe reactions.[4,12,31–33,38] The specificity of skin tests is 95% for undiluted SPT, 91% to 96% for 1:10 diluted IDT in IHR, and close to 100% for delayed skin tests in NIHR.[12,31] The sensitivity is higher when testing IHR undiluted in IDT, but specificity is reduced.[4,33] Cross-sensitivity does occur between RCM, more in NIHR than in IHR.[12,44] The pattern of cross reactivity of different RCMs is under observation.[44–46]

Box 1
Clinical indications for radiocontrast media allergy work-up

Indications:
Urticaria, angioedema, flushing, isolated bronchospasm, anaphylaxis, delayed-appearing urticaria or angioedema (although causal relationship remains questionable), maculopapular exanthema, fixed drug eruption symmetric drug-related intertriginous, acute generalized exanthematous pustulosis. For severe bullous skin reactions (Stevens-Johnson syndrome, toxic epidermal necrolysis, drug reaction with eosinophilia, and systemic symptoms) only skin tests, generally no drug provocation test are indicated, individual decisions possible.

Examples for no indication:
Patients labeled as "iodine allergic." Patients with food, insect venom, drug allergies, but no previous reaction to radiocontrast media. Patients with subjective or unspecific symptoms, such as generalized pruritus, feeling of warmth, flushing, erythema at injection site, nausea, paresthesia, rhinorrhea, headache, or dizziness.

In NIHR, cross reactivity of iobitridol (a nonionic monomer, low-osmolar contrast agent available in the United Kingdom and Europe but not available in the United States) to other RCM has been reported to be low, which may be related to its R_1 chain being different from that of other RCMs.[47] For IHR, the iso-osmolar RCM iodixanol seems to have a low rate of IHRs and among low osmolar RCM some agents (eg, iomeprol) have recently been associated with higher reaction rates than others (eg, iohexol).[48,49]

In Vitro Tests

Measuring increased tryptase levels over baseline levels in serum 1 to 4 hours after the onset of an IHR can support the diagnosis of anaphylaxis.[50] The basophil activation test has confirmed the diagnosis of IHR to RCM in few studies with high specificity (88% [4%–100%]) and moderate sensitivity (46%–62%).[51–53] Lymphocyte transformation tests may be positive in NIHR and RCM-reactive T cell lines and clones have been demonstrated, although the sensitivity seems to be lower as compared with skin tests.[54] None of these functional tests for immediate or delayed hypersensitivity is routinely available or has been validated in large studies.

Drug Provocation Test

Drug provocation test (DPT) with RCM has been shown to be safe in the hands of experienced centers; however, protocols are diverse and require standardization.[41,44,45,51,55–57] Intravenous DPT has been done with the skin test–negative culprit to exclude RCM allergy or with an alternative skin test–negative RCM to be used in the next contrasted examination.[36] Alternatively, a skin test–negative RCM is re-exposed at a radiology department without prior DPT, because this seems to be safe.[32,33,36,38] DPT with a skin test–negative alternative substance may be particularly considered after severe anaphylaxis.[36] Contraindications are renal insufficiency, hyperthyroidism, radioactive iodine therapy, and pregnant and breast-feeding women. RCM-induced nephropathy has to be avoided.[58] The decision requires a risk-benefit analysis in each patient.

DISCUSSION
Management in Acute Need for Imaging

Principal options for patients with previous RCM HR are shown in **Table 1**. In patients who developed mild IHR (urticaria ± angioedema) or mild NIHR (maculopapular exanthem) after RCM exposition and immediate and urgent need of another RCM-based imaging, contrast with a nonculprit RCM is given under emergency preparedness, because of the low risk of an allergic reaction (**Fig. 1**).[36,43] Premedication may be considered, because it suppresses most mild or moderate severity nonallergic reactions.[36,59] Diagnostic accuracy of noncontrast computed tomograms is often not a suitable imaging alternative (eg, magnetic resonance tomography, native computed tomography, or MRI scan).[60] Changing the RCM from the culprit to a different RCM in a patient with previous RCM reaction was more effective than premedication with single-dose antihistamine or with single-dose corticosteroid at least in countries that may have access to structurally disparate radiocontrast agents.[61,62] Different premedication protocols have been published for IHR. A combination of H_1 antihistamine (eg, 50 mg of diphenhydramine 1 hour before application) and corticosteroids (eg, 50 mg of prednisone 13, 7, and 1 hours before application) is most often used.[40] After mild reactions, however, corticosteroid in addition to antihistamine prophylaxis did not show an additional benefit and may not be required.[63] Premedication is getting increasingly controversial, because the efficacy is likely to be low, mostly suppressing

Table 1
Overview of management options in patients with radiocontrast media hypersensitivity reaction

Management	Discussion	Patient Selection
Avoidance	Safest approach, but RCM examination may be urgently needed and diagnosis remains unresolved.	Patients with other diagnostic options (eg, magnet resonance tomography). Patients without urgent need for RCM.
Premedication	Well-established; however, benefit remains uncertain and not sufficiently demonstrated. Premedication reduces reaction rate particularly of nonsevere reactions, less reliable in severe allergic HR and breakthrough reactions do occur. Gives a false sense of security. Different regimes do exist. Adverse effects to corticosteroids have to be considered.	Patients where skin tests cannot be performed. Patients with nonallergic reactions without positive skin test. Patients with very severe reactions as additional safety measure.
Use of a nonculprit alternative by history	Weak but growing evidence for easy and uncomplicated reduction of reaction rates. Cross-reactivity patterns for selection of alternative not well studied.	Patients with immediate urgent need of RCM without possibility of skin tests. Patients with nonsevere reactions.
Use of skin test–negative alternative RCM	Expertise needed and time consuming. Dissects allergic from nonallergic reactions with different risk prognosis. Applicable in only a few patients with IHR-positive skin test. In those, good negative predictive value. Omission of skin test–positive RCM indicates tolerance and largely reduces/eliminates risk of anaphylaxis.	Patients with suspicion of IHR or NIHR where skin tests can be performed.

nonallergic cutaneous reactions, and because corticosteroids may lead to adverse events (eg, increased blood pressure, elevated glucose levels, and disruption of diabetic control), their use is being questioned.[64] The setting for RCM exposition should be as safe as possible (eg, taking place in hospitals with code teams and with close observation, possibly using pulse oximetry). Mastocytosis has not been reported to be associated with a higher frequency of IHRs.[65] Recent results indicate that reducing injection speed and using lower dose of the RCM is associated with a lower relative risk of an IHR to RCM.[66] In one study, a reduced dose of contrast media achieved by lowering the computed tomography tube voltage to 100 kVp, a contrast material dose of 1.5 mL/kg (maximum, 130 mL), and an injection speed of 2.5 or 3 mL/s led to a reduced rate of IHR of 1.42% as compared with 1.86% in the conventional control subjects, with a multivariable-adjusted relative risk of 0.85 ($P = .03$). Extrinsic warming of the RCM has been reported to be associated with a reduced IHR rate, although this finding should be confirmed.[67] These general measures should be applied to further reduce the reaction risk.

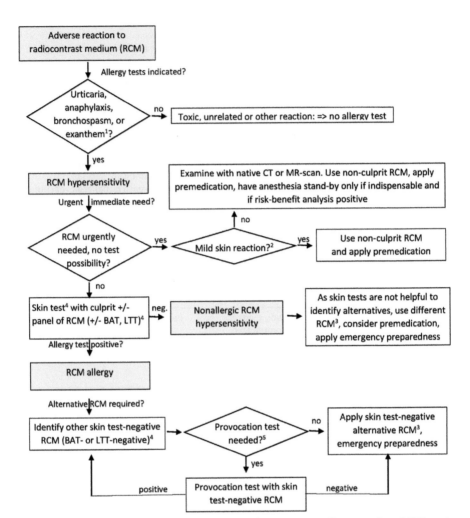

Fig. 1. Management of patients with previous radiocontrast medium reaction. AGEP, acute generalized exanthematous pustulosis; BAT, basophil activation test; CT, computed tomography; DRESS, drug reaction with eosinophilia and systemic symptoms; LTT, lymphocyte transformation test; SDRIFE, symmetrical drug-related intertriginous and flexural exanthema; SJS, Stevens-Johnson syndrome; TEN, toxic epidermal necrolysis. [1]including exanthem variants, such as SDRIFE, AGEP, DRESS, SJS, TEN. After severe bullous exanthems or after reactions with systemic symptoms, but future total RCM avoidance is generally recommended; [2]such as urticaria or "benign" maculopapular exanthema; [3]not after severe bullous exanthems or after drug reaction with systemic symptoms; [4]BAT= basophil activation test, and LTT= lymphocyte transformation test may be helpful in some cases; [5]decided on a risk-benefit analysis, e.g. patients with urgent need, higher risk and severe reactions. (*Adapted from* Brockow K. Medical Algorithm: Diagnosis and Treatment of Radiocontrast Media Hypersensitivity. Allergy. 2020 May; 75(5):1278-80.)

In patients after severe anaphylaxis, RCM should be avoided and an allergy work-up is warranted. If RCM is considered indispensable, a risk-benefit analysis may result in giving a nonculprit RCM, normally after premedication and with emergency preparedness including anesthesia stand-by. In immediate need, desensitization may be considered.[68–70] In patients with severe bullous or systemic NIHR beyond medical control, RCM has to be avoided and other alternative procedures, such as MRI with gadolinium-based contrast agents, are preferred.

Management with Time for Allergy Work-up

Normally an allergy work-up is recommended (see **Fig. 1**). In patients with IHR being skin test–positive to the culprit RCM, a skin test–negative alternative should be administered without premedication, but with emergency preparedness and tolerance is expected,[32,33,38,41,42,71] with only a few exceptions.[72] Applying premedication is added in severe IHRs as an additional precaution, but its efficacy is unclear and adverse effects have to be considered. The culprit and other skin test-positive RCMs should be avoided. If available, basophil activation test or lymphocyte transformation tests may supplement allergy testing, although cutoff values for positive results remain nonvalidated. Whether DPT or direct re-exposure is preferable can be decided on an individual basis (eg, depending on the severity of the reaction, availability of DPT, emergency preparedness, and experience of the center). A negative DPT with a skin test–negative agent has a high negative predictive value of greater than 90% in the real-life setting.[71,73] In patients with negative skin tests to the culprit, a nonculprit RCM is applied with or without premedication under emergency preparedness.

SUMMARY

Evidence is accumulating to support that skin tests may be positive particularly in those patients with severe RCM hypersensitivity and that skin tests in these patients are helpful to indicate severe allergic reactions and to direct the choice of alternative RCM in the future. In most patients, avoidance of the culprit and change of the RCM directed by allergy tests increases the safety of subsequent RCM exposures in patients with previous RCM hypersensitivity.

CLINICS CARE POINTS

- In patients with previous HR to RCM, avoid the culprit RCM.
- In patients with IHR, most reactions are mild and nonallergic. If skin tests to the culprit result negative, there is a risk for a future reaction, but severe future reactions are highly unlikely when using a nonculprit alternative ± premedication.
- In patients with moderate to severe IHR, skin tests are more often positive and can then direct the choice of RCM to be used in the future by using an alternative to which skin testing is negative. In this case premedication in these skin test–positive patients is generally not needed.
- Drug provocation tests are done to expose patients with previous RCM IHR in a setting experienced with drug HR and treatment of anaphylaxis.
- As per other types of non-IgE-mediated reactions, general measures of reducing injection speed, using a lower dose, and extrinsic warming of the RCM is associated with a lower relative risk of an IHR to RCM and should be applied in patients with previous severe IHR to RCM.

DISCLOSURE

No conflict of interest, no funding.

REFERENCES

1. Christiansen C. X-ray contrast media: an overview. Toxicology 2005;209:185–7.
2. Katayama H, Yamaguchi K, Kozuka T, et al. Adverse reactions to ionic and nonionic contrast media. A report from the Japanese Committee on the Safety of Contrast Media. Radiology 1990;175:621–8.
3. Brockow K, Christiansen C, Kanny G, et al. Management of hypersensitivity reactions to iodinated contrast media. Allergy 2005;60:150–8.
4. Clement O, Dewachter P, Mouton-Faivre C, et al. Immediate hypersensitivity to contrast agents: the French 5-year CIRTACI Study. EClinicalMedicine 2018;1:51–61.
5. Schonmann C, Brockow K. Adverse reactions during procedures: hypersensitivity to contrast agents and dyes. Ann Allergy Asthma Immunol 2020;124:156–64.
6. Bircher AJ, Brockow K, Grosber M, et al. Late elicitation of maculopapular exanthemas to iodinated contrast media after first exposure. Ann Allergy Asthma Immunol 2013;111:576–7.
7. Brockow K, Ardern-Jones MR, Mockenhaupt M, et al. EAACI position paper on how to classify cutaneous manifestations of drug hypersensitivity. Allergy 2019;74:14–27.
8. Cha MJ, Kang DY, Lee W, et al. Hypersensitivity reactions to iodinated contrast media: a multicenter study of 196 081 patients. Radiology 2019;293:117–24.
9. Endrikat J, Michel A, Kolbach R, et al. Risk of hypersensitivity reactions to iopromide after intra-arterial versus intravenous administration: a nested case-control analysis of 133,331 patients. Invest Radiol 2020;55:38–44.
10. Kim YS, Choi YH, Cho YJ, et al. Incidence of breakthrough reaction in patients with prior acute allergic-like reactions to iodinated contrast media according to the administration route. Korean J Radiol 2018;19:352–7.
11. Smith MA, Newton LP, Barcena Blanch MA, et al. Risk for anaphylactic reaction from cardiac catheterization in patients receiving beta-adrenergic blockers or angiotensin-converting enzyme-inhibitors. J Allergy Clin Immunol Pract 2020;8:1900–5.
12. Brockow K, Romano A, Aberer W, et al. Skin testing in patients with hypersensitivity reactions to iodinated contrast media: a European multicenter study. Allergy 2009;64:234–41.
13. Tasker F, Fleming H, McNeill G, et al. Contrast media and cutaneous reactions. Part 1. Immediate hypersensitivity reactions to contrast media and gadolinium deposition. Clin Exp Dermatol 2019;44:839–43.
14. Tasker F, Fleming H, McNeill G, et al. Contrast media and cutaneous reactions. Part 2. Delayed hypersensitivity reactions to iodinated contrast media. Clin Exp Dermatol 2019;44:844–60.
15. Brockow K, Vieluf D, Puschel K, et al. Increased postmortem serum mast cell tryptase in a fatal anaphylactoid reaction to nonionic radiocontrast medium. J Allergy Clin Immunol 1999;104:237–8.
16. Sapra A, Bhandari P, Manek M, et al. Fatal anaphylaxis to contrast a reality: a case report. Cureus 2019;11:e6214.
17. Yang Z, Li R, Yue J, et al. Fatal contrast medium-induced adverse response to iohexol in carotid artery angioplasty: a case report. Medicine (Baltimore) 2019;98:e16758.
18. Wakabayashi T, Sasaoka Y, Sakai Y, et al. Transient angioedema of the small bowel because of intravenous nonionic iodinated contrast media. J Pediatr 2021;230:264–5.
19. Shibuya K, Kasama S, Funada R, et al. Kounis syndrome induced by contrast media: a case report and review of literature. Eur J Radiol Open 2019;6:91–6.

20. Dorniak K, Galaska R, Fijalkowski M, et al. Severe left ventricular outflow tract obstruction associated with Kounis syndrome following iodinated contrast administration. Pol Arch Intern Med 2019;129:924–6.
21. Machet P, Marce D, Ziyani Y, et al. Acute generalized exanthematous pustulosis induced by iomeprol with cross-reactivity to other iodinated contrast agents and mild reactions after rechallenge with iopromide and oral corticosteroid premedication. Contact Dermatitis 2019;81:74–6.
22. Tan CM, Zipursky JS. Acute generalized exanthematous pustulosis caused by an intravenous radiocontrast medium. CMAJ 2020;192:E1097.
23. Soria A, Bernier C, Veyrac G, et al. Drug reaction with eosinophilia and systemic symptoms may occur within 2 weeks of drug exposure: a retrospective study. J Am Acad Dermatol 2020;82:606–11.
24. Pop M, Hemenway A, Shakeel F. Probable parenteral and oral contrast-induced Stevens Johnson syndrome/toxic epidermal necrolysis. Am J Emerg Med 2021; 45:684 e5–e6.
25. Alamri Y, Hsu B. DRESS syndrome due to iodinated contrast medium. N Z Med J 2020;133:93–5.
26. Cunha IM, Maganinho P, Marques ML, et al. Recurrent neck swelling after iodinated contrast media administration. Radiol Case Rep 2021;16:1508–10.
27. Brockow K, Sanchez-Borges M. Hypersensitivity to contrast media and dyes. Immunol Allergy Clin N Am 2014;34:547–64, viii.
28. Jiang W, Hu S, Che D, et al. A mast-cell-specific receptor mediates iopamidol induced immediate IgE-independent anaphylactoid reactions. Int Immunopharmacol 2019;75:105800.
29. Yuan F, Zhang C, Sun M, et al. MRGPRX2 mediates immediate-type pseudoallergic reactions induced by iodine-containing iohexol. Biomed Pharmacother 2021;137:111323.
30. Brockow K. Immediate and delayed reactions to radiocontrast media: is there an allergic mechanism? Immunol Allergy Clin North Am 2009;29:453–68.
31. Yoon SH, Lee SY, Kang HR, et al. Skin tests in patients with hypersensitivity reaction to iodinated contrast media: a meta-analysis. Allergy 2015;70:625–37.
32. Sohn KH, Seo JH, Kang DY, et al. Finding the optimal alternative for immediate hypersensitivity to low-osmolar iodinated contrast. Invest Radiol 2021;56:480–5.
33. Kim SR, Park KH, Hong YJ, et al. Intradermal testing with radiocontrast media to prevent recurrent adverse reactions. AJR Am J Roentgenol 2019;213:1187–93.
34. Chung SJ, Kang DY, Lee W, et al. HLA-DRB1*15: 02 is associated with iodinated contrast media-related anaphylaxis. Invest Radiol 2020;55:304–9.
35. Kim EY, Choi SJ, Ghim JL, et al. Associations between HLA-A, -B, and -C alleles and iodinated contrast media-induced hypersensitivity in Koreans. Transl Clin Pharmacol 2021;29:107–16.
36. Torres MJ, Trautmann A, Böhm I, et al. Practice parameters for diagnosing and managing iodinated contrast media hypersensitivity. Allergy 2020;76(5):1325–39.
37. Lee JH, Kwon OY, Park SY, et al. Validation of the prescreening intradermal skin test for predicting hypersensitivity to iodinated contrast media: a prospective study with ICM Challenge. J Allergy Clin Immunol Pract 2020;8:267–72.
38. Gamboa P, Sanchez de Vicente J, Galan C, et al. Tolerance to iopamidol in patients with confirmed allergic immediate hypersensitivity to iomeprol. J Allergy Clin Immunol Pract 2021;9:2101–2103 e1.
39. Broyles AD, Banerji A, Barmettler S, et al. Practical guidance for the evaluation and management of drug hypersensitivity: specific drugs. J Allergy Clin Immunol Pract 2020;8:S16–116.

40. Sánchez-Borges M, Aberer W, Brockow K, et al. Controversies in drug allergy: radiographic contrast media. J Allergy Clin Immunol In Pract 2019;7(1):61–5.

41. Trautmann A, Brockow K, Behle V, et al. Radiocontrast media hypersensitivity: skin testing differentiates allergy from nonallergic reactions and identifies a safe alternative as proven by intravenous provocation. J Allergy Clin Immunol Pract 2019;7:2218–24.

42. Kwon OY, Lee JH, Park SY, et al. Novel strategy for the prevention of recurrent hypersensitivity reactions to radiocontrast media based on skin testing. J Allergy Clin Immunol Pract 2019;7:2707–13.

43. Brockow K. Medical algorithm: diagnosis and treatment of radiocontrast media hypersensitivity. Allergy 2020;75:1278–80.

44. Lerondeau B, Trechot P, Waton J, et al. Analysis of cross-reactivity among radio-contrast media in 97 hypersensitivity reactions. J Allergy Clin Immunol 2016;137: 633–5.e4.

45. Gracia-Bara MT, Moreno E, Laffond E, et al. Tolerability of iobitridol in patients with non-immediate hypersensitivity reactions to iodinated contrast media. Allergy 2018;74(1):195–7.

46. Gaudin O, Deschamps O, Duong TA, et al. Cutaneous tests and interest of iobi-tridol in non-immediate hypersensitivity to contrast media: a case series of 43 pa-tients. J Eur Acad Dermatol Venereol 2020;34:e178–80.

47. Borras J, El-Qutob D, Lopez R, et al. Hypothesized epitope localization in hyper-sensitivity reactions to iodinated contrast media. J Investig Allergol Clin Immunol 2019;29:82–3.

48. Lee SY, Kang DY, Kim JY, et al. Incidence and risk factors of immediate hypersen-sitivity reactions associated with low-osmolar iodinated contrast media: a longitu-dinal study based on a real-time monitoring system. J Investig Allergol Clin Immunol 2019;29:444–50.

49. An J, Jung H, Kwon OY, et al. Differences in adverse reactions among iodinated contrast media: analysis of the KAERS database. J Allergy Clin Immunol Pract 2019;7:2205–11.

50. Valent P, Bonadonna P, Hartmann K, et al. Why the 20% + 2 tryptase formula is a diagnostic gold standard for severe systemic mast cell activation and mast cell activation syndrome. Int Arch Allergy Immunol 2019;180:44–51.

51. Salas M, Gomez F, Fernandez TD, et al. Diagnosis of immediate hypersensitivity reactions to radiocontrast media. Allergy 2013;68:1203–6.

52. Pinnobphun P, Buranapraditkun S, Kampitak T, et al. The diagnostic value of basophil activation test in patients with an immediate hypersensitivity reaction to radiocontrast media. Ann Allergy Asthma Immunol 2011;106:387–93.

53. Trcka J, Schmidt C, Seitz CS, et al. Anaphylaxis to iodinated contrast material: nonallergic hypersensitivity or IgE-mediated allergy? AJR Am J Roentgenol 2008;190:666–70.

54. Lerch M, Keller M, Britschgi M, et al. Cross-reactivity patterns of T cells specific for iodinated contrast media. J Allergy Clin Immunol 2007;119:1529–36.

55. Torres MJ, Gomez F, Dona I, et al. Diagnostic evaluation of patients with nonim-mediate cutaneous hypersensitivity reactions to iodinated contrast media. Allergy 2012;67:929–35.

56. Vernassiere C, Trechot P, Commun N, et al. Low negative predictive value of skin tests in investigating delayed reactions to radio-contrast media. Contact Derma-titis 2004;50:359–66.

57. Vega F, Mugica MV, Bazire R, et al. Adverse reactions to iodinated contrast media: safety of a study protocol that includes fast full-dose parenteral challenge tests searching for an alternative contrast media. Clin Exp Allergy 2020;50:271–4.
58. Vega F, Mugica MV, Argiz L, et al. Protocol to prevent contrast-induced nephropathy in parenteral challenge tests for allergy evaluation of hypersensitivity reactions to iodinated contrast media. Clin Exp Allergy 2020;50(10):1200–3.
59. Kim JH, Choi SI, Lee YJ, et al. Pharmacological prevention of delayed hypersensitivity reactions caused by iodinated contrast media. World Allergy Organ J 2021;14:100561.
60. Nam SY, Ahn SJ, Jang YR, et al. Diagnostic accuracy of non-contrast abdomino-pelvic computed tomography scans in follow-up of breast cancer patients. Br J Radiol 2021;94:20201087.
61. Park HJ, Park JW, Yang MS, et al. Re-exposure to low osmolar iodinated contrast media in patients with prior moderate-to-severe hypersensitivity reactions: a multicentre retrospective cohort study. Eur Radiol 2017;27:2886–93.
62. Park SJ, Kang DY, Sohn KH, et al. Immediate mild reactions to CT with iodinated contrast media: strategy of contrast media readministration without corticosteroids. Radiology 2018;288:710–6.
63. Park SJ, Lee SY, Yoon SH, et al. Corticosteroid prophylaxis may be not required for patients with mild hypersensitivity reaction to low-osmolar contrast media. Eur J Radiol 2020;130:109152.
64. Amr BS, Lippmann M, Tobbia P, et al. Impact of short term oral steroid use for intravenous contrast media hypersensitivity prophylaxis in diabetic patients undergoing nonemergent coronary angiography or interventions. Catheter Cardiovasc Interv 2019;96(7):1392–1398..
65. Carter MC, Metcalfe DD, Matito A, et al. Adverse reactions to drugs and biologics in patients with clonal mast cell disorders: a Work Group Report of the Mast Cells Disorder Committee, American Academy of Allergy, Asthma & Immunology. J Allergy Clin Immunol 2019;143:880–93.
66. Park HJ, Son JH, Kim TB, et al. Relationship between Lower dose and injection speed of iodinated contrast material for CT and acute hypersensitivity reactions: an observational Study. Radiology 2019;293:565–72.
67. Zhang B, Liu J, Dong Y, et al. Extrinsic warming of low-osmolality iodinated contrast media to 37 degrees C reduced the rate of allergic-like reaction. Allergy Asthma Proc 2018;39:e55–63.
68. Gandhi S, Litt D, Chandy M, et al. Successful rapid intravenous desensitization for radioiodine contrast allergy in a patient requiring urgent coronary angiography. J Allergy Clin Immunol Pract 2014;2:101–2.
69. Brockow K. Reply to: "Include desensitization to radiocontrast media in the diagnostic algorithm". Allergy 2021;76:1304–5.
70. Khan S, Kamani A, Strauss BH, et al. Successful coronary angiography following rapid intravenous desensitization for refractory contrast allergy. Can J Cardiol 2020;36:1161.e1-2.
71. Schrijvers R, Breynaert C, Ahmedali Y, et al. Skin testing for suspected iodinated contrast media hypersensitivity. J Allergy Clin Immunol Pract 2018;6:1246–54.
72. Dona I, Bogas G, Salas M, et al. Hypersensitivity reactions to multiple iodinated contrast media. Front Pharmacol 2020;11:575437.
73. Meucci E, Radice A, Fassio F, et al. Diagnostic approach to hypersensitivity reactions to iodinated contrast media: a single-center experience on 98 patients. Eur Ann Allergy Clin Immunol 2020;52:220–9.

The Who, What, Where, When, Why, and How of Drug Desensitization

Barbara C. Yang, MD*, Mariana C. Castells, MD, PhD

KEYWORDS

- Desensitization • Drug allergy • Hypersensitivity • Adverse drug reaction
- Infusion reaction

KEY POINTS

- Rapid drug desensitization is a clinical procedure that allows for the safe administration of a drug in patients who have a history of hypersensitivity reaction to that drug.
- The procedure of rapid desensitization is the embodiment of personalized medicine, being both standardized and fully customized to meet the needs of each individual patient.
- Desensitization using first-line therapy leads to higher efficacy, has fewer side effects, is more cost-effective, and results in increased quality of life and life expectancy when compared with second-line therapy.

INTRODUCTION

Hypersensitivity reactions to drugs have increased in the past 25 years due to increased exposures and availability of efficient, targeted, and personalized medications. Patients with cancer live longer and are exposed to multiple cycles of classical and new chemotherapeutic drugs, including checkpoint inhibitors. Patients with chronic inflammatory diseases, such as rheumatoid arthritis, Crohn disease, and others are repeatedly exposed to targeted monoclonal antibodies. Patients with cystic fibrosis (CF) have prolonged lives and require increased antibiotic exposures. Patients react after multiple exposures due to sensitization or at the first exposure due to diluents or nonimmune activation of target cells. New phenotypes and endotypes such as cytokine release reactions have been uncovered, challenging old paradigms of drug hypersensitivity. Safely overcoming these new complex drug allergies is the goal of rapid drug desensitizations.

Division of Allergy and Clinical Immunology, Department of Medicine, Harvard Medical School, Brigham and Women's Hospital, 60 Fenwood Road, Hale Building for Transformative Medicine, Room 5002-B, Boston, MA 02115, USA
* Corresponding author.
E-mail address: bcyang@bwh.harvard.edu

Immunol Allergy Clin N Am 42 (2022) 403–420
https://doi.org/10.1016/j.iac.2021.12.004
0889-8561/22/© 2021 Elsevier Inc. All rights reserved.

immunology.theclinics.com

Abbreviations	
DNP	2,4-dinitrophenyl bound to human serum albumin
OVA	chicken egg ovalbumin

CLASSIFICATION OF HYPERSENSITIVITY REACTIONS AND PREMISE AND DEFINITIONS OF DESENSITIZATION

Rapid drug desensitization is an individually tailored procedure to administer a medication safely and effectively to patients who have experienced an acute or delayed hypersensitivity reaction. In desensitization, the patient is risk stratified to determine eligibility, is premedicated appropriately, and increasing doses of a medication are administered at specific rapid intervals with management of any breakthrough reactions during the procedure until a total therapeutic dose has been administered.[1–3] The procedure induces an incremental unresponsiveness of the immune response in exposure to a medication.[4,5] As long as subsequent doses of the same medication continue to be administered at regular intervals to maintain a stable pharmacokinetic state, the immune tolerance can be maintained. If 3 to 4 half-lives of the medication have elapsed, desensitization would need to be performed again.[6,7]

The initial hypersensitivity reaction a patient may experience can be classified into 1 of 7 types: type I immediate hypersensitivity (both IgE mediated and non-IgE mediated), cytokine release, mixed, type II cytotoxic hypersensitivity, type III immune complex mediated, delayed type IV hypersensitivity, and infusion-related reaction (**Fig. 1**).[8] The new nomenclature relies on the description of a reaction's clinical presentation (phenotype) and a reaction's underlying mechanism and biomarkers (endotype). The phenotype of a type I hypersensitivity reaction involves occurrence within minutes after exposure (usually less than 1 hour). The signs and symptoms include possible cutaneous (urticaria, pruritus, flushing, angioedema), respiratory (dyspnea, wheezing, desaturations, airway tightening), cardiovascular (hypotension, tachycardia, and even cardiovascular collapse), gastrointestinal (nausea, vomiting, diarrhea), and neurologic (syncope, seizure) manifestations.[9] Biomarkers include serum tryptase and serum interleukin (IL)-6 levels obtained during a drug reaction.[10]

The endotype of type I reactions can be either IgE mediated or non-IgE mediated. If IgE mediated, there must have been some initial exposure to the medication leading to the formation of drug-specific IgE. Cross-linking of the IgE on mast cells upon reexposure leads to mast cell degranulation. If non-IgE mediated, the same mast cell

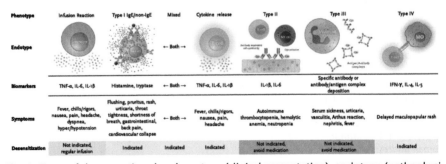

Fig. 1. Types of drug reactions by phenotype (clinical presentation), endotype (pathophysiology), biomarkers, symptoms, and whether desensitization is indicated. (*Created with* BioRender.com.)

degranulation occurs, but through a mechanism leading to direct mast cell degranulation without the formation or cross-linking of IgE. Such direct degranulation can occur because of the medication's activation of specific proteases, activation of complement, activation of Toll-like receptors, release of neuropeptides, the release of other cytokines, the chemical structure of the medication having a tetrahydroisoquinolone motif, or cationic mediators and substances directly activating the Mas-related G protein-coupled receptor-X2 (MRGPRX2) on mast cells.[11–13] MRGPRX2 is an orphan receptor (meaning its physiologic ligand has yet to be identified) whose activity has been identified as causal in anywhere from 5% to 70% of type I endotype reactions during administration of numerous drugs, such as vancomycin, nondepolarizing neuromuscular blockers, morphine, and fluoroquinolones.[14] Many chemotherapeutic drugs may cause infusion reactions in a non-IgE-mediated manner. Paclitaxel, for example, is solubilized in Cremophor, a kind of castor oil, which can cause direct histamine release from mast cells.[15]

The mediators released upon mast cell degranulation can be directly traced to each sign or symptom of this reaction's phenotype. In the early phase of mast cell degranulation, histamine is responsible for vasodilation, secretion of mucus, and smooth muscle contraction. The release of tryptase generates C3a and C5a—the anaphylatoxins, and the alpha chain of fibrinogen can be broken by β-tryptase, which can increase bleeding risk.[16] Tryptase is also used as a blood biomarker for identifying this type of reaction. Activation of factors V and VIII in the coagulation pathway can lead to disseminated intravascular coagulation, further increasing bleeding risk. Prostaglandin D_2 and leukotrienes B_4, C_4, and D_4 lead to smooth muscle spasm and increased vasodilation. Activation of the complement cascade by released chymase-cleaving C3 leads to hypotension. Release of neuropeptides further degranulate nearby mast cells. The release of chemokines leads to the recruitment of other effector cells (Th2 cells, eosinophils, and basophils). In the late phase of degranulation, tumor necrosis factor (TNF) is released, and its concentration has been associated with the severity of the event.[11]

Cytokine release reactions are differentiated from the others in phenotype by the rapid onset of fever, chills, rigors, hypertension or hypotension, chest pain, back pain, pelvic pain, or myalgias during medication administration.[8] Cytokine release reactions were first described with the murine monoclonal antibody OKT3, but can occur more recently with many chimeric and humanized monoclonal antibodies, such as rituximab or trastuzumab.[17] These types of reactions are mediated by antibody-mediated cell cytotoxicity and/or are complement-mediated leading to a release of IL-6 and TNF-α, the measurement of the former being a useful biomarker for this type of reaction if drawn at the time of reaction.[10,18]

The primary driver of cytokine release reactions is the release of IL-6.[18,19] The primary mediators of fever are IL-1, IL-6, and TNF-α, and IL-1R antagonist (anakinra) reduces both IL-1 and IL-6, showing that IL-1 seems to induce IL-6. IL-6 works directly on the central nervous system at the level of the hypothalamus to reset one's temperature to a higher set point, resulting in fever.[20] Serum concentrations of IL-6 are elevated in cytokine release reactions, making IL-6 a good biomarker to help differentiate this type of reaction.[8] Steroids have also been shown to be effective in reducing the severity of symptoms of cytokine release, and the use of tocilizumab, an antibody against the IL-6R, is likely to have a role in mitigating the symptoms of cytokine-release.[21]

Mixed reactions include features of both type I hypersensitivity reactions and cytokine-release reactions.[8] These patients may have a positive skin test result, which is highly suggestive of type I reaction; have elevated tryptase levels; and have elevated

IL-6 levels during breakthrough reactions that may occur during desensitization. More than half of all mixed reactions seem to change from primarily type I phenotype to cytokine release phenotype. One possible explanation is that the premedications given during the desensitization protocol may prevent symptoms primarily related with a type I reaction and unmask the symptoms primarily related with the cytokine release phenotype. In addition, it has also yet to be determined whether multiple exposures of certain medications induce or predispose a switch from type I to cytokine release (eg, with repeated exposures to oxaliplatin and a change in tumor burden, if a portion of tumor is escaping the oxaliplatin, the greater tumor burden may lead to greater IL-6 release).[22]

Type II hypersensitivity reactions are mediated by IgG and complement-dependent cytotoxicity and most often present as cytopenia (eg, autoimmune thrombocytopenia, hemolytic anemia, or neutropenia).[1,23] Type III hypersensitivity reactions are mediated by the deposition of soluble IgG/IgM immune complexes in tissues leading to possible serum sickness, urticaria, or even vasculitis (such as Arthus reaction).[24] In general, the timeframe of presentation for type II and type III reactions occurs at least 5 to 7 days after first exposure to the drug.

Delayed type IV hypersensitivity reactions present with a time course that is typically several days to even weeks after the initial exposure to the drug and is primarily characterized by cutaneous involvement ranging anywhere from a benign maculopapular rash to severe cutaneous adverse reactions (SCARs) often involving mucosal surfaces (drug eruption with eosinophilia and systemic symptoms [DRESS], Stevens-Johnson syndrome, toxic epidermal necrolysis, or acute generalized exanthematous pustulosis [AGEP]).[6] Occasionally the reaction can start several hours after exposure to the drug as in the case of fixed drug eruption. The endotype of delayed reactions is primarily mediated by T cells, macrophages, and monocytes.

Last, the phenotype of infusion-related reactions is like that of a milder phenotype of cytokine release reactions, typically do not involve increase in levels of serum IL-6 or other cytokines, and are self-limited.[8] These types of reactions do not require desensitization and can be managed by decreasing the rate of infusion of the original medication with or without premedication including steroids targeted to control the symptoms of the reaction.

Specifically in an IgE-mediated type I hypersensitivity reaction, IgE bound to FcεRI cross-links when exposed to antigen, leading to the activation of intracellular Src family tyrosine kinases Lyn and Fyn, and then the recruitment and activation of the tyrosine kinase Syk, which phosphorylates LAT, leading to the activation of phospholipase Cγ1, which catalyzes phosphatidylinositol-4,5-phosphate to the second messengers inositol triphosphate and diacylglycerol, the binding of which to the endoplasmic reticulum results in the emptying of intracellular Ca^{2+} into the cytosol and the sustained elevation of intracellular Ca^{2+}, leading to the reorganization of cortical actin to the polymerized actin necessary for the anchoring and trafficking of secretory vesicles to fuse with the cell membrane, leading to their exocytosis (degranulation) (**Fig. 2**).[25,26]

Mechanisms of Desensitization

There are many proposed mechanisms for rapid desensitization, some of which may be complementary.[27] The first proposed mechanism for IgE-mediated type I hypersensitivity reactions involves increased internalization of IgE/FcεRI complexes through increasing cross-linking starting at low antigen concentrations. These complexes are initially internalized during desensitization and the remaining antigen-laden IgE bound to the alpha chain of the FcεRI remains at the membrane level after

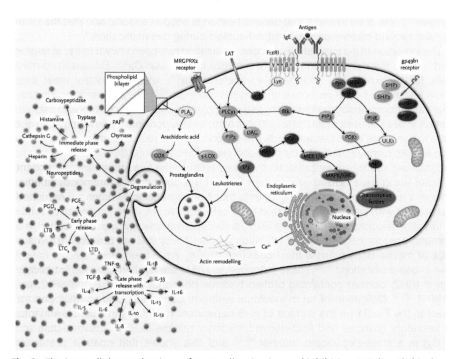

Fig. 2. The intracellular mechanisms of mast cell activation and inhibition. IgE directly binds to the α subunit of the high-affinity FcεR1, which becomes activated when cross-linked; this phosphorylates Src homology tyrosine kinases Lyn and Fyn, which downstream activates phospholipase Cγ (PLCγ1)-driven hydrolyzation of phosphatidylinositol 4,5-bisphosphate (PIP$_2$) to inositol triphosphate (IP$_3$), releasing calcium ions from the endoplasmic reticulum into the cytosol, causing actin remodeling and degranulation of premade, immediate-phase mediators (tryptase, heparin, chymase, histamine, platelet-activating factor, neuropeptides, cathepsin G, and carboxypeptidase). This also activates the mitogen-activated protein kinase (MAPK) pathway of transcription factors that lead to early-phase arachidonic acid synthesis (prostaglandins D$_2$ and E$_2$, leukotrienes B$_4$, C$_4$, and D$_4$), transcription of late-phase cytokines (TNF-α and transforming growth factor [TGF]-β) and interleukins (IL-4, 5, 6, 8, 10, 12, 13, 16, and 33), and mast cell survival. The Mas-related G protein-coupled receptor-X2 (MRGPRX2) leads to direct mast cell activation primarily by cationic drugs without the presence of preformed IgE. A transmembrane glycoprotein called gp49b1 has 2 immunoreceptor tyrosine-based inhibitory motifs (ITIMs) that recruit Src homology domain type 2-containing tyrosine phosphates (SHP-1 and SHP-2) and members of the Src homology domain type 2-containing inositol polyphosphate 5-phosphates (SHIP-1 and SHIP-2), decreasing the levels of the second messenger phosphatidylinositol 3′ kinase (PI3K) and dephosphorylating second messengers that would have otherwise led to mobilization of calcium, resulting in inhibition of mast cell degranulation. PLA2, phospholipase A2; COX, cyclooxygenase 1 & 2 enzyme pathway; 5-LOX, 5-lipoxygenase enzyme pathway. (*Created with* BioRender.com.)

desensitization.[28,29] Desensitization is not due to depletion of histamine or other mediators, because desensitized mast cells still contain large amounts of their mediators.[4,30] Desensitization does not cause the subthreshold depletion of common intracellular second messengers because when mast cells were sensitized in vitro to both DNP and OVA, DNP-desensitized cells responded with full degranulation to OVA antigen and OVA-desensitized cells responded with full degranulation to DNP antigen.[29] This goes to show that desensitization is antigen specific and that the intracellular second messengers are not exhausted during desensitization.[31]

The inhibition of degranulation after desensitization has been shown to be, at least in part, due to the mast cell's inability to mobilize intracellular Ca^{2+}. Desensitized mast cells fail to exhibit any change in intracellular Ca^{2+}, whereas control mast cells show a sustained Ca^{2+} response on antigen challenge.[32] Artificially elevating intracellular Ca^{2+} concentration with ionomycin is sufficient to overcome the block to degranulation in desensitized mast cells. Cofilin is a protein responsible for severing actin and thus making free actin filament ends available for further reorganization. Desensitization inhibits turnover of cofilin by phosphorylation at the serine 3 position; this seems to block out the movement of actin that is specific to the Fcε receptor related to the antigen being desensitized—more than 75% of the degranulation response to other antigens is preserved, and this suggests that the aggregates of actin are somehow associated with specifically activated IgE/FcεRI complexes.

Inhibitor receptors, such as gp49B1, a transmembrane glycoprotein that has 2 immunoreceptor tyrosine-based inhibition motifs (ITIMs) that are present on the surface of mouse bone marrow mast cells (mBMMCs), have been postulated to have a role in desensitization.[33–35] These cytoplasmic ITIMs are binding sites for Src homology 2 (SH2) domain containing protein tyrosine phosphatases, SHP-1, SHP-2, and SHIP-1.[36,37] Coligation of rat monoclonal antibody B23.1 bound to gp49B1 and IgE fixed to the FcεR1 on the surface of IL-3-dependent mBMMCs inhibited exocytosis of secretory granules and lipid-derived mediator release (ie, β-hexosaminidase and LTC_4) in a dose-dependent manner,[38,39] and this shows that gp49B1 prevented antigen-induced, IgE-mediated mast cell degranulation and may be involved in the pathophysiology of desensitization.[40]

WHAT ARE THE GOALS OF DESENSITIZATION?

Why subject patients to a medication to which they have already experienced a hypersensitivity reaction strong enough to prevent them from getting it again on its own? Many medications to which hypersensitivity reactions occur are cancer chemotherapeutic drugs, monoclonal antibodies, or even antibiotics. These medications are first-line therapies, improving quality of life and life expectancy.[9] First-line therapies are recommended due to higher efficacy, fewer side effects, and unique mechanisms of action that give the greatest benefit to patients. Sometimes there is no alternative to a specific drug. With appropriate risk stratification, desensitization can make these drugs available again to the patient, even in cases of severe anaphylaxis.[41]

Desensitization is cost effective when compared with a second-line therapy (if one even exists). Millions of people in the United States have no health insurance, and in 2009, an estimated 58.7 million (19.5% of the population) people had no health insurance for at least part of the year.[42] Drugs that are used for chemotherapy can cost hundreds or even thousands of dollars per dose. In a cohort study of 2523 people receiving chemotherapy for lung cancer, the monthly overall costs of care were substantially higher for those receiving second- and third-line therapy versus first-line therapy.[43] Specifically, the cost per patient per month for those on first-line therapy ranged on average from $3500 to $3900, whereas the cost for those on second- or third–line therapy was on average $7200 to $9600. In another study with 357 patients with a history of ovarian cancer and hypersensitivity reaction to carboplatin, 171 of whom were desensitized to carboplatin, the other 186 not desensitized to carboplatin, the average costs for each hospital encounter were 31% higher in those patients who did not receive desensitization ($8700 to $7800 greater in the controls).[44] In this same study and others, there was also a nonsignificant increase in life expectancy (cohort survival) in allergic, desensitized patients when compared with nonallergic, nondesensitized patients.[44,45]

WHO SHOULD OR SHOULD NOT RECEIVE DESENSITIZATION?

To both determine eligibility for desensitization and customize the protocol thereof, each patient should first be risk stratified (**Fig. 3**).[46] If the initial reaction involved anaphylaxis, even when severe enough to require endotracheal intubation, this is not a contraindication, but there would be a higher risk of breakthrough reaction during desensitization.[44] Patients with severe respiratory or cardiovascular disease (eg, severe chronic obstructive pulmonary disease or heart failure) or those who are pregnant are candidates for desensitization, but in a higher risk category. Although not contraindicated, β-blockers can mask the tachycardia of anaphylaxis and may prevent the activity of epinephrine, and both β-blockers and angiotensin-converting enzyme inhibitors can worsen hypotension during an episode of anaphylaxis.[47]

Patients with CF are repeatedly exposed to multiple antibiotics and tend to have a higher prevalence of allergic reactions to antibiotics.[48] First-line therapy in patients with CF is very important to fight pseudomonal infections.[49] Normally, such severe obstructive lung disease (forced expiratory volume in the first second of expiration < 50% of predicted value with chronic lung disease) would be a contraindication, but desensitization has been shown to be safe and effective for maintaining first-line therapy in patients with CF.[50] Desensitization has even been repeatedly performed successfully for patients with a history of anaphylaxis to β-lactam antibiotics while on extracorporeal membrane oxygenation.[51]

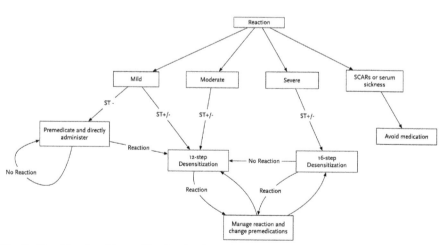

Fig. 3. Algorithm for risk stratification for desensitization. Severe cutaneous adverse reactions (SCARs) include toxic epidermal necrolysis (TEN), Stevens-Johnson syndrome (SJS), drug eruption with eosinophilia and systemic symptoms (DRESS), or acute generalized exanthematous pustulosis (AGEP) and are absolute contraindications to desensitization. (*Adapted from* Yang BC, Castells MC. Rituximab hypersensitivity and desensitization: a personalized approach to treat cancer and connective tissue diseases. Ann Allergy Asthma Immunol 2019;123(1):11–5; with permission.)

Absolute contraindications to desensitization are SCARs, such as Stevens-Johnson syndrome and toxic epidermal necrolysis, DRESS, or AGEP.[52,53] Some of these reactions occur in individuals who already have genetic risk factors such as carriage of a specific HLA class I allele, and the risk of reexposure, even through desensitization, can induce a severe reaction.[54] If the initial reaction is a Gell and Coombs type II (immunocytotoxic), type III reaction (immune complex mediated, such as serum sickness), or vasculitis, desensitization is also contraindicated because reexposure of any kind can be fatal.[6]

TMP-SMX is a first-line drug in prophylaxis against *Pneumocystis jirovecii* pneumonia in immunocompromised patients and is associated with delayed exanthematous maculopapular type IV hypersensitivity reaction, which is also amenable to desensitization in a safe and effective fashion with a rapid desensitization protocol.[55–59]

A modified Brown classification is used next to determine the severity of the initial reaction to the medication: mild, moderate, or severe.[60,61] Mild reactions involve only 1 organ system and are usually only cutaneous in nature. Moderate reactions involve 2 organ systems or more, but there are no changes in vital signs (ie, hypotension or oxygen desaturation). Severe reactions involve 2 or more organ systems and involve changes in vital signs.

Risk stratification involves skin testing when possible. The testing is performed at least 2 to 3 weeks after the initial reaction to minimize false-negative results. Skin testing can yield insight into the pathophysiology of the reaction. If a skin prick or intradermal test result is immediately positive, it reinforces that the reaction is an IgE-mediated type I hypersensitivity and would be extremely amenable to desensitization.[5] A delayed reaction to skin testing (hours to days later) would be a type IV hypersensitivity. These delayed reactions, if they do not involve mucosal surfaces, are still amenable to desensitization. A negative skin test result does not necessarily mean that the pathophysiology was not due to a type I or type IV hypersensitivity. Many drugs either need to be conjugated with a carrier protein through their normal route of administration before becoming an allergen or the allergen is a metabolite of the original drug.[62] If skin testing is positive, desensitization is indicated. If skin testing result is negative and the initial reaction was moderate or severe, desensitization may also be indicated. If skin testing result was negative and the initial reaction was mild, a standard infusion with or without premedication may be recommended.[63]

Other biomarkers for risk stratification may be available in the future. Directly testing for specific IgE to platins has also been shown to be more specific than skin testing and may be a helpful tool for diagnosis.[64,65] The basophil activation test successfully identifies patients more likely to have a reaction to platins during desensitization—increased expression of CD203c was associated with increased risk of reactions and increased expression of CD63 was associated with more severe reactions.[66] Most recently, a test using nanoallergens—phospholipids displaying small drug metabolites as haptens—involves mixing mast cell-like cells (RBL-SX38) in vitro with patient serum to identify specific IgE-FcεRI cross-linking and degranulation response, all without subjecting a patient to the risks and delays inherent to skin testing.[67]

WHEN TO PERFORM DESENSITIZATION?

Explicitly, desensitization is indicated whenever there is evidence of a type I reaction by skin test positivity and/or by symptoms, cytokine release type, mixed type, type IV reaction except for SCARs, if the drug is more effective and/or associated with fewer side effects, or if the drug has a unique mechanism of action.[6] The patient would then have to be risk stratified as previously described. There are special considerations for specific circumstances, however.

When a patient presents with the need for β-lactam therapy and has a history of allergy to β-lactams, risk stratification is done through a pathway (**Fig. 4**).[68] Most patients with a reported penicillin allergy tolerate penicillin. Patients who avoid penicillin therapy without true allergy are at significantly greater risk of treatment failure and have an increased incidence of antibiotic resistance. To prevent these outcomes, a unified penicillin and cephalosporin pathway algorithm has been published. The patient's primary team follows the pathway, involving infectious disease specialists to identify the most optimum antibiotic and allergy and immunology specialists and pharmacists to perform procedures as necessary. Those patients with type II through IV reactions are advised drug avoidance and to use alternative agents. Patients with other types of reactions may be amenable to test dose procedure in a monitored setting versus penicillin skin testing. If positive, these patients would be good candidates for desensitization.

It is recommended that all patients who are to undergo desensitization should have a baseline serum tryptase level to be performed 2 to 3 weeks outside of a reaction to screen for mastocytosis, other mast cell activation diseases, and more recently, for hereditary α-tryptasemia.[69,70] Also, drug-specific tests should also be performed, such as for preformed IgE against galactose-α-1,3-galactose for those who are to undergo cetuximab therapy.[71]

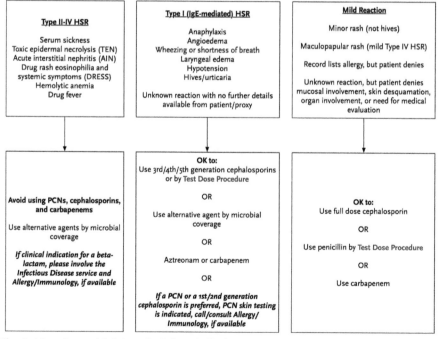

Fig. 4. Mass General Brigham (MGB) penicillin hypersensitivity pathway (Boston, MA, USA). PST, penicillin skin test; HSR, hypersensitivity reaction; PCN, penicillin. (*From* Wolfson AR, Huebner EM, Blumenthal KG. Acute care beta-lactam allergy pathways: approaches and outcomes. Ann Allergy Asthma Immunol 2019;123(1):16–34; with permission.)

WHERE TO PERFORM DESENSITIZATION?

Most desensitizations can be performed outside of an intensive care unit (ICU) setting, which reduces use of resources and costs. As of 2010, ICU costs in the United States were on average $4300 per day.[72] What is required is the availability of appropriate concentrations of the medication to be administered in accordance with the desensitization plan, continuous telemetry monitoring, and 1:1 nursing for the duration of the desensitization. The nurse can then follow existing standing orders for changing IV fluid rates and performing medication administration for predetermined possible reactions.

In a study of 2177 desensitization procedures by Sloane and colleagues,[44] those with a history of severe reactions had their initial desensitization procedures performed in a medical ICU setting, but their subsequent desensitizations were all performed safely in an outpatient setting. If the initial reaction was severe and a 16-bag desensitization is to be performed, an ICU setting may not be unreasonable given the increased risk of subsequent severe reaction. In our experience, even if the initial desensitization is performed in an ICU setting, subsequent desensitizations can be performed in an outpatient setting.[5]

HOW TO PERFORM DESENSITIZATION?

The first step in desensitization is arranging the appropriate customized premedication before beginning the procedure (**Fig. 5**). The medications are chosen specifically to prevent the symptoms identified in the patient's original reaction to the drug to which to be desensitized.[46,47] Most patients receive famotidine and cetirizine—these drugs are of less benefit to those with predominantly cytokine release reactions. If the initial reaction involved fevers or chills, we use a combination of acetaminophen and meperidine. For nausea, patients receive ondansetron. For symptoms of anxiety, we administer lorazepam. If the patient experienced flushing, we add aspirin. If there was a history of bronchospasm, we give inhaled β-agonists and montelukast or zileuton.[73]

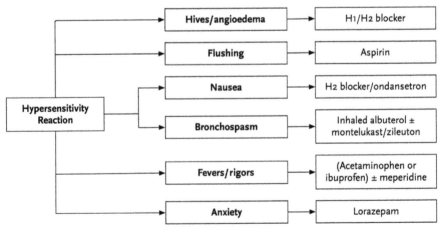

Fig. 5. Premedication is personally tailored for each patient. The exact medications used are selected based on the symptoms the patient experienced during the initial reaction to the desensitization drug. (*From* Yang BC, Castells M. Diagnosis and treatment of drug hypersensitivity reactions to biologicals: medical algorithm. Allergy 2020; doi:10.1111/all.14432; with permission.)

Table 1
Example of a 3-bag, 12-step desensitization to oxaliplatin

Name of medication:		Oxaliplatin
Target dose (mg)		135
Standard volume per bag (mL)		250
Final rate of infusion (mL/h)		80
Calculated target concentration (mg/mL)		0.54
Standard time of infusion (minutes)		188

		Total mg Per Bag	Amount of Bag Infused (mL)
Solution 1	250 mL 0.0054 mg/mL	1.35	9.38
Solution 2	250 mL 0.054 mg/mL	13.5	18.8
Solution 3	250 mL 0.54 mg/mL	134	250

Step	Solution	Rate (mL/h)	Time (min)	Volume Infused Per Step (mL)	Dose Administered with This Step (mg)	Cumulative Dose (mg)
1	1	2.5	15	0.625	0.003	0.003
2	1	5	15	1.25	0.007	0.01
3	1	10	15	2.5	0.01	0.02
4	1	20	15	5	0.03	0.05
5	2	5	15	1.25	0.07	0.12
6	2	10	15	2.5	0.14	0.25
7	2	20	15	5	0.27	0.52
8	2	40	15	10	0.54	1.06
9	3	10	15	2.5	1.34	2.40
10	3	20	15	5	2.68	5.08
11	3	40	15	10	5.36	10.4
12	3	80	174	233	125	135
	Total time (minutes) =		339			

After premedication, the desensitization itself is performed (**Tables 1** and **2**). The medication is split up into a 1- to 4-bag series (the 4-bag series is reserved for those with a history of severe reactions).[9,45] Each bag has an increasing concentration of the medication. The desensitization process is performed with one-to-one nursing under continuous telemetry monitoring with vital signs taken every 15 minutes, before proceeding to each next step. The beginning concentration of the medication is many orders of magnitude less than that of a normal dose, with the final dose being administered at the target concentration for normal administration. Every 15 minutes, the rate of administration for each bag is roughly doubled, proceeding from one bag to the next throughout the entire desensitization until the final step completes administration of an entire dose of the medication.

At any step of desensitization, or even at multiple steps, a breakthrough reaction may occur. The most common time for a breakthrough reaction to occur is during

Table 2
Example of a 3-bag, 12-step desensitization to infliximab

Name of medication:						Infliximab
Target dose (mg)						610
Standard volume per bag (mL)						250
Final rate of infusion (mL/h)						80
Calculated target concentration (mg/mL)						2.44
Standard time of infusion (minutes)						188

				Total mg per bag	Amount of bag infused (mL)
Solution 1	250 mL 0.0244 mg/mL			6.1	9.25
Solution 2	250 mL 0.244 mg/mL			61	18.8
Solution 3	250 mL 2.42 mg/mL			605	250

Step	Solution	Rate (mL/h)	Time (min)	Volume Infused Per Step (mL)	Dose Administered with This Step (mg)	Cumulative Dose (mg)
1	1	2	15	0.5	0.01	0.01
2	1	5	15	1.25	0.03	0.04
3	1	10	15	2.5	0.06	0.10
4	1	20	15	5	0.12	0.23
5	2	5	15	1.25	0.3	0.53
6	2	10	15	2.5	0.6	1.14
7	2	20	15	5	1.2	2.36
8	2	40	15	10	2.4	4.8
9	3	10	15	2.5	6.1	10.9
10	3	20	15	5	12.1	23
11	3	40	15	10	24.2	47.2
12	3	80	174	233	563	610
	Total time (minutes) =		339			

the final step. We have standing orders in place throughout the procedure so that the nurse can deal with each reaction symptom in a customized manner (**Fig. 6**). As soon as a breakthrough reaction is identified, the infusion is held and the rate of intravenous fluids is increased dramatically to dilute mediators (>500 mL/h). If there is a change in vital signs concerning for anaphylaxis (hypotension, desaturation, syncope) then intramuscular epinephrine is administered with the possibility of supplementation with corticosteroids at a later time. If there is no change in vital signs concerning for anaphylaxis, the individual medications that would have been given in premedication are administered to manage the individual symptoms involved. Once the reaction has resolved, the infusion is continued at the current step. The desensitization proceeds, dealing with breakthrough reactions as they occur, until the entire dose of the medication is finally administered in the last bag.

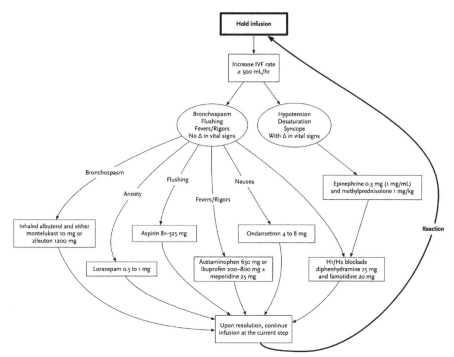

Fig. 6. Algorithm for the management of breakthrough reactions during desensitization. *(From* Yang BC, Castells MC. Rituximab hypersensitivity and desensitization: a personalized approach to treat cancer and connective tissue diseases. Ann Allergy Asthma Immunol 2019;123(1):11–5; with permission.)

SUMMARY

Rapid drug desensitization is an established, useful, and powerful tool of modern allergy and clinical immunology that allows the treatment of allergic patients with first-line medications that promote their increased quality of life, and in many cases decreases cost and increases life expectancy. Who: the patient in need of first-line medical therapy; What: stimulating cellular inhibitory mechanisms; When: at the time of need; Where: in the safest environment; Why: to promote increased quality of life and life expectancy; How: using standardized protocols validated by many successful cases in the hands of desensitization-trained allergists, nurses, and pharmacists.

CLINICS CARE POINTS

- What: Hypersensitivity reactions can be classified into 1 of 7 types based on clinical symptoms and serum biomarkers. During a reaction, it may help to draw serum tryptase and IL-6 levels to aid in classification.

- Who: For most medications, patients risk stratified to a higher risk category benefit from fewer breakthrough reactions with more desensitization steps than those risk-stratified to a lower risk category.

- Where: The selection of the safest environment for desensitization should be based on risk stratification. Most desensitizations occur in an outpatient setting.

- When: Desensitization is especially indicated when skin testing result is positive, indicating a type I reaction. Desensitization is not indicated for patients with a history of type II reactions, type III reactions, and SCARs.
- Why: As long as a medication's doses can be closely measured (ie, through dilutions or compounding), it may be amenable for use in desensitization.
- How: A standardized protocol should be followed that includes premedication, steady increases in the rate of administration of a drug until the target dose has been reached, one-to-one nursing during the time of the desensitization, and protocols in place to manage breakthrough reactions.

ACKNOWLEDGMENTS

Graphics are, in part, created with Biorender.com.

DISCLOSURE

The authors have nothing to disclose.

REFERENCES

1. Demoly P, Adkinson NF, Brockow K, et al. International Consensus on drug allergy. Allergy 2014;69(4):420–37.
2. Cernadas JR, Brockow K, Romano A, et al. General considerations on rapid desensitization for drug hypersensitivity - a consensus statement. Allergy 2010;65(11):1357–66.
3. Joint Task Force on Practice P, American Academy of Allergy A, Immunology, et al. Drug allergy: an updated practice parameter. Ann Allergy Asthma Immunol 2010;105(4):259–73.
4. Shalit M, Levi-Schaffer F. Challenge of mast cells with increasing amounts of antigen induces desensitization. Clin Exp Allergy 1995;25(9):896–902.
5. Castells MC, Tennant NM, Sloane DE, et al. Hypersensitivity reactions to chemotherapy: outcomes and safety of rapid desensitization in 413 cases. J Allergy Clin Immunol 2008;122(3):574–80.
6. Castells M. Drug hypersensitivity and anaphylaxis in cancer and chronic inflammatory diseases: the role of desensitizations. Front Immunol 2017;8:1472.
7. Diaferio L, Giovannini M, Clark E, et al. Protocols for drug allergy desensitization in children. Expert Rev Clin Immunol 2020;16(1):91–100.
8. Isabwe GAC, Garcia Neuer M, de Las Vecillas Sanchez L, et al. Hypersensitivity reactions to therapeutic monoclonal antibodies: Phenotypes and endotypes. J Allergy Clin Immunol 2018;142(1):159–70.e2.
9. Castells M, Sancho-Serra Mdel C, Simarro M. Hypersensitivity to antineoplastic agents: mechanisms and treatment with rapid desensitization. Cancer Immunol Immunother 2012;61(9):1575–84.
10. Picard M, Galvao VR. Current knowledge and management of hypersensitivity reactions to monoclonal antibodies. J Allergy Clin Immunol Pract 2017;5(3):600–9.
11. Lieberman P, Garvey LH. Mast cells and anaphylaxis. Curr Allergy Asthma Rep 2016;16(3):20.
12. McNeil BD, Pundir P, Meeker S, et al. Identification of a mast-cell-specific receptor crucial for pseudo-allergic drug reactions. Nature 2015;519(7542):237–41.
13. Porebski G, Kwiecien K, Pawica M, et al. Mas-Related G Protein-Coupled Receptor-X2 (MRGPRX2) in drug hypersensitivity reactions. Front Immunol 2018;9:3027.

14. McNeil BD. MRGPRX2 and adverse drug reactions. Front Immunol 2021;12: 676354.
15. Hong DIC. Desensitization for allergic reactions to chemotherapy. Yonsei Med J 2019;60(2):119–25.
16. Guilarte M, Sala-Cunill A, Luengo O, et al. The mast cell, contact, and coagulation system connection in anaphylaxis. Front Immunol 2017;8:846.
17. Doessegger L, Banholzer ML. Clinical development methodology for infusion-related reactions with monoclonal antibodies. Clin Transl Immunol 2015;4(7):e39.
18. Jakubovic BD, Sanchez-Sanchez S, Hamadi S, et al. Interleukin-6: A novel biomarker for monoclonal antibody and chemotherapy-associated hypersensitivity confirms a cytokine release syndrome phenotype-endotype association. Allergy 2020. https://doi.org/10.1111/all.14644.
19. Kruger-Krasagakes S, Moller A, Kolde G, et al. Production of interleukin-6 by human mast cells and basophilic cells. J Invest Dermatol 1996;106(1):75–9.
20. Luheshi GN. Cytokines and fever. Mechanisms and sites of action. Ann N Y Acad Sci 1998;856:83–9.
21. Lee DW, Gardner R, Porter DL, et al. Current concepts in the diagnosis and management of cytokine release syndrome. Blood 2014;124(2):188–95.
22. Silver J, Garcia-Neuer M, Lynch DM, et al. Endophenotyping oxaliplatin hypersensitivity: personalizing desensitization to the atypical platin. J Allergy Clin Immunol Pract 2020;8(5):1668–80.e2.
23. O'Meara S, Nanda KS, Moss AC. Antibodies to infliximab and risk of infusion reactions in patients with inflammatory bowel disease: a systematic review and meta-analysis. Inflamm Bowel Dis 2014;20(1):1–6.
24. Bavbek S, Ataman S, Akinci A, et al. Rapid subcutaneous desensitization for the management of local and systemic hypersensitivity reactions to etanercept and adalimumab in 12 patients. J Allergy Clin Immunol Pract 2015;3(4):629–32.
25. MacGlashan DW Jr. IgE-dependent signaling as a therapeutic target for allergies. Trends Pharmacol Sci 2012;33(9):502–9.
26. Metcalfe DD, Peavy RD, Gilfillan AM. Mechanisms of mast cell signaling in anaphylaxis. J Allergy Clin Immunol 2009;124(4):639–46 [quiz: 647-8].
27. Liu A, Fanning L, Chong H, et al. Desensitization regimens for drug allergy: state of the art in the 21st century. Clin Exp Allergy 2011;41(12):1679–89.
28. Oka T, Rios EJ, Tsai M, et al. Rapid desensitization induces internalization of antigen-specific IgE on mouse mast cells. J Allergy Clin Immunol 2013;132(4): 922–32.e1-16.
29. Sancho-Serra Mdel C, Simarro M, Castells M. Rapid IgE desensitization is antigen specific and impairs early and late mast cell responses targeting FcepsilonRI internalization. Eur J Immunol 2011;41(4):1004–13.
30. de Las Vecillas Sanchez L, Alenazy LA, Garcia-Neuer M, et al. Drug hypersensitivity and desensitizations: mechanisms and new approaches. Int J Mol Sci 2017; 18(6). https://doi.org/10.3390/ijms18061316.
31. Morales AR, Shah N, Castells M. Antigen-IgE desensitization in signal transducer and activator of transcription 6-deficient mast cells by suboptimal doses of antigen. Ann Allergy Asthma Immunol 2005;94(5):575–80.
32. Ang WX, Church AM, Kulis M, et al. Mast cell desensitization inhibits calcium flux and aberrantly remodels actin. J Clin Invest 2016;126(11):4103–18.
33. Castells MC, Wu X, Arm JP, et al. Cloning of the gp49B gene of the immunoglobulin superfamily and demonstration that one of its two products is an early-expressed mast cell surface protein originally described as gp49. J Biol Chem 1994;269(11):8393–401.

34. Bulfone-Paus S, Nilsson G, Draber P, et al. Positive and negative signals in mast cell activation. Trends Immunol 2017;38(9):657–67.

35. Katz HR. Inhibition of anaphylactic inflammation by the gp49B1 receptor on mast cells. Mol Immunol 2002;38(16–18):1301–5.

36. Fujioka Y, Matozaki T, Noguchi T, et al. A novel membrane glycoprotein, SHPS-1, that binds the SH2-domain-containing protein tyrosine phosphatase SHP-2 in response to mitogens and cell adhesion. Mol Cell Biol 1996;16(12):6887–99.

37. Huber M, Helgason CD, Damen JE, et al. The src homology 2-containing inositol phosphatase (SHIP) is the gatekeeper of mast cell degranulation. Proc Natl Acad Sci U S A 1998;95(19):11330–5.

38. Katz HR, Vivier E, Castells MC, et al. Mouse mast cell gp49B1 contains two immunoreceptor tyrosine-based inhibition motifs and suppresses mast cell activation when coligated with the high-affinity Fc receptor for IgE. Proc Natl Acad Sci U S A 1996;93(20):10809–14.

39. McCormick MJ, Castells MC, Austen KF, et al. The gp49A gene has extensive sequence conservation with the gp49B gene and provides gp49A protein, a unique member of a large family of activating and inhibitory receptors of the immunoglobulin superfamily. Immunogenetics 1999;50(5–6):286–94.

40. Castells MC, Klickstein LB, Hassani K, et al. gp49B1-alpha(v)beta3 interaction inhibits antigen-induced mast cell activation. Nat Immunol 2001;2(5):436–42.

41. Caiado J, Bras R, Paulino M, et al. Rapid desensitization to antineoplastic drugs in an outpatient immunoallergology clinic: Outcomes and risk factors. Ann Allergy Asthma Immunol 2020;125(3):325–33.e1.

42. Centers for Disease C, Prevention. Vital signs: health insurance coverage and health care utilization — United States, 2006–2009 and January-March 2010. MMWR Morb Mortal Wkly Rep 2010;59(44):1448–54.

43. Ramsey SD, Martins RG, Blough DK, et al. Second-line and third-line chemotherapy for lung cancer: use and cost. Am J Manag Care 2008;14(5):297–306.

44. Sloane D, Govindarajulu U, Harrow-Mortelliti J, et al. Safety, costs, and efficacy of rapid drug desensitizations to chemotherapy and monoclonal antibodies. J Allergy Clin Immunol Pract 2016;4(3):497–504.

45. Bonamichi-Santos R, Castells M. Diagnoses and management of drug hypersensitivity and anaphylaxis in cancer and chronic inflammatory diseases: reactions to taxanes and monoclonal antibodies. Clin Rev Allergy Immunol 2018;54(3):375–85.

46. Yang BC, Castells MC. Rituximab hypersensitivity and desensitization: a personalized approach to treat cancer and connective tissue diseases. Ann Allergy Asthma Immunol 2019;123(1):11–5.

47. Yang BC, Castells M. Diagnosis and treatment of drug hypersensitivity reactions to biologicals: medical algorithm. Allergy 2020. https://doi.org/10.1111/all.14432.

48. Koch C, Hjelt K, Pedersen SS, et al. Retrospective clinical study of hypersensitivity reactions to aztreonam and six other beta-lactam antibiotics in cystic fibrosis patients receiving multiple treatment courses. Rev Infect Dis 1991;13(Suppl 7):S608–11.

49. Burrows JA, Nissen LM, Kirkpatrick CM, et al. Beta-lactam allergy in adults with cystic fibrosis. J Cyst Fibros 2007;6(4):297–303.

50. Legere HJ 3rd, Palis RI, Rodriguez Bouza T, et al. A safe protocol for rapid desensitization in patients with cystic fibrosis and antibiotic hypersensitivity. J Cyst Fibros 2009;8(6):418–24.

51. Foer D, Marquis K, Romero N, et al. Challenges and safety of beta-lactam desensitization during extracorporeal membrane oxygenation. Ann Allergy Asthma Immunol 2019;122(6):661–3.

52. Bachot N, Roujeau JC. Differential diagnosis of severe cutaneous drug eruptions. Am J Clin Dermatol 2003;4(8):561–72.

53. Pirmohamed M, Friedmann PS, Molokhia M, et al. Phenotype standardization for immune-mediated drug-induced skin injury. Clin Pharmacol Ther 2011;89(6): 896–901.

54. Mezzano V, Giavina-Bianchi P, Picard M, et al. Drug desensitization in the management of hypersensitivity reactions to monoclonal antibodies and chemotherapy. BioDrugs 2014;28(2):133–44.

55. Kitazawa T, Seo K, Yoshino Y, et al. Efficacies of atovaquone, pentamidine, and trimethoprim/sulfamethoxazole for the prevention of Pneumocystis jirovecii pneumonia in patients with connective tissue diseases. J Infect Chemother 2019;25(5): 351–4.

56. Yoshizawa S, Yasuoka A, Kikuchi Y, et al. A 5-day course of oral desensitization to trimethoprim/sulfamethoxazole (T/S) in patients with human immunodeficiency virus type-1 infection who were previously intolerant to T/S. Ann Allergy Asthma Immunol 2000;85(3):241–4.

57. Gluckstein D, Ruskin J. Rapid oral desensitization to trimethoprim-sulfamethoxazole (TMP-SMZ): use in prophylaxis for Pneumocystis carinii pneumonia in patients with AIDS who were previously intolerant to TMP-SMZ. Clin Infect Dis 1995;20(4):849–53.

58. Absar N, Daneshvar H, Beall G. Desensitization to trimethoprim/sulfamethoxazole in HIV-infected patients. J Allergy Clin Immunol 1994;93(6):1001–5.

59. Pyle RC, Butterfield JH, Volcheck GW, et al. Successful outpatient graded administration of trimethoprim-sulfamethoxazole in patients without HIV and with a history of sulfonamide adverse drug reaction. J Allergy Clin Immunol Pract 2014; 2(1):52–8.

60. Brown SG. Clinical features and severity grading of anaphylaxis. J Allergy Clin Immunol 2004;114(2):371–6.

61. Picard M, Pur L, Caiado J, et al. Risk stratification and skin testing to guide reexposure in taxane-induced hypersensitivity reactions. J Allergy Clin Immunol 2016;137(4):1154–64.e2.

62. Brockow K, Romano A, Blanca M, et al. General considerations for skin test procedures in the diagnosis of drug hypersensitivity. Allergy 2002;57(1):45–51.

63. Brennan PJ, Rodriguez Bouza T, Hsu FI, et al. Hypersensitivity reactions to mAbs: 105 desensitizations in 23 patients, from evaluation to treatment. J Allergy Clin Immunol 2009;124(6):1259–66.

64. Caiado J, Castells M. Presentation and diagnosis of hypersensitivity to platinum drugs. Curr Allergy Asthma Rep 2015;15(4):15.

65. Caiado J, Venemalm L, Pereira-Santos MC, et al. Carboplatin-, oxaliplatin-, and cisplatin-specific IgE: cross-reactivity and value in the diagnosis of carboplatin and oxaliplatin allergy. J Allergy Clin Immunol Pract 2013;1(5):494–500.

66. Giavina-Bianchi P, Galvao VR, Picard M, et al. Basophil activation test is a relevant biomarker of the outcome of rapid desensitization in platinum compounds-allergy. J Allergy Clin Immunol Pract 2017;5(3):728–36.

67. Deak PE, Kim B, Adnan A, et al. Nanoallergen platform for detection of platin drug allergies. J Allergy Clin Immunol 2019;143(5):1957–60.e12.

68. Wolfson AR, Huebner EM, Blumenthal KG. Acute care beta-lactam allergy pathways: approaches and outcomes. Ann Allergy Asthma Immunol 2019;123(1): 16–34.
69. Hsu Blatman KS, Castells MC. Desensitizations for chemotherapy and monoclonal antibodies: indications and outcomes. Curr Allergy Asthma Rep 2014; 14(8):453.
70. Lyons JJ. Hereditary alpha tryptasemia: genotyping and associated clinical features. Immunol Allergy Clin North Am 2018;38(3):483–95.
71. Chung CH, Mirakhur B, Chan E, et al. Cetuximab-induced anaphylaxis and IgE specific for galactose-alpha-1,3-galactose. N Engl J Med 2008;358(11):1109–17.
72. Halpern NA, Pastores SM. Critical care medicine beds, use, occupancy, and costs in the United States: a methodological review. Crit Care Med 2015; 43(11):2452–9.
73. Breslow RG, Caiado J, Castells MC. Acetylsalicylic acid and montelukast block mast cell mediator-related symptoms during rapid desensitization. Ann Allergy Asthma Immunol 2009;102(2):155–60.

Aspirin-Exacerbated Respiratory Disease: A Unique Case of Drug Hypersensitivity

Kristen B. Corey, MD[a], Katherine N. Cahill, MD[b],*

KEYWORDS

- Aspirin-exacerbated respiratory disease • Aspirin • Desensitization • Eicosanoids
- Mast cells • Anaphylaxis

KEY POINTS

- A clinical history of aggressive or difficult-to-control CRSwNP or asthma and/or acute upper or lower airway reactions with cyclooxygenase-1 (COX-1) inhibitor ingestion should prompt evaluation for AERD.
- COX-1 inhibitor-induced reactions in AERD are characterized by the onset of upper and/or lower respiratory reactions within minutes-to-hours of exposure resulting from a decrease in prostaglandin E_2 levels triggering mast cell activation and eicosanoid production.
- AERD and IgE-mediated hypersensitivity share many clinical features secondary to their shared chemical mediator production; however, AERD is a unique process that has important differentiating features with regard to disease chronicity, timeline of acute reaction, and therapeutic options.

INTRODUCTION

Aspirin-exacerbated respiratory disease (AERD) is a unique form of drug hypersensitivity that differs fundamentally from classic IgE-mediated and cell-mediated drug hypersensitivities. Many of the clinical signs and symptoms of an acute reaction are similar to those experienced with an immediate hypersensitivity, as are the chemical mediators; however, unique features of the baseline pathophysiology of cyclooxygenase-1 (COX-1) inhibitor-induced reactions require specialized attention on the part of the practicing clinician.

[a] Division of Allergy, Pulmonary, and Critical Care Medicine, Department of Medicine, Vanderbilt University Medical Center, 2611 West End Avenue, Suite 210, Nashville, TN 37203, USA;
[b] Division of Allergy, Pulmonary, and Critical Care Medicine, Department of Medicine, Vanderbilt University Medical Center, 2525 West End Avenue, Suite 450, Room 418, Nashville, TN 32703, USA
* Corresponding Author.
E-mail address: katherine.cahill@vumc.org

Immunol Allergy Clin N Am 42 (2022) 421–432
https://doi.org/10.1016/j.iac.2021.12.005
0889-8561/22/© 2021 Elsevier Inc. All rights reserved.

Abbreviations	
AERD	aspirin-exacerbated respiratory disease
CRSwNP	chronic rhinosinusitis with nasal polyposis
COX	cyclooxygenase
cysLT	cysteinyl leukotriene(s)
5-LO	5-lipooxygenase
LT	leukotriene
NSAID	Nonsteroidal anti-inflammatory drug
PG	prostaglandin

Background

AERD consists of a clinical triad of chronic rhinosinusitis with nasal polyposis (CRSwNP), asthma, and acute upper and/or lower respiratory reactions after the ingestion of COX-1 inhibitors (aspirin sensitivity). Other common identifiers in the medical literature include Samter's triad, nonsteroidal antiinflammatory (NSAID)-exacerbated respiratory disease (N-ERD), or aspirin-induced asthma. As a chronic, acquired, and progressive disorder characterized by type 2 eosinophilic inflammation of the airways, patients with AERD often present with persistent upper and/or lower airway symptoms that are difficult-to-control. However, both acute and chronic disease are marked by a spectrum of signs and symptoms. For example, some patients experience aggressive upper airway sinusitis and nasal polyposis with only mild lower airway symptoms; other patients struggle with severe, difficult-to-control asthma and have relatively quiescent sinus disease.[1] Even acute reactions differ among individuals, with some experiencing only asthmatic responses to COX-1 inhibitors, some only naso-ocular reactions, and still others with both.[2,3] The hallmark histologic finding in samples of nasal tissue is robust eosinophilic infiltration mixed with mast cells, both important effector cells in the pathophysiology of AERD. In general, AERD is thought to be underdiagnosed. Among adults with asthma, the prevalence of AERD is estimated to be about 7%, and even higher in adults with CRSwNP (10%) and severe asthma (15%).[4]

DISCUSSION
Clinical Characteristics

AERD possesses many clinical characteristics that set it apart from classic immediate-type hypersensitivity reactions (**Fig. 1**). The most striking difference is that AERD is a chronic disease with evident clinical symptoms that are augmented with acute ingestion of the drug in question, compared with immediate hypersensitivity whereby underlying disease is unlikely to predict clinical allergy. AERD has a predilection for adults and typically presents in the third to fourth decade of life, though symptom onset in peripubescent children can occur a rate of 3.5% in one study.[5,6] Even in the absence of COX-1 inhibitor ingestion, AERD often is marked by aggressive, difficult-to-control disease compared with aspirin-tolerant CRSwNP and asthma. Study of a large cohort of patients with these diagnoses revealed that patients with AERD had more severe sinus disease, decreased baseline forced expiratory volume in 1 second (FEV1), and were more likely to have systemic steroid-dependent disease in comparison to their non-AERD counterparts.[7] These patients have rapid regrowth of polyp tissue after resection, requiring more sinus surgeries than their counterparts, and chronic hyposmia or anosmia can be quite profound.[5,7] Severe, eosinophilic, and/or corticosteroid-dependent asthma and aggressive CRSwNP requiring repeat surgical intervention should prompt further investigation into the diagnosis of AERD.

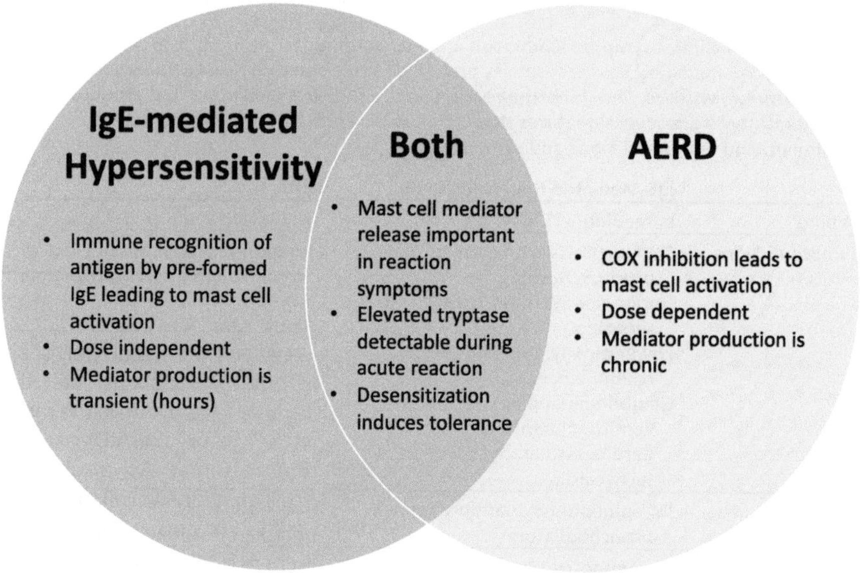

Fig. 1. General comparisons between IgE-mediated Hypersensitivity and AERD. IgE-mediated hypersensitivity and AERD share some features with regard to mediator release and desensitization as an appropriate therapy; however, there are many unique features that differentiate the two diagnoses.

In addition to the chronic, persistent aspects of AERD, the disease is also characterized by acute upper and/or lower respiratory reactions after the ingestion of aspirin and NSAID medications, the key clinical feature of AERD. These reactions have elements that can be found in classic IgE-mediated hypersensitivity, but they also are unique in timing and symptoms (**Table 1**). Baseline findings of hyposmia, nasal congestion, and lower airway obstruction are augmented by the administration of COX-1 inhibitors. Typically, patients describe the onset of symptoms within 30 to 90 minutes of ingestion, though sometimes outside this window, and many reactions prompt urgent or emergent evaluation and treatment. The patient will most often describe upper airway symptoms of acute conjunctivitis, rhinorrhea, and nasal congestion, along with lower airway signs and symptoms of wheeze, shortness of breath, and obstruction that necessitate medical intervention with bronchodilators. Extrarespiratory symptoms involving the skin or gastrointestinal tract occur in a subset of patients; however, hypotension and anaphylaxis are rare findings. Appearance of a macular eruption differs in appearance and mechanism from the urticaria that is often seen in immediate hypersensitivity reactions.[8–10] Additionally, patients with AERD report mild-to-moderate respiratory symptoms within minutes of ingestion of alcohol, though this is not universal.[11] Interestingly, symptom severity is largely dose-dependent, with some individuals tolerating small doses of aspirin on a regular basis (eg, daily aspirin 81 mg) but reporting reactions with higher doses of COX-1 inhibitors. This dose dependence also distinguishes AERD from classic IgE-mediated hypersensitivity.[12]

Diagnosis

Like traditional drug hypersensitivity to NSAIDs, no sensitive or specific in vitro testing is available for the diagnosis of AERD. The diagnostic gold standard is the aspirin

Table 1
Comparison of clinical symptoms between IgE-mediated hypersensitivity and AERD. While immediate IgE-mediated hypersensitivity and AERD share some clinical features such as bronchospasm, wheeze, and rhinorrhea as well as the chemical mediators that produce these symptoms, there are several features that differ between the 2 including the timing, treatment, and additional signs and symptoms.

	IgE-Mediated Hypersensitivity	AERD
Timing	Immediate (15–60 min)	Usually delayed (up to 3 h)
Symptoms/Signs	Skin: urticaria, angioedema, pruritus, flushing Upper airway: rhinorrhea, sneezing Lower airway: bronchospasm, cough, wheeze GI: abdominal pain, nausea, vomiting, diarrhea Cardiovascular: hypotension, tachycardia	Commonly: bronchospasm, ocular conjunctivitis, nasal congestion, rhinorrhea Others: cutaneous eruption, abdominal pain, diarrhea Rarely: anaphylaxis
Treatment	IM epinephrine ± antihistamines, bronchodilators	Bronchodilators, LT blockers ± antihistamines
Major Chemical Mediator(s)	Histamine, cysLTs Produced acutely	cysLTs, PGD_2 Produced chronically, increased acutely with COX-inhibitor exposure
Minor Chemical Mediator(s)	PGD_2	Histamine

Abbreviations: COX, cyclooxygenase; cysLT, cysteinyl leukotrienes; LT, leukotriene; PGD_2, Prostaglandin D_2.

provocation challenge. History is the most important tool for diagnosis, as this will provide an index of suspicion for the clinician. Clear or documented history of a clinical respiratory reaction to an NSAID, particularly to 2 or more class members, may eliminate the need for an observed challenge. The goal of an aspirin provocation challenge is to elicit a respiratory reaction in those with AERD. There exist several published protocols detailing the steps of aspirin challenge, and they vary based on location, timing, and type of COX-1 inhibitor/route of administration, and all are completed once respiratory symptoms develop or the patient tolerates 325 mg of aspirin without respiratory symptoms—a negative challenge.[13,14] Most commonly, oral aspirin is used due to its availability and low cost; however, protocols using intranasal ketorolac or a combination of the 2 are available.[14,15] A challenge may be completed in a single day in the outpatient clinic, or the provider may elect to perform it over a couple of days in the outpatient clinic, both of which have been proven safe and effective.[13,16,17] One may consider the resources available as well as the support staff onsite when determining the appropriate procedure. Regardless of the chosen protocol, it is important to practice caution in patients with severe or uncontrolled asthma, as symptom provocation may lead to life-threatening lower airway obstruction. The AAAAI Workgroup suggests that patients should have a baseline FEV1 of at least 70% predicted and good control of symptoms in the weeks preceding challenge.[14] In patients who are unable to meet this criterion, NSAID avoidance is recommended and the challenge should be deferred to the time at which asthma is under good control.

A reaction occurs when the patient develops an increase in 2 or more upper respiratory symptoms or there is at least a 15% decline in FEV1 from baseline or at least

20% decline from baseline on peak flow measurement.[14] A clinical reaction during the challenge is diagnostic for AERD. If a patient tolerates 325 mg of aspirin without the development of any respiratory symptoms, the challenge is negative and an AERD diagnosis excluded.

Management with Daily Aspirin Therapy

Treatment of AERD as a chronic disease is focused on managing symptoms and preventing the recurrence of polyposis and progression of airway disease along with improving quality of life. There exist various medical therapies, including intranasal corticosteroids, oral antihistamines, and oral leukotriene (LT) blockers, that help to achieve control. However, in comparison to immediate hypersensitivity whereby drug avoidance is the mainstay of treatment, a key therapeutic approach, safe and effective in improving quality of life and disease progression, is aspirin desensitization followed by daily aspirin therapy.[14,18] While the terminology is the same, aspirin desensitization for AERD differs fundamentally from traditional desensitization for IgE-mediated hypersensitivity. Aspirin desensitization protocols for AERD follow directly from protocols used for aspirin challenge in AERD but differ in goal. The goal of aspirin desensitization for AERD is to safely overcome a respiratory reaction to aspirin and achieve tolerance of 325 mg of aspirin. Protocols vary in the starting dose of aspirin, typically between 20.25 mg and 60 mg, and in the timing of dosing increase. In general, no matter the starting dose, the dose is doubled over the predetermined timing interval, typically between 1 and 3 hours, to a target dose of 325 mg, at which point the patient is considered desensitized. Studies show that patients will most often react after the 40.5 mg or the 81 mg dose, with an average time to the reaction of approximately 60 minutes.[13] Naso-ocular symptoms are the most commonly experienced symptom during desensitization, followed by bronchial symptoms.[17] Acute symptoms should be treated according to the involved system with oral antihistamines, inhaled bronchodilators, and intramuscular epinephrine in rare cases of systemic reactions. When the clinical reaction symptoms have stabilized, the provocative dose should be readministered, at which point it is generally well-tolerated, and the desensitization continues to a target dose of 325 mg of aspirin. If higher daily dosing of aspirin is desired, the patient may continue to increase the dose of aspirin at home up to 1300 mg total daily dose. Daily doses between 325 and 1300 mg are associated with improvement in severity and regrowth of nasal polyposis, number of episodes of sinusitis and systemic steroids, sense of smell, and quality of life.[14,19]

It is important to make distinctions between desensitization for a classic immediate drug hypersensitivity and desensitization for AERD (**Fig. 2**). A key difference lies in the known mechanisms of desensitization between IgE-mediated hypersensitivity and aspirin desensitization in AERD, which is discussed in further detail later. Simply put, in IgE-mediated allergy, it is thought that desensitization causes low-level cross-linking of IgE on the surface of mast cells and impairs receptor internalization, inhibiting mast cell degranulation and clinical effects of the reaction.[20] In aspirin desensitization in AERD, the major mechanism is thought to center around decreased production of prostaglandin (PG)D_2 and downregulation of cysteinyl leukotriene (cysLT) receptors on the airway epithelium that lead to an improvement in clinical symptoms with long-term use.[21] While effects of desensitization for IgE-mediated drug allergy occur immediately, individuals undergoing aspirin desensitization for AERD may not experience the complete benefit of symptom improvement for a full 6 to 12 months after desensitization is completed and daily therapy is continued. Additionally, it is commonplace to premedicate desensitization for IgE-mediated hypersensitivity to prevent any symptoms that may occur at various doses of the chosen medication. Premedication with leukotriene

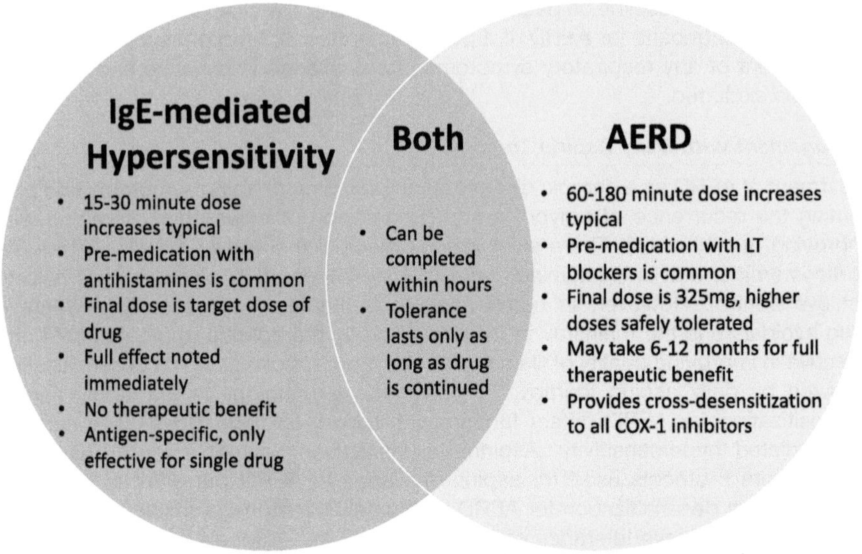

Fig. 2. Comparison of Desensitization between IgE-mediated hypersensitivity and AERD. Desensitization induces tolerance in both IgE-mediated hypersensitivity and AERD; however, the protocols, target doses, and implications differ between the 2 diagnoses as highlighted above.

(LT) blockers in individuals undergoing aspirin desensitization has been shown to decrease or even completely eliminate or the severity of lower airway bronchial reactions during desensitization.[3] Seemingly, the symptoms are shifted to the upper airway, thereby making desensitization an even safer procedure, especially in individuals who have had severe reactions in the past.[3] One must consider the intended purpose and individual patient if choosing to use LT blockers before aspirin challenge or desensitization. There are reports of individuals on LT blockers who did not display respiratory reactions after previously documented reaction with COX-1 inhibitors, a so-called "silent desensitization."[3] If aspirin challenge is performed to confirm the diagnosis of AERD, it is prudent to withhold any LT modifying drugs; however, if the diagnosis is known and desensitization is the sole purpose, LT blockers have a role in creating a safer and more tolerable procedure for the patient.

With the availability of targeted biologic agents for patients with eosinophilic asthma and nasal polyposis, their use in AERD is increasing in frequency. Anti-IgE omalizumab and anti-IL-4Rα dupilumab are approved for moderate-to-severe asthma in children, adolescents, and adults and nasal polyposis in adults. Anti-IL-5 pathway monoclonal antibodies are approved for moderate-to-severe eosinophilic asthma in adolescents and adults; mepolizumab was recently approved and others are in phase III trials for use in nasal polyposis as well. These are appropriate alternatives in patients who are not candidates for aspirin desensitization or otherwise do not tolerate aspirin therapy, including patients with uncontrolled asthma or those with contraindications to daily aspirin therapy (eg, peptic ulcer disease, bleeding diathesis).

Pathophysiology of Chronic Disease and Cyclooxygenase-Inhibitor-Induced Reactions

Though the mechanisms are not fully understood, both the chronic disease state and acute aspirin sensitivity center around dysregulated eicosanoid homeostasis with evidence of a depressed PGE_2 pathway and subsequent chronic mast cell activation and induction of type 2 inflammation. PGE_2 is an important negative regulator of 5-lipoxygenase (5-LO) activity and downstream production of cysteinyl leukotrienes (cysLTs). Additionally, PGE_2 is known to restrain mast cell activation and subsequent production of preformed and synthesized mediator release, including PGD_2, histamine, tryptase, and additional cysLTs.[22] Release of mast cell mediators creates a robust environment for type 2 inflammation involving eosinophils, T helper 2 (T_H2) lymphocytes, and type 2 innate lymphoid cells (ILC2s) acting through PGD_2 binding to chemoattractant receptor homologous molecule expressed on T_H2 (CRTH2) receptor on these cells.[21,23] Individuals with AERD have decreased PGE_2 expression at baseline, possibly due to decreased COX-2 expression, combined with the upregulation of type 1 cysLT receptors ($CysLTR_1$) on inflammatory cells of the airway that lead to chronic type 2 inflammation. Clinically, this inflammation results in asthma, often severe, and CRSwNP.

In addition to the chronic defects in PGE_2 expression, $CysLTR_1$ expression, and type 2 inflammation, ingestion of COX-1 inhibitors results in acute upper and/or lower airway reactions thought to be due to similar mechanisms. Likely due to decreased expression of COX-2 in individuals with AERD, ingestion of aspirin and other COX-1 inhibitors results in significant decreases in PGE_2 that release the brakes on mast cell activation and allow for unregulated production of cysLTs via 5-LO activity. The clinical effects of this are seen locally with nasal congestion and rhinorrhea, ocular conjunctivitis, and bronchospasm. PGD_2 production in the airway tissue acts as a chemoattractant for type 2 inflammatory cells such as eosinophils, basophils, ILC2s, and T_H2 lymphocytes to the airway epithelium via CRTH2, contributing further to the acute reaction.[21,23] These mediators are also produced on a systemic level as evidenced by elevated urinary LTE_4 and PGD_2 metabolites in the hours following acute reaction (**Fig. 3**). High levels of PGD_2 metabolites following aspirin exposure are associated with systemic symptoms such as abdominal pain, nausea, vomiting, diarrhea, and skin rash.[9] There is increasing evidence for a role of platelet activation in the pathogenesis of aspirin reactions. Activated platelets are an abundant source of arachidonic acid that can be rapidly converted to lipid mediators[24]; platelets release PGD_2 and thromboxane (TX)A_2 that can mediate effects of bronchoconstriction and promote inflammatory cell chemotaxis to the airway. Additionally, platelets through direct interactions with granulocytes, specifically neutrophils, can increase the production of cysLTs, further contributing to the acute and chronic pathologies of AERD.[25]

Acute reactions due to COX-1 inhibitor sensitivity in AERD differ in timeline and mechanism from classic IgE-mediated hypersensitivity (see **Fig. 3**). Immediate hypersensitivity is mediated by cross-linking of IgE bound to FcεR1 receptors on the surface of mast cells and basophils, leading to degranulation and activation of these cells, producing the clinical signs and symptoms. Mechanistically, the process is divided into two phases—the early phase and the late phase—separated by the timing and the significant chemical mediators and cells involved.[26] The current knowledge of AERD pathogenesis does not delineate a role for cross-linking of IgE on mast cells in either acute reactions or chronic inflammation.[23] However, small studies whereby omalizumab was administered to individuals with AERD revealed symptomatic improvement in chronic upper and lower airway disease as well as decreased lipid mediator production during aspirin challenge.[27,28] It is proposed that low-level activation of mast cells by an antigen that has not yet been identified possibly contributes to the chronic mediator production in the disease process.[23]

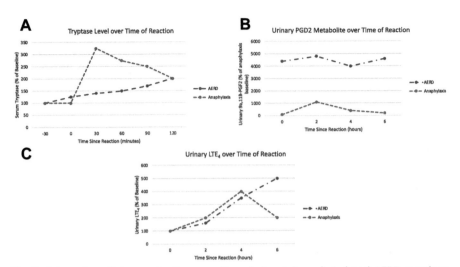

Fig. 3. Selected mediator production over time during IgE mediated and AERD reactions. Production of contributory chemical mediators of each reaction over time adapted from previously modeled data in individuals experiencing confirmed reactions of each pathology. (*A*) Serum tryptase level from the onset of reaction to 120 minutes, revealing that tryptase levels in anaphylaxis peak around 30 minutes and subsequently fall slowly[30] whereas, tryptase levels in AERD rise slowly after the onset of reaction.[35] (*B*) Urinary 9α,11b-PGF$_2$, a metabolite of PGD2 starting from the time of reaction to 6 hours, demonstrates similar trends between anaphylaxis[31] and AERD[35] but with significantly higher levels at baseline and during a reaction for individuals with AERD. (*C*) Urinary LTE$_4$ over the course of a reaction declines between 4 and 6 hours in anaphylaxis,[31] while the levels continue to rise during this same time in individuals with AERD.[35]

The acute, early phase of IgE-mediated reactions is due to rapid mast cell release of histamine upon activation and activation of histamine receptors leading to the cutaneous, respiratory, and GI signs and symptoms[29]; however, despite non-IgE-mediated mast cell activation and histamine release in COX-1 inhibitor reactions, histamine does not seem to play an important role in disease manifestations and is not considered a significant disease mediator.[23,24] A hallmark of immediate hypersensitivity reactions is acute elevations in serum tryptase peaking 60 to 90 minutes following reaction and falling slowly for the hours thereafter.[26] Tryptase elevations may also be seen in individuals experiencing acute reactions with COX-1 inhibitors. Interestingly, in individuals with AERD on daily aspirin therapy, tryptase levels paradoxically remain elevated from baseline after weeks of daily therapy, a differentiating factor from IgE-mediated reactions whereby tryptase levels fall to baseline hours after reaction and desensitization.[26,30,31] Similar to an acute aspirin reaction in AERD, in immediate reactions, there are also rapid elevations in lipid mediators such as cysLTs and PGD$_2$ that are synthesized by mast cells; after the early phase, PGD$_2$ continues to be synthesized for several hours via COX-1 activity in cell mediators.[26,32] It is thought that these mediators act as chemoattractants that contribute to the late phase of anaphylaxis involving the recruitment of eosinophils, basophils, and T$_H$2 lymphocytes, a similar process to what is seen in airway epithelial tissue in individuals with AERD after aspirin ingestion.[21,23,26] Overall, there are similar mediators produced after classic IgE-mediated hypersensitivity and COX-1 respiratory reactions in AERD; however, the timeline of production and the initial triggers differ between the 2 processes.

Mechanisms of Daily Aspirin Therapy

The exact mechanism(s) by which aspirin desensitization followed by daily aspirin therapy is effective in quality of life and symptom improvement in AERD are not clear. Several mechanisms have been proposed including cysLTR1 downregulation on airway mucosal epithelium,[33] inhibition of IL-4/STAT6 pathway,[34] and inhibition of PGD_2 production and effector cell chemotaxis to the respiratory tract.[30] It may be that a combination of these mechanisms is responsible for the improvement in polyp and asthma severity, number of systemic steroid courses, and tolerance of higher doses of COX-1 inhibitors. It is known that daily aspirin therapy does not correct the dysregulation of PGE_2, as levels are uniquely suppressed in those with AERD on aspirin therapy, while they remain at baseline levels in aspirin-tolerant patients with asthma on 1300 mg of aspirin daily after 8 weeks.[30] This continued suppression of PGE_2 leads to the enhancement of the 5-LO pathway with increases in cysLT production, which is balanced by the downregulation of cysLTR1 on airway epithelium that can lead to an improvement in symptoms.[30,33] The decline in PGE_2 contributes to increased mast cell activation as measured by increased plasma tryptase levels on high-dose aspirin, though this does not seem to have a significant effect on symptoms.[30] Importantly, inhibition of COX-1 leads to a decrease in PGD_2 production that diminishes the chemotaxis of CRTH2+ inflammatory cells, such as eosinophils and T_H2 lymphocytes, to the upper and lower airway mucosa, resulting in an improvement in symptoms as well as a decrease in airway remodeling associated with chronic inflammation.[21] Paradoxically, some of the mechanisms of improvement associated with daily aspirin therapy—decreased PGD_2 production and downregulation of cysLTR1 on airway mucosal tissue—are not associated with improvement in a key feature of AERD—the derangement of PGE_2.

The mechanisms described above are in contrast to desensitization mechanisms in classic immediate hypersensitivity. Desensitization for IgE-mediated hypersensitivity is antigen-specific, meaning that the effects are only for the drug of choice; however, in AERD, the effects of desensitization apply across all classes of COX-1 inhibitors.[20] Mechanisms of desensitization in classic IgE-mediated hypersensitivity are equally unclear; however, proposed mechanisms of inhibited mast cell degranulation include the downregulation of FcεR1 on mast cells, calcium channel dysregulation, and inhibition of actin polymerization of mast cells.[20] In both, successful desensitization is followed by clinical tolerance to the desensitized drug which is maintained through chronic exposure.

SUMMARY

AERD is a chronic, progressive disease of the upper and lower respiratory tract characterized by asthma, CRSwNP, and acute aspirin sensitivity that differs in the mechanism, diagnosis, treatment, and effect on the quality of life from classic immediate drug hypersensitivity. The pathophysiology centers on the dysregulation of PGE_2 that is further impaired by the ingestion of COX-1 inhibitors. Individuals with AERD experience a spectrum of upper and lower airway symptoms, from minimal to aggressive nasal polyposis and mild to severe, difficult-to-control asthma. Diagnosis of AERD is accomplished using an aspirin challenge procedure and documentation of a reaction with naso-ocular, asthmatic, or combination of symptoms. Aspirin desensitization and continuation of daily therapy provide many patients with improvement in systemic steroid dependence, regrowth of polyps, and quality of life.

CLINICS CARE POINTS

- A clinical history of aggressive or difficult-to-control CRSwNP or asthma or acute upper or lower airway reactions with COX-1 inhibitor ingestion should prompt evaluation for AERD.

- Multiple protocols for aspirin challenge and desensitization can be performed rapidly over several hours or spread out over 2 days; the clinician should consider the available resources, comfort of staff, and burden on the patient when choosing the proper protocol.

- Premedication with leukotriene blockers can prevent severe lower respiratory tract reactions, but caution should be given to the risk of "silent desensitization."

- Aspirin desensitization and daily aspirin therapy is a cost-effective, well-tolerated management strategy for patients with AERD that can decrease the severity of sinus disease, polyp growth, steroid dependence, and asthma and improve the quality of life and sense of smell in patients with AERD.

- AERD and IgE mediated hypersensitivity share many clinical features secondary to their shared chemical mediator production; however, AERD is a unique process that has important differentiating features with regard to disease chronicity, timeline of acute reaction, and therapeutic options.

DISCLOSURE

K.N. Cahill has severed on scientific advisory boards for Teva, GlaxoSmithKline, Blueprint Medicines, Regeneron, Genentech, Sanofi-Pasteur and reports personal fees from Novartis, Third Harmonic Bio, Ribon Therapeutics, and Verantos outside the submitted work and reports funding from NIH U01AI155299 and U19AI095227. K.B. Corey has no disclosures to report.

REFERENCES

1. White AA, Stevenson DD. Aspirin-Exacerbated Respiratory Disease. N Engl J Med 2018;379(11):1060–70.

2. Pleskow WW, Stevenson DD, Mathison DA, et al. Aspirin-sensitive rhinosinusitis/asthma: spectrum of adverse reactions to aspirin. J Allergy Clin Immunol 1983;71(6):574–9.

3. White A, Ludington E, Mehra P, et al. Effect of leukotriene modifier drugs on the safety of oral aspirin challenges. Ann Allergy Asthma Immunol 2006;97(5):688–93.

4. Rajan JP, Wineinger NE, Stevenson DD, et al. Prevalence of aspirin-exacerbated respiratory disease among asthmatic patients: a meta-analysis of the literature. J Allergy Clin Immunol 2015;135(3):676–81.e1.

5. Berges-Gimeno MP, Simon RA, Stevenson DD. The natural history and clinical characteristics of aspirin-exacerbated respiratory disease. Ann Allergy Asthma Immunol 2002;89(5):474–8.

6. Tuttle KL, Schneider TR, Henrickson SE, et al. Aspirin-exacerbated respiratory disease: not always "adult-onset". J Allergy Clin Immunol Pract 2016;4(4):756–8.

7. Stevens WW, Peters AT, Hirsch AG, et al. Clinical Characteristics of Patients with Chronic Rhinosinusitis with Nasal Polyps, Asthma, and Aspirin-Exacerbated Respiratory Disease. J Allergy Clin Immunol Pract 2017;5(4):1061–70.e3.

8. Buchheit KM, Cahill KN, Katz HR, et al. Thymic stromal lymphopoietin controls prostaglandin D2 generation in patients with aspirin-exacerbated respiratory disease. J Allergy Clin Immunol 2016;137(5):1566–76.e5.

9. Cahill KN, Bensko JC, Boyce JA, et al. Prostaglandin D(2): a dominant mediator of aspirin-exacerbated respiratory disease. J Allergy Clin Immunol 2015;135(1):245–52.

10. Laidlaw TM, Gakpo DH, Bensko JC, et al. Leukotriene-Associated Rash in Aspirin-Exacerbated Respiratory Disease. J Allergy Clin Immunol Pract 2020;8(9):3170–1.

11. Cardet JC, White AA, Barrett NA, et al. Alcohol-induced respiratory symptoms are common in patients with aspirin exacerbated respiratory disease. J Allergy Clin Immunol Pract 2014;2(2):208–13.

12. Lee-Sarwar K, Johns C, Laidlaw TM, et al. Tolerance of daily low-dose aspirin does not preclude aspirin-exacerbated respiratory disease. J Allergy Clin Immunol Pract 2015;3(3):449–51.

13. DeGregorio GA, Singer J, Cahill KN, et al. A 1-Day, 90-Minute Aspirin Challenge and Desensitization Protocol in Aspirin-Exacerbated Respiratory Disease. J Allergy Clin Immunol Pract 2019;7(4):1174–80.

14. Stevens WW, Jerschow E, Baptist AP, et al. The role of aspirin desensitization followed by oral aspirin therapy in managing patients with aspirin-exacerbated respiratory disease: A Work Group Report from the Rhinitis, Rhinosinusitis and Ocular Allergy Committee of the American Academy of Allergy, Asthma & Immunology. J Allergy Clin Immunol 2021;147(3):827–44.

15. Lee RU, White AA, Ding D, et al. Use of intranasal ketorolac and modified oral aspirin challenge for desensitization of aspirin-exacerbated respiratory disease. Ann Allergy Asthma Immunol 2010;105(2):130–5.

16. Pelletier T, Roizen G, Ren Z, et al. Comparable safety of 2 aspirin desensitization protocols for aspirin exacerbated respiratory disease. J Allergy Clin Immunol Pract 2019;7(4):1319–21.

17. Williams AN, Simon RA, Woessner KM, et al. The relationship between historical aspirin-induced asthma and severity of asthma induced during oral aspirin challenges. J Allergy Clin Immunol 2007;120(2):273–7.

18. Walters KM, Waldram JD, Woessner KM, et al. Long-term Clinical Outcomes of Aspirin Desensitization With Continuous Daily Aspirin Therapy in Aspirin-exacerbated Respiratory Disease. Am J Rhinol Allergy 2018;32(4):280–6.

19. Berges-Gimeno MP, Simon RA, Stevenson DD. Long-term treatment with aspirin desensitization in asthmatic patients with aspirin-exacerbated respiratory disease. J Allergy Clin Immunol 2003;111(1):180–6.

20. de Las Vecillas Sanchez L, Alenazy LA, Garcia-Neuer M, et al. Drug hypersensitivity and desensitizations: mechanisms and new approaches. Int J Mol Sci 2017;18(6). https://doi.org/10.3390/ijms18061316.

21. Cahill KN. Immunologic effects of aspirin desensitization and high-dose aspirin therapy in aspirin-exacerbated respiratory disease. J Allergy Clin Immunol 2021;148(2):344–7.

22. Sestini P, Armetti L, Gambaro G, et al. Inhaled PGE2 prevents aspirin-induced bronchoconstriction and urinary LTE4 excretion in aspirin-sensitive asthma. Am J Respir Crit Care Med 1996;153(2):572–5.

23. Boyce JA. Aspirin sensitivity: lessons in the regulation (and dysregulation) of mast cell function. J Allergy Clin Immunol 2019;144(4):875–81.

24. Laidlaw TM. Pathogenesis of NSAID-induced reactions in aspirin-exacerbated respiratory disease. World J Otorhinolaryngol Head Neck Surg 2018;4(3):162–8.

25. Laidlaw TM, Kidder MS, Bhattacharyya N, et al. Cysteinyl leukotriene overproduction in aspirin-exacerbated respiratory disease is driven by platelet-adherent leukocytes. Blood 2012;119(16):3790–8.

26. Ogawa Y, Grant JA. Mediators of anaphylaxis. Immunol Allergy Clin N Am 2007; 27(2):249–60, vii.

27. Hayashi H, Fukutomi Y, Mitsui C, et al. Omalizumab for Aspirin Hypersensitivity and Leukotriene Overproduction in Aspirin-exacerbated Respiratory Disease. A Randomized Controlled Trial. Am J Respir Crit Care Med 2020;201(12):1488–98.

28. Hayashi H, Mitsui C, Nakatani E, et al. Omalizumab reduces cysteinyl leukotriene and 9alpha,11beta-prostaglandin F2 overproduction in aspirin-exacerbated respiratory disease. J Allergy Clin Immunol 2016;137(5):1585–7.e4.

29. Reber LL, Hernandez JD, Galli SJ. The pathophysiology of anaphylaxis. J Allergy Clin Immunol 2017;140(2):335–48.

30. Cahill KN, Cui J, Kothari P, et al. Unique Effect of Aspirin Therapy on Biomarkers in Aspirin-exacerbated Respiratory Disease. A Prospective Trial. Am J Respir Crit Care Med 2019;200(6):704–11.

31. Vadas P, Perelman B, Liss G. Platelet-activating factor, histamine, and tryptase levels in human anaphylaxis. J Allergy Clin Immunol 2013;131(1):144–9.

32. Ono E, Taniguchi M, Mita H, et al. Increased production of cysteinyl leukotrienes and prostaglandin D2 during human anaphylaxis. Clin Exp Allergy 2009;39(1): 72–80.

33. Sousa AR, Parikh A, Scadding G, et al. Leukotriene-receptor expression on nasal mucosal inflammatory cells in aspirin-sensitive rhinosinusitis. N Engl J Med 2002; 347(19):1493–9.

34. Katial RK, Martucci M, Burnett T, et al. Nonsteroidal anti-inflammatory-induced inhibition of signal transducer and activator of transcription 6 (STAT-6) phosphorylation in aspirin-exacerbated respiratory disease. J Allergy Clin Immunol 2016; 138(2):579–85.

35. Bochenek G, Nagraba K, Nizankowska E, et al. A controlled study of 9alpha,11-beta-PGF2 (a prostaglandin D2 metabolite) in plasma and urine of patients with bronchial asthma and healthy controls after aspirin challenge. J Allergy Clin Immunol 2003;111(4):743–9.

Pediatric Drug Allergy

Connor Prosty, MD(c), BSc[a],*, Ana M. Copaescu, MD, PhD(c)[b],
Sofianne Gabrielli, MD(c), MSc[c], Pasquale Mule, MSc(c), BSc[c],
Moshe Ben-Shoshan, MD, MSc[c]

KEYWORDS

- Drug • Antibiotic • Nonsteroidal anti-inflammatory drug • Hypersensitivity • Allergy
- Pediatric • Children

KEY POINTS

- Self-reported drug allergies are common among children and these labels carry significant clinical and economic implications.
- Most self-reported drug allergies are not confirmed by a diagnostic workup.
- Direct challenge tests can be safely and effectively used to evaluate penicillin derivative allergies in children.
- The best diagnostic approaches for patients presenting with the most severe cutaneous adverse reactions are unknown.
- Evidence on the best diagnostic approaches in cases whereby the culprit drug may be protopathic and not truly implicated are unknown.

Abbreviations	
NSAID	non steroidal anti-inflammatory drug
SSLR	serum sickness-like reaction
SJS	stevens-Johnson syndrome
AGEP	acute generalised exanthematous pustulosis
SCAR	severe cutaneous adverse reaction
DRESS	drug reaction with eosinophilia and systemic symptoms
SPT	skin prick test
IDT	intradermal test
sIgE	specific IgE test
NPV	negative predictive value
PPV	positive predictive value
TEN	toxic epidermal necrolysis

[a] Faculty of Medicine, McGill University, 1001 Decarie Boulevard, Montréal, Québec H4A 3J1, Canada; [b] Department of Medicine, Division of Allergy and Clinical Immunology, McGill University Health Centre (MUHC), McGill University, 1001 Decarie Boulevard, Montréal, Québec H4A 3J1, Canada; [c] Division of Allergy, Immunology, and Dermatology, Montreal Children's Hospital, 1001 Decarie Boulevard, Montréal, Québec H4A 3J1, Canada
* Corresponding author.
E-mail address: connor.prosty@mail.mcgill.ca

Immunol Allergy Clin N Am 42 (2022) 433–452
https://doi.org/10.1016/j.iac.2022.01.001
0889-8561/22/© 2022 Elsevier Inc. All rights reserved.
immunology.theclinics.com

ADR	adverse drug reaction
PT	patch test
LTT	lymphocyte transformation test

INTRODUCTION

True drug allergies are relatively rare among children; however, children are often incorrectly labeled at the time of an acute viral infection. Urticaria or a delayed exanthem associated with an antibiotic is rarely followed-up in children with an appropriate diagnostic workup. Drug allergy labels are common and have significant associated cost and health implications.[1,2] The prevalence of self-reported drug allergies among children ranges from 2.9% to 16.8%, whereas as few as 4% of these suspected drug allergies are confirmed after appropriate diagnostic work-up.[3] Antibiotics and NSAIDs account for the majority of reported drug allergies in children.[4] In the following sections, we will review current data related to the prevalence, diagnosis, and management of common pediatric drug allergies.

BETA-LACTAM ANTIBIOTICS
Prevalence, Cross-Reactivity, and Natural History

Beta-lactams are among the safest, most effective, and widely used antibiotics for treating community and hospital-acquired pediatric infections. The prevalence of self-reported penicillin-class and cephalosporin allergy among children range from 5% to 10% and 0.5% to 1.1%,[5,6] respectively, but true allergies to beta-lactams are rare. A recent study established that among the 1914 children assessed for suspected amoxicillin allergy only 5.4% (2.2% immediate and 3.2% nonimmediate) had a true allergy.[7] Among children with confirmed penicillin class allergies, cross-reactivity to cephalosporins with dissimilar R1 side chains is low (approximately 2%), but cross-reactivity increases with R1 side chain similarity.[8] The prevalence of confirmed cephalosporin allergy among children evaluated for a suspected allergy ranges from 14.3% to 28.9%.[9–11] Additionally, data suggest that in children, true beta-lactam allergy typically resolves in children by adulthood. Among children with a history of positive direct ingestion challenge to beta-lactams, 89% tolerated a subsequent direct ingestion challenge after a mean of 3.5 years after the initial evaluation.[12] Given these findings, it is suggested that the majority of children presenting

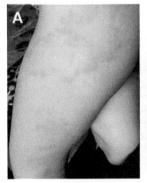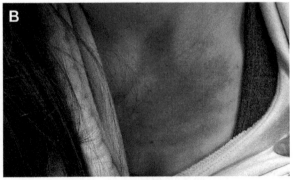

Fig. 1. (A) Child presenting with urticaria after amoxicillin challenge. (B) Child presenting with maculopapular rash after cefixime challenge.

with benign skin rashes should not avoid future treatment even in the absence of drug challenges.

Presentation

In children, reactions to beta-lactams most commonly occur between 1 and 3 years of age, with amoxicillin being the most frequent culprit, followed by third-generation cephalosporins,[7,13] likely due to their relative usage in children. Nonimmediate reactions (occurring more than 1 hour after exposure) to beta-lactams are more common than immediate reactions.[7,11,13] Among patients presenting with a suspected drug allergy, the most common symptoms are urticaria (**Fig. 1**A) and maculopapular rashes (**Fig. 1**B), followed by angioedema and gastrointestinal symptoms (vomiting and diarrhea). One study of 1431 pediatric patients documented that 7% of patients with a suspected allergy to beta-lactams reported anaphylaxis to the culprit drug, and of these reactions, 50% were confirmed as true allergy based on skin testing and challenge.[14] In most patients, symptoms from suspected beta-lactam allergies resolve within 3 days of onset, whereas in approximately 10% to 20% symptoms persist for more than 7 days.[7,13]

Serum-sickness-like reaction (SSLR) is a subtype of nonimmediate reaction presenting with arthralgia and a rash (often with hemorrhagic components) with or without fever (**Fig. 2**). SSLRs are benign and often occur several days to weeks after starting antibiotic treatment. SSLRs are reported to occur more often in children,[15] are more common after treatment with cefaclor versus amoxicillin,[16] and occur in approximately 1% to 2% of patients with suspected drug allergy.[14]

Beta-lactams trigger up to 30% to 40% of all severe cutaneous adverse reactions (SCARs) in children, the most common reaction being Stevens–Johnson syndrome (SJS).[17,18] Penicillin derivatives are reported to cause the majority of pediatric acute generalized exanthematous pustulosis (AGEP) and drug reaction with eosinophilia and systemic symptoms (DRESS).[19] However, the proportion of cases of SCARs attributed to beta-lactams may be confounded by protopathic bias, whereby beta-lactams are administered at the onset of SCAR symptoms and are misattributed as the cause.[20]

Approach

When assessing a patient with a suspected beta-lactam allergy, antibiotic treatment should be ceased and an alternative antibiotic with a low risk of cross-reactivity should be prescribed. A thorough history should be taken to establish the nature of the

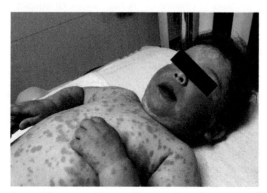

Fig. 2. Child presenting with serum sickness-like reaction after amoxicillin treatment.

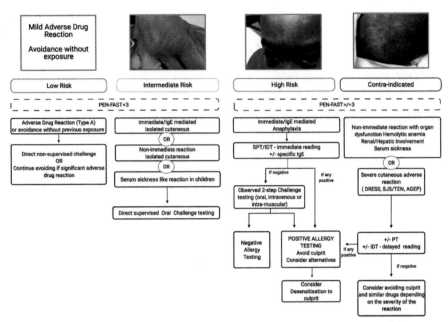

Fig. 3. Algorithm for diagnostic approach in pediatric patients with suspected beta-lactam allergy. Abbreviations: AGEP, acute generalized exanthematous pustulosis; DRESS, drug reaction with eosinophilia and systemic symptoms; IDT, intradermal testing; PT, patch testing; SJS, Steven-Johnson syndrome; SPT, skin prick testing; TEN, toxic epidermal necrolysis; Note 1: Delayed reactions are defined as reactions that occur more than 1 hour after drug administration. Note 2: In severe cutaneous adverse reactions and serum sickness reaction, drug provocation is contraindication, and the culprit drug should be avoided.

reaction (immediate/nonimmediate and allergic/hypersensitivity) and the likelihood of the antibiotic being the cause. History taking should assess the timeframe of the reaction, past exposure/reactions to the antibiotic, indication for antibiotic prescription, symptoms of the reaction, and concurrent medication use.[21] As most drug reactions involve a rash, the skin should be evaluated to assess the morphology of the rash (macular and/or papular vs urticarial vs vesicular/bullous). Recently, the PEN-FAST approach was developed and validated in adults to identify low-risk penicillin hypersensitivities reactions amenable to direct delabeling or direct oral challenge; however, this has not been validated in children.[22] A high index of suspicion for SCARs and SSLRs should be maintained for patients presenting with systemic symptoms and/or severe cutaneous symptoms. The recommended approach to the diagnosis of a beta-lactam allergy is summarized in **Fig. 3**.

Diagnosis

There has been a recent paradigm shift in the diagnosis of beta-lactam allergy, mainly amoxicillin, in children not presenting with anaphylaxis or SCARs. Several studies support the safety and diagnostic value of the direct ingestion challenge (without prior skin or blood tests).[7,13,23] Classically, skin prick tests (SPT) and intradermal tests (IDT) using various antigenic determinants of penicillin, and, infrequently, specific IgE tests (sIgE) have been used in the diagnosis of pediatric drug allergies. Despite the high specificity and negative predictive value (NPV) of these tests, recent pediatric studies suggest poor sensitivity and low positive predictive value (PPV), which limits their

Table 1
Diagnostic properties of available tests for suspected beta-lactam and non–beta-lactam allergies in children

Drug	Test	Patients Evaluated with the Test and Gold Standard	Index Reaction Timing	Author, Year	Sensitivity (%)	Specificity (%)	PPV (%)	NPV (%)
Amoxicillin/ Penicillin	SPT	732	Nonimmediate and Immediate	Ibáñez et al,[107] 2018	9.1	98.3	20.0	95.8
Amoxicillin/ Penicillin	SPT (Penicillin G only)	562	Nonimmediate and Immediate	Picard et al,[30] 2014	–	–	–	95.2
Amoxicillin/ Penicillin	SPT	337	Nonimmediate	Barni et al,[108] 2015	8	99.7	–	–
Amoxicillin/ Penicillin	SPT	168	Immediate	Celik et al,[109] 2020	–	–	–	92.2
Amoxicillin/ Penicillin	IDT	732	Nonimmediate and Immediate	Ibáñez et al,[107] 2018	0.0	100.0	–	95.0
Amoxicillin/ Penicillin	IDT	77	Nonimmediate	Caubet et al,[26] 2010	50	91.8	25	97.1
Amoxicillin/ Penicillin	sIgE	732	Nonimmediate and Immediate	Ibáñez et al,[107] 2018	2.9	99	12.5	95.3
Amoxicillin/ Penicillin	SPT and IDT	17	Nonimmediate and Immediate	Mill et al,[13] 2016	5.9	–	–	–
Amoxicillin/ Penicillin	Ingestion challenge	55	Nonimmediate and Immediate	Mill et al,[13] 2016	–	100	100	89.1
Amoxicillin/ Penicillin	Ingestion challenge	265	Nonimmediate and Immediate	Exius et al,[7] 2021	–	–	–	85.3
Cephalosporin	SPT and IDT	136	Nonimmediate and Immediate	Touati et al,[9] 2021	–	–	–	91.9
Cephalosporin	SPT and IDT	96	Nonimmediate and Immediate	Romano et al,[27] 2008	72.1	–	–	–

(continued on next page)

Table 1
(continued)

Drug	Test	Patients Evaluated with the Test and Gold Standard	Index Reaction Timing	Author, Year	Sensitivity (%)	Specificity (%)	PPV (%)	NPV (%)
Cephalosporin	IDT	11	Nonimmediate	Caubet et al,[26] 2010	100	88.9	33.3	100
Cephalosporin	sIgE	23	Immediate	Mori et al,[10] 2019	20	95.6	50	84.6
Cephalosporin	Ingestion challenge	6	Nonimmediate and Immediate	Attari et al,[29] 2019 (Conference Abstract)	-	-	-	83.3
Clarithromycin	SPT	89	Nonimmediate and Immediate	Suleyman et al,[62] 2021	-	73.9	-	92.1
Azithromycin	SPT	6	Immediate	Barni et al,[54] 2015	-	-	75	50
Clarithromycin	SPT	32 (nonimmediate) and 19 (immediate)	Nonimmediate and Immediate	Barni et al,[54] 2015	-	-	-	94 (nonimmediate) and 100 (immediate)

diagnostic value (**Table 1**). No standardized protocol exists for direct ingestion challenge in children; however, amoxicillin challenges have been used successfully using 10% of the therapeutic dose followed by a 90% of the therapeutic dose 20 minutes later, with a subsequent 1-hour observation period.[7,13] Two large pediatric studies using amoxicillin challenge reported only mild reactions.[7,13] Both these studies assessed the NPV of the direct ingestion challenge and determined it to be 85.3% to 89.1%.[7,13] Moreover, one of these studies determined that the PPV of the direct ingestion challenge was 100% (95%CI: 86.3%, 100.0%) and that the specificity was 100% (95%CI: 90.9%, 100.0%).[13] More recently, a study on children presenting with SSLRs after amoxicillin treatment revealed that direct ingestion challenge may be an appropriate strategy in these cases.[24] Of the patients challenged, 2.7% reacted immediately (within 1 hour) and 4.0% had a nonimmediate reaction.[24] Among the 43 patients successfully contacted, 20 reported subsequent culprit antibiotic use, of whom 25.0% had a subsequent mild reaction (macular/papular rash) not in keeping with the original SSLR.[24]

Unlike penicillin, no commercially standardized reagents exist for cephalosporin skin testing. For parenteral forms, dilution of native cephalosporins into nonirritating concentrations is suggested.[25] There are currently no skin tests based diagnostic strategies for oral cephalosporins that are not available in a parenteral formulation. The data on the diagnostic properties of skin tests and sIgE in the diagnosis of cephalosporin allergies are limited (see **Table 1**). Current data may suggest that skin tests have much better sensitivities in the diagnosis of cephalosporin than penicillin allergies (sensitivity: 72.1%–100%).[26,27] In contrast, a large study of adults and adolescents found the sensitivity of IDT in the diagnosis of immediate cephalosporin allergy to be 0%.[28] However, this study is confounded by the restricted range of cephalosporins tested and the study design, which tested participants for cephalosporin allergy without a history of reaction to cephalosporins. Scarce data on direct ingestion challenge for the diagnosis of a cephalosporin allergy in children are available. A conference abstract reported that among 89 children with suspected cephalosporin allergies undergoing direct ingestion challenge, only 6.7% reacted and all reactions were mild and limited to the skin.[29] Of the 42 patients with negative cephalosporin challenge who responded to the follow-up questionnaire, 6 reported subsequent cephalosporin use and one of which had a mild reaction.[29] Further studies on large patient populations are necessary to validate the diagnostic properties and safety of direct cephalosporin challenges.

For patients with a history of anaphylaxis or SCAR to beta-lactams, direct ingestion challenge is contraindicated. A negative skin test should be elicited before direct ingestion challenge in patients with a history of anaphylaxis to beta-lactams.[21,30]

Management

Because of low cross-reactivity between penicillin derivatives and cephalosporins, most cases of true penicillin allergy can safely be administered cephalosporins with dissimilar side chains.[31] In one study of 30 children with nonimmediate allergies to penicillin, all patients tolerated cephalosporin on challenge.[32] In these patients, third generation cephalosporins are often recommended.[33] For patients with immediate reactions to penicillin, some studies suggest that skin testing with second/third generation cephalosporins with dissimilar side chains should precede antibiotic challenge.[33–35] Other studies indicate that a structurally dissimilar cephalosporin, such as cefixime, could be used safely with no prior skin test in children with confirmed amoxicillin allergies.[13] There is an increased risk for reactions (10%, involving mild cutaneous reactions) with first generation cephalosporins containing similar side chains, such as cephalexin.[7] Alternatively, in children with a cephalosporin allergy, without a known history of penicillin allergy, penicillin can be safely administered following a negative cephalosporin skin test and negative cephalosporin challenge.[36] While most patients with cephalosporin and/or penicillin allergies can safely be prescribed aztreonam,[21] patients allergic to ceftazidime should avoid aztreonam without specific allergy testing due their identical side chains.[37] Penicillin allergic patients may also undergo carbapenem challenges, as there is low cross-reactivity between these antibiotic types.[21,38] In a study of 104 adolescent and adult patients allergic to penicillin, one patient had a positive IDT to meropenem, and the remaining patients with negative skin tests tolerated meropenem challenge.[38] Alternatives to beta-lactams depend on the type of infection being treated but for common community-acquired infections could include azithromycin or clindamycin for IgE-mediated reactions. Since resistance is common among community-acquired infections delabeling beta-lactam allergy is an important antimicrobial stewardship strategy in children that has positive benefits into adulthood.[39] Cefdinir has been suggested as an alternative for non-IgE mediated reactions to penicillin; however, the cross-reactivity between cefdinir and penicillin for IgE-mediated reactions would be less than 2%.[40] These alternative medications are associated with a 2- to 5-fold cost increase compared with amoxicillin providing an additional incentive for penicillin testing and delabeling approaches in childhood.[39]

Desensitization provides temporary antibiotic tolerance by diminishing the immune response to a given medication and may be used when alternative antibiotics are contraindicated, unavailable, and/or less effective. These situations occur most often in patients with life-threatening infections whereby a beta-lactam is the drug of choice or multidrug-resistant infections and/or chronic conditions.[41]

Desensitization has been proposed for suspected IgE-mediated reactions, as well as nonsevere type IV reactions.[42] Contraindications include type II hypersensitivity reactions, type III reactions, and SCARs.[42] Importantly, a careful risk/benefit analysis should be performed before performing desensitization.

Studies and standardized protocols on pediatric desensitization are lacking. Given the paucity of the data, adult protocols are frequently adapted for use in children. The penicillin desensitization protocol published by Sullivan and colleagues is the most widely used or adapted protocol in clinical practice.[43] This protocol involves an initial dose of penicillin beginning at 1/10000 to 1/1000 of the target therapeutic dose, and doses are doubled at 15- to 20-min intervals.[41] Oral desensitization for penicillin has been suggested to be safer and is favored for children.[41] A study on oral penicillin desensitization in 24 adults and 2 children successfully desensitized 25 out of 26 participants.[44] Cessation of protocol occurred in a 15-year-old participant with cystic fibrosis and severe pulmonary disease due to gradual worsening of wheezing. Sparse data exist describing successful desensitization to non–penicillin beta-lactams in children.[45]

Importantly, desensitization should be performed by well-trained specialists in a setting equipped to treat adverse reactions (e.g., anaphylaxis). There is a need for more data on its safety and efficacy in the pediatric population. Given that most drug allergies are desensitized empirically and not based on a positive skin test, it is recommended that patients follow-up with an allergist for further testing and potential delabeling 6 weeks either following the procedure or completion of therapy.

Impact of Drug Allergy Label on Cost and Care in Children

Antibiotic allergy labels in the pediatric population are associated with adverse health and economic outcomes. In a study of 1718 hospitalized children, those labeled as penicillin-allergic had a longer duration of hospital stay and a higher comorbidity index compared with control patients.[46] Another study determined that beta-lactam allergic patients were more likely to receive broad-spectrum antibiotics compared with nonallergic patients.[47] Broad-spectrum antibiotics may be less effective, have more side effects, and contribute to antibiotic resistance.[21]

Drug allergy labels increase the cost of care for both patients and health care systems. Treatment with alternative antibiotics is more expensive than the standard of care. The use of alternative antibiotics among 48 pediatric patients was found to be associated with an average additional cost of $326.50 CAD per patient compared with beta-lactam standard-of-care.[48]

Drug Allergy Delabeling

Appropriate diagnostic workup is essential in preventing erroneous drug allergy labeling. However, both pediatric emergency medicine and primary care providers were found to infrequently refer children for detailed penicillin allergy assessment.[49]

Following a negative challenge, the beta-lactam allergy label should be entirely removed from a patient's medical record. However, failure to adequately update medication allergy records has been estimated to occur in more than one in 5 patients,[50] which impedes future beta-lactam prescriptions.

Patients who tolerate beta-lactam challenges, as well as their families, should be educated that they are not allergic to the medication and can safely take it in the future. Picard and colleagues report that 18% of parents are reluctant to give their children penicillin despite removal of the allergy label due to fear of subsequent reaction.[51] Several strategies have been proposed to improve the efficacy of delabeling beta-lactam allergies. A study of an extended versus a short ingestion challenge protocol (7 days vs 1 day) for suspected beta-lactam allergy in adults demonstrated increased beta-lactam usage at follow-up in patients on the extended protocol.[52] Further, Jeimy and colleagues have proposed written instructions to reiterate a patient's successful challenge and educate on anaphylaxis.[21] Taken together, a thorough evaluation, proper documentation, and patient education may improve drug allergy delabeling and mitigate the negative impacts of a drug allergy label.

NON–BETA-LACTAM ANTIBIOTICS
Prevalence of Hypersensitivity Among Children

Non–beta-lactam antibiotics, mainly macrolides, are often used in clinical practice to treat children for a variety of infections. The prevalence of self-reported macrolide allergy is low and ranges from 0.3% to 0.8% in children.[5,33] Sulfonamide antibiotics can be prescribed to treat urinary tract infections, as prophylaxis therapy for acute otitis media, and for the prevention of meningococcal infections. Due to its known toxicity, sulfonamides are not recommended for children below the age of 2 months.[53] The self-reported allergy prevalence of these antibiotics among children ranges from 0.5% to 2.7%.[5]

Other non–beta-lactam antibiotic allergic reactions reported in children include fluoroquinolones, tetracyclines, clindamycin, aminoglycosides, glycopeptides, and nitroimidazoles. The prevalence of self-reported allergic reactions for fluoroquinolones and tetracyclines among children was 0.004% to 0.04% and 0% to 0.3%, respectively.[5] There are limited data on the prevalence of allergic reactions to all other antibiotics due to their infrequent prescription and application in the pediatric population.

Presentation

Allergic reactions to macrolides can present as either immediate or nonimmediate reactions. Among nonimmediate reactions to clarithromycin, the majority (over 90%)

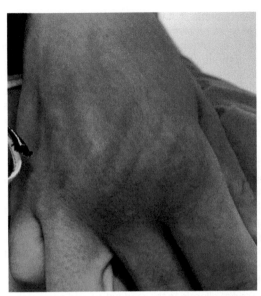

Fig. 4. Maculopapular exanthema in a child with a positive challenge to azithromycin.

present with cutaneous manifestations, such as urticaria, angioedema, and/or maculopapular rash (**Fig. 4**).[54] Immediate reactions to clarithromycin also commonly present as cutaneous manifestations, with a smaller proportion reporting gastrointestinal symptoms.[54] Anaphylaxis to clarithromycin is rare, reported to be one case per one million per year in pediatric studies.[55] Nonimmediate reactions to azithromycin present similarly to nonimmediate reactions to clarithromycin listed above; however, immediate reactions have been reported to be more severe. In a comparative study of azithromycin versus clarithromycin, it was found that among children presenting with immediate reactions to azithromycin, half had history of anaphylaxis.[54]

Allergic reactions to sulfonamide antibiotics can present as a variety of reaction severities and can be immediate or nonimmediate.[56] Cutaneous manifestations, including maculopapular rash and fixed drug eruption, are the most common presentations.[57] More severe presentations can include cell-mediated reactions such as DRESS, SJS, or toxic epidermal necrolysis (TEN).

Allergic reactions to other antibiotics, such as fluoroquinolones and tetracyclines, occur mostly among those with chronic diseases.[6] Similarly, allergic reactions to aminoglycosides and glycopeptides (vancomycin, teicoplanin) are infrequent in children but can include both immediate and nonimmediate reactions, including anaphylaxis.[58,59] Vancomycin is now the most common antibiotic associated with DRESS in many series.[60]

Approach and Diagnosis

The therapeutic approach following a suspected allergic reaction to non–beta-lactam antibiotics includes avoidance of the culprit drug and assessment by a specialist to properly identify a true hypersensitivity reaction.[61] For non–beta-lactam antibiotics, validated skin tests are not available; therefore, an ingestion challenge is frequently required.

Studies assessing the validity of skin tests to diagnose macrolide allergy report that predictive values of SPT are highly variable and are much lower and less accurate compared with beta-lactam antibiotics (see **Table 1**). In a recent study of 160 children with suspected clarithromycin allergy, the specificity of SPT was 73.9% (95%CI: 64.7%, 81.8%) and sensitivity was negligible. The NPV was 92.1% (95%CI: 60.3%, 77.6%) and PPV was negligible.[62] This is in line with a study by Mori and colleagues, assessing clarithromycin allergy in children, which reports a sensitivity and specificity of 75% and 90%, respectively.[63] Predictive values for azithromycin have been assessed by Barni and colleagues, reporting a PPV of 75% and an NPV of 50%, which is much lower compared with clarithromycin.[54] It has been demonstrated that SPT results were not compatible with ingestion challenge results, emphasizing the important role of the ingestion challenge in diagnosing macrolide allergy. There are no studies assessing the predictive values for the ingestion challenge of macrolides in children.

Similarly, skin tests and in vitro tests for sulfonamide antibiotic allergy are reported to be unreliable.[64] Undergoing a direct ingestion challenge should be considered on an individual basis based on patient need and risk-benefit ratio. Recent data support the use of an ingestion challenge as an effective mechanism to delabel sulfa antibiotic allergy[64,65].

It was suggested that SPT and IDT for fluoroquinolones and tetracyclines are associated with high risk for false-positive results due to the potential for mast cell activation.[66] Hence, the ingestion challenge for quinolones and tetracyclines is currently the most appropriate diagnostic tool.

Management

The management of macrolide antibiotic allergy includes avoidance of the culprit drug. Macrolides are unlikely to be cross-reactive; however, there are few published case reports describing cross-reactivity among different macrolides, possibly due to similarities in the chemical structure.[66] Cross-reactivity among the macrolides is less commonly reported than other antibiotic categories, such as beta-lactams.[33] Desensitization to macrolide hypersensitivity has been shown to be successful in a few cases.[66]

Sulfonamide antibiotic allergy management involves immediate withdrawal of the culprit drug and prescription of a safe alternative. While there is limited evidence on the cross-reactivity between sulfonamides, it seems unlikely that sulfonamide antimicrobials and sulfonamide nonantimicrobials would cross-react due to differences in chemical structure.[64] Desensitization is possible among patients with mild reactions and is especially indicated among patients with human immunodeficiency virus who require prophylactic sulfonamides. Multiple different protocols have been published, with the majority updosing over the span of several days.[66] Desensitization for patients with anaphylaxis is rare. However, there has been one successful published protocol to date.[64] When possible, attempts should be made to delabel the patient of sulfa antibiotic allergy.[65]

For other non–beta-lactam antibiotics, there is lack of data on potential cross-reactivity. The safest approach among patients with tetracycline hypersensitivity is to change to an alternative drug with a similar antibiotic spectrum.[67] Desensitization protocols have been described for patients allergic to tetracycline.[67] Cross-reactivity among fluoroquinolones has been demonstrated in a handful of published case reports.[66] Given that there is some evidence, other fluoroquinolone antibiotics should be avoided. Desensitization is also a management option for patients with hypersensitivity to fluoroquinolones; however, many of these can also be delabeled using ingestion challenge.[66] Fluoroquinolones often cause hives and symptoms that mimic IgE-mediated reactions; however, they are known to interact with MRGPRX2 and cause non–IgE-mediated mast cell activation. If the latter, antihistamines are helpful to allow continued dosing.

NONSTEROIDAL ANTI-INFLAMMATORY DRUGS
Presentation

Following antibiotics, NSAIDs are one of the most common reported causes for adverse drug reaction (ADR) in children, with a self-reported prevalence of 0.7%[68] In a cohort of 211 Thai children with a median age of 4, NSAIDs were considered causal in 4.7% of ADR,[69] while in a cohort from Latin America that included 862 patients (178 children), NSAIDs represented the majority of culprit agents at 52.3% with an increase incidence in children and adults compared with an elderly population.[70] Differences in prevalence may be attributed to a difference in populations, differences in existing types of prescribed and over-the-counter used NSAIDS and/or due to differences in diagnostic strategies.[71]

The most commonly implicated NSAID is ibuprofen.[72–76] The main identified risk factors for NSAID hypersensitivity are older age, atopy, chronic urticaria, a previous anaphylaxis history, the number of concomitant drugs, and a family history of NSAID allergy.[72,75–82]

Approach and Diagnosis

Because of the low accuracy of the available skin testing for NSAIDs, various authors do not employ these investigational tools.[74,76,83] In general, SPT has been described with approximately 5% to 33% positivity rate.[70,73,75,80,81,84,85]

Ingestion challenge remains the gold standard for NSAID assessment allowing to confirm or rule out the allergy. The rate of positive ingestion challenge reported in the literature varies from 11%[74,80] to 30%[70,72,73,75,81,85] for the majority of the studies. There is no consensus among the different studies regarding the number of steps required for ingestion challenge with some studies indicating only a maximum of steps performed for drug challenge (e.g., less than 5 escalating steps).[72,73,86] Furthermore, a negative drug challenge might not necessarily predict tolerance as reported in some pediatric cohorts whereby 4% to 12% of the patients described a reaction following a negative challenge test,[86,87] allowing the calculation of an NPV of 96.3%.[87] Following allergy confirmation to a COX-1 NSAID, alternative agents can be considered such as acetaminophen (at <1 g/d, when it has minimal COX-1 inhibition[88]) as well as COX-2 agents.[89] Following this literature review, we believe that a direct ingestion challenge in children in a well-supervised and equipped setting is the preferred diagnostic strategy.

SEVERE CUTANEOUS ADVERSE REACTIONS IN CHILDREN
Presentation

In the pediatric population, the most common SCAR phenotypes were reported are SJS/TEN,[19,70,74,83,90–95] DRESS,[19,92,93,96–98] and AGEP.[92,93,97] Some reports suggest, however, that SCARs are less prevalent and have a better prognosis being less associated with comorbidities in the pediatric population compared with an adult population.[70,92,95,96]

The main reported culprit drugs for SJS/TEN in children are antibiotics such as beta-lactams and sulfonamides[19,74,90,92,95,99,100] followed by anticonvulsant drugs such as phenobarbital, carbamazepine, and phenytoin.[90–92,95] Besides drugs, *Mycoplasma pneumoniae,* cytomegalovirus, and adenovirus were considered causal in pediatric cases of SJS/TEN.[19,90,92,93,101] While the literature described a mortality of up to 5% for SJS and up to 35% for TEN,[93,95] in some pediatric cohorts this was reported at 1.5%[90]–2.9%.[92] Antibiotics such as amoxicillin-clavulanate,[92,93] vancomycin,[74] and antiepileptics[93] such as phenytoin,[19] carbamazepine[92,96] are then main culprits associated with DRESS syndrome in children. Antibiotics, such as amoxicillin, were the most commonly suspected cause of AGEP in the pediatric population.[92]

Because of the increased prevalence of infections and inflammatory manifestations such as Kawasaki disease in children, the diagnosis of SCAR may be challenging.[96] During the acute phase, skin biopsy can help confirm the diagnosis.[92] In terms of acute management, similar to adults, besides adequate bedside care, SJS/TEN is often treated with systemic corticosteroids and intravenous immunoglobulins.[92,93,95] DRESS and AGEP are treated with drug withdrawal and oral antihistamines with some of the DRESS cases also receiving systemic corticosteroids[93] and intravenous immunoglobulins.[92,96]

Approach and Diagnosis

Six months after the complete resolution of the skin condition, these reactions can be evaluated in the allergy clinic by IDT and patch testing (PT) as well as immunologic assays such as the lymphocyte transformation tests (LTT), enzyme-linked ImmunoSpot, and flow cytometric lymphocyte activation tests.[19,93,102,103] PT has been used in various pediatric studies with concentrations of 5%, 10%, 20%, 30%, and 50% in petrolatum (e.g., beta-lactams such as benzyl-penicillin, ampicillin, amoxicillin, and anticonvulsants such as carbamazepine, phenobarbital, and lamotrigine).[73,83,92,93] Various pediatric reports showed positive PT results in cases of SJS[74] as well as positive PT and delayed IDT for DRESS.[74,104] However, in larger cohorts, PT has shown poor sensitivity in children (<5%).[73] Further studies are required to establish the validity of PT in the pediatric population. IDT with delayed reading is rarely described in the pediatric population.[93] Similar to the adult population, delayed IDT was positive in DRESS.[93] In cases of SCAR, ingestion challenge is considered contra-indicated. However, recent reports questioned this practice allowing rechallenge in specific situations in resource-poor settings whereby there are no alternative drugs.[105]

In terms of *in vitro* testing, reports are limited to case reports and case series. For example, LTT was a valuable tool in various pediatric reports such as a case of phenytoin associated with DRESS,[19] a case of amoxicillin and ibuprofen associated TEN.[19] A large pediatric cohort demonstrated 12/15 (80%) positive LTT in a cohort of varied phenotypes including DRESS and SJS/TEN.[93]

Genetic associations have been established that have both a preventive and diagnostic role. In a Thai pediatric population, an association has been described between carbamazepine-induced SJS/TEN and HLA-B*1502.[90] This has led to preventive genotyping before treatment with carbamazepine in these regions. As more genetic associations are described in association with SCAR, HLA testing may become increasingly useful for screening testing and diagnosis.

SUMMARY

In the last decade, there has been a paradigm shift in the diagnosis of drug allergy, mainly penicillin derivatives, in the pediatric population. Cases of reported nonsevere reactions (defined as the presence of rash with no vesicles/bullous lesions and no mucosal involvement) to penicillin derivatives should be assessed with a direct ingestion challenge.[106] However, there is still a lack of sufficient evidence regarding the best diagnostic approach for non–beta-lactam antibiotics and NSAIDs, and scarce data on the best diagnostic tests for SCAR. Our review will assist allergists and physicians treating children to appropriately diagnose and manage drug allergy. Appropriate diagnosis is crucial to prevent mislabeling, increase the use of appropriate first-line antibiotics, and decrease the use of alternative broad-spectrum antibiotics.

CLINICS CARE POINTS

- Drug allergy labels in children are costly and are correlated with adverse health outcomes.
- Children presenting with adverse drug reactions potentially allergic in nature should be assessed by an allergist, as true drug allergies are uncommon.
- Cases of nonsevere reactions to penicillin derivatives can be appropriately assessed by a direct ingestion test.
- In cases of negative diagnostic workup for drug allergy, patient/parent education, and medical record delabeling are crucial.
- In cases of positive diagnostic workup for drug allergy, the use of that drug is contraindicated, and an appropriate alternative or, in certain cases, desensitization can be considered.

DISCLOSURE

The authors have nothing to disclose.

REFERENCES

1. Macy E, Contreras R. Health care use and serious infection prevalence associated with penicillin "allergy" in hospitalized patients: A cohort study. J Allergy Clin Immunol 2014;133(3):790–6.
2. Mattingly TJ 2nd, Fulton A, Lumish RA, et al. The Cost of Self-Reported Penicillin Allergy: A Systematic Review. J Allergy Clin Immunol Pract 2018;6(5):1649–1654 e1644.
3. Park JS, Suh DI. Drug Allergy in Children: What Should We Know? Clin Exp Pediatr 2020;63(6):203–10.
4. Gabrielli S, Clarke AE, Eisman H, et al. Disparities in rate, triggers, and management in pediatric and adult cases of suspected drug-induced anaphylaxis in Canada. Immun Inflamm Dis 2018;6(1):3–12.
5. Macy E, Poon K-YT. Self-reported Antibiotic Allergy Incidence and Prevalence: Age and Sex Effects. Am J Med 2009;122(8):778.e771–7.
6. Norton AE, Konvinse K, Phillips EJ, et al. Antibiotic Allergy in Pediatrics. Pediatrics 2018;141(5):e20172497.
7. Exius R, Gabrielli S, Abrams EM, et al. Establishing amoxicillin allergy in children through direct graded oral challenge (GOC): evaluating risk factors for positive challenges, safety, and risk of cross reactivity to cephalosporines. J Allergy Clin Immunol Pract 2021;9(11):4060–6.
8. Picard M, Robitaille G, Karam F, et al. Cross-Reactivity to Cephalosporins and Carbapenems in Penicillin-Allergic Patients: Two Systematic Reviews and Meta-Analyses. J Allergy Clin Immunol Pract 2019;7(8):2722–38.e2725.
9. Touati N, Cardoso B, Delpuech M, et al. Cephalosporin Hypersensitivity: Descriptive Analysis, Cross-Reactivity, and Risk Factors. J Allergy Clin Immunol Pract 2021;9(5):1994–2000.e1995.
10. Mori F, Liccioli G, Piccorossi A, et al. The Diagnosis of Ceftriaxone Hypersensitivity in a Paediatric Population. Int Arch Allergy Immunol 2019;178(3):272–6.
11. Yilmaz Topal O, Kulhas Celik I, Turgay Yagmur I, et al. Evaluation of Clinical Properties and Diagnostic Test Results of Cephalosporin Allergy in Children. Int Arch Allergy Immunol 2021;182(8):709–15.

12. Tonson la Tour A, Michelet M, Eigenmann PA, et al. Natural History of Benign Nonimmediate Allergy to Beta-Lactams in Children: A Prospective Study in Re-treated Patients After a Positive and a Negative Provocation Test. J Allergy Clin Immunol Pract 2018;6(4):1321–6.

13. Mill C, Primeau M-N, Medoff E, et al. Assessing the Diagnostic Properties of a Graded Oral Provocation Challenge for the Diagnosis of Immediate and Nonim-mediate Reactions to Amoxicillin in Children. JAMA Pediatr 2016;170(6): e160033.

14. Ponvert C, Perrin Y, Bados-Albiero A, et al. Allergy to betalactam antibiotics in children: results of a 20-year study based on clinical history, skin and challenge tests. Pediatr Allergy Immunol 2011;22(4):411–8.

15. Gomes ER, Brockow K, Kuyucu S, et al. Drug hypersensitivity in children: report from the pediatric task force of the EAACI Drug Allergy Interest Group. Allergy 2016;71(2):149–61.

16. Heckbert SR, Stryker WS, Coltin KL, et al. Serum sickness in children after anti-biotic exposure: Estimates of occurrence and morbidity in a health maintenance organization population. Am J Epidemiol 1990;132(2):336–42.

17. Esmaeilzadeh H, Farjadian S, Alyasin S, et al. Epidemiology of Severe Cuta-neous Adverse Drug Reaction and Its HLA Association among Pediatrics. Iran J Pharm Res 2019;18(1):506–22.

18. Oh HL, Kang DY, Kang HR, et al. Severe Cutaneous Adverse Reactions in Korean Pediatric Patients: A Study From the Korea SCAR Registry. Allergy Asthma Immunol Res 2019;11(2):241–53.

19. Belver MT, Michavila A, Bobolea I, et al. Severe delayed skin reactions related to drugs in the paediatric age group: A review of the subject by way of three cases (Stevens-Johnson syndrome, toxic epidermal necrolysis and DRESS). Allergol Immunopathol (Madr) 2016;44(1):83–95.

20. Lebrun-Vignes B, Guy C, Jean-Pastor M-J, et al. Is acetaminophen associated with a risk of Stevens-Johnson syndrome and toxic epidermal necrolysis? Anal-ysis of the French Pharmacovigilance Database. Br J Clin Pharmacol 2018; 84(2):331–8.

21. Jeimy S, Ben-Shoshan M, Abrams EM, et al. Practical guide for evaluation and management of beta-lactam allergy: position statement from the Canadian So-ciety of Allergy and Clinical Immunology. Allergy Asthma Clin Immunol 2020; 16(1):95.

22. Trubiano JA, Vogrin S, Chua KYL, et al. Development and Validation of a Peni-cillin Allergy Clinical Decision Rule. JAMA Intern Med 2020;180(5):745–52.

23. Vezir E, Dibek Misirlioglu E, Civelek E, et al. Direct oral provocation tests in non-immediate mild cutaneous reactions related to beta-lactam antibiotics. Pediatr Allergy Immunol 2016;27(1):50–4.

24. Delli Colli L, Gabrielli S, Abrams EM, et al. Differentiating Between β-Lactam-Induced Serum Sickness-Like Reactions and Viral Exanthem in Children Using a Graded Oral Challenge. J Allergy Clin Immunol Pract 2021;9(2):916–21.

25. Drug Allergy: An Updated Practice Parameter. Ann Allergy Asthma Immunol 2010;105(4):259–73.e278.

26. Caubet J-C, Kaiser L, Lemaître B, et al. The role of penicillin in benign skin rashes in childhood: a prospective study based on drug rechallenge. J Allergy Clin Immunol 2011;127(1):218–22.

27. Romano A, Gaeta F, Valluzzi RL, et al. Diagnosing Hypersensitivity Reactions to Cephalosporins in Children. Pediatrics 2008;122(3):521.

28. Yoon SY, Park SY, Kim S, et al. Validation of the cephalosporin intradermal skin test for predicting immediate hypersensitivity: a prospective study with drug challenge. Allergy 2013;68(7):938–44.

29. Attari Z, Gabrielli S, Torabi B, et al. Diagnosis Of Cephalosporin Allergy Through Graded Oral Challenge. J Allergy Clin Immunol 2019;143(2):AB195.

30. Picard M, Paradis L, Bégin P, et al. Skin testing only with penicillin G in children with a history of penicillin allergy. Ann Allergy Asthma Immunol 2014;113(1): 75–81.

31. Cernadas JR. Desensitization to antibiotics in children. Pediatr Allergy Immunol 2013;24(1):3–9.

32. Callero A, Berroa F, Infante S, et al. Tolerance to cephalosporins in nonimmediate hypersensitivity to penicillins in pediatric patients. J Investig Allergol Clin Immunol 2014;24(2):134–6.

33. Calamelli E, Caffarelli C, Franceschini F, et al. A practical management of children with antibiotic allergy. Acta Biomed 2019;90(3-S):11–9.

34. Mirakian R, Leech SC, Krishna MT, et al. Management of allergy to penicillins and other beta-lactams. Clin Exp Allergy 2015;45(2):300–27.

35. Zagursky RJ, Pichichero ME. Cross-reactivity in β-Lactam Allergy. J Allergy Clin Immunol Pract 2018;6(1):72–81.e71.

36. Abrams E, Netchiporouk E, Miedzybrodzki B, et al. Antibiotic Allergy in Children: More than Just a Label. Int Arch Allergy Immunol 2019;180(2):103–12.

37. Frumin J, Gallagher JC. Allergic cross-sensitivity between penicillin, carbapenem, and monobactam antibiotics: what are the chances? Ann Pharmacother 2009;43(2):304–15.

38. Romano A, Viola M, Guéant-Rodriguez RM, et al. Brief communication: tolerability of meropenem in patients with IgE-mediated hypersensitivity to penicillins. Ann Intern Med 2007;146(4):266–9.

39. Vyles D, Antoon JW, Norton A, et al. Children with reported penicillin allergy: Public health impact and safety of delabeling. Ann Allergy Asthma Immunol 2020;124(6):558–65.

40. Pichichero ME. Cephalosporins can be prescribed safely for penicillin-allergic patients. J Fam Pract 2006;55(2):106–12.

41. Caimmi S, Caffarelli C, Saretta F, et al. Drug desensitization in allergic children. Acta Biomed 2019;90(3-s):20–9.

42. Diaferio L, Giovannini M, Clark E, et al. Protocols for drug allergy desensitization in children. Expert Rev Clin Immunol 2020;16(1):91–100.

43. Sullivan TJ, Yecies LD, Shatz GS, et al. Desensitization of patients allergic to penicillin using orally administered beta-lactam antibiotics. J Allergy Clin Immunol 1982;69(3):275–82.

44. Stark BJ, Earl HS, Gross GN, et al. Acute and chronic desensitization of penicillin-allergic patients using oral penicillin. J Allergy Clin Immunol 1987; 79(3):523–32.

45. De Maria C, Lebel D, Desroches A, et al. Simple intravenous antimicrobial desensitization method for pediatric patients. Am J Health Syst Pharm 2002; 59(16):1532–6.

46. Sousa-Pinto B, Araújo L, Freitas A, et al. Hospitalizations in Children with a Penicillin Allergy Label: An Assessment of Healthcare Impact. Int Arch Allergy Immunol 2018;176(3–4):234–8.

47. Jones TW, Fino N, Olson J, et al. The impact of beta-lactam allergy labels on hospitalized children. Infect Control Hosp Epidemiol 2021;42(3):318–24.

48. Picard M, Bégin P, Bouchard H, et al. Treatment of patients with a history of penicillin allergy in a large tertiary-care academic hospital. J Allergy Clin Immunol Pract 2013;1(3):252–7.

49. Vyles D, Mistry RD, Heffner V, et al. Reported Knowledge and Management of Potential Penicillin Allergy in Children. Acad Pediatr 2019;19(6):684–90.

50. Shenoy ES, Macy E, Rowe T, et al. Evaluation and Management of Penicillin Allergy: A Review. JAMA 2019;321(2):188–99.

51. Picard M, Paradis L, Nguyen M, et al. Outpatient penicillin use after negative skin testing and drug challenge in a pediatric population. Allergy Asthma Proc 2012;33(2):160–4.

52. Ratzon R, Reshef A, Efrati O, et al. Impact of an extended challenge on the effectiveness of β-lactam hypersensitivity investigation. Ann Allergy Asthma Immunol 2016;116(4):329–33.

53. Burgos RM, Reynolds KM, Williams J, et al. Trimethoprim-Sulfamethoxazole Associated Drug-Induced Liver Injury in Pediatrics: A Systematic Review. Pediatr Infect Dis J 2020;39(9):824–9.

54. Barni S, Butti D, Mori F, et al. Azithromycin is more allergenic than clarithromycin in children with suspected hypersensitivity reaction to macrolides. J Investig Allergol Clin Immunol 2015;25(2):128–32.

55. Lebel M. Pharmacokinetic properties of clarithromycin: A comparison with erythromycin and azithromycin. Can J Infect Dis 1993;4(3):148–52.

56. Guvenir H, Dibek Misirlioglu E, Capanoglu M, et al. Proven Non-β-Lactam Antibiotic Allergy in Children. Int Arch Allergy Immunol 2016;169(1):45–50.

57. Schnyder B, Pichler WJ. Allergy to sulfonamides. J Allergy Clin Immunol 2013; 131(1). 256-257.e251-255.

58. Childs-Kean LM, Shaeer KM, Varghese Gupta S, et al. Aminoglycoside Allergic Reactions. Pharmacy (Basel) 2019;7(3).

59. Huang V, Clayton NA, Welker KH. Glycopeptide Hypersensitivity and Adverse Reactions. Pharmacy (Basel). 2020;8(2).

60. Lam BD, Miller MM, Sutton AV, et al. Vancomycin and DRESS: A retrospective chart review of 32 cases in Los Angeles, California. J Am Acad Dermatol 2017;77(5):973–5.

61. Grinlington L, Choo S, Cranswick N, et al. Non-β-Lactam Antibiotic Hypersensitivity Reactions. Pediatrics 2020;145(1).

62. Suleyman A, Yucel E, Sipahi Cimen S, et al. Clarithromycin hypersensitivity in children: Is there a link with β-lactam hypersensitivity? Pediatr Allergy Immunol 2021;32(8):1781–7.

63. Mori F, Barni S, Pucci N, et al. Sensitivity and specificity of skin tests in the diagnosis of clarithromycin allergy. Ann Allergy Asthma Immunol 2010; 104(5):417–9.

64. Khan DA, Knowles SR, Shear NH. Sulfonamide Hypersensitivity: Fact and Fiction. J Allergy Clin Immunol Pract 2019;7(7):2116–23.

65. Krantz MS, Stone CA Jr, Abreo A, et al. Oral challenge with trimethoprim-sulfamethoxazole in patients with "sulfa" antibiotic allergy. J Allergy Clin Immunol Pract 2020;8(2):757–60.e754.

66. Sánchez-Borges M, Thong B, Blanca M, et al. Hypersensitivity reactions to non beta-lactam antimicrobial agents, a statement of the WAO special committee on drug allergy. World Allergy Organ J 2013;6(1):18.

67. Maciag MC, Ward SL, O'Connell AE, et al. Hypersensitivity to tetracyclines: Skin testing, graded challenge, and desensitization regimens. Ann Allergy Asthma Immunol 2020;124(6):589–93.

68. Rebelo Gomes E, Fonseca J, Araujo L, et al. Drug allergy claims in children: from self-reporting to confirmed diagnosis. Clin Exp Allergy 2008;38(1): 191–8.

69. Indradat S, Veskitkul J, Pacharn P, et al. Provocation proven drug allergy in Thai children with adverse drug reactions. Asian Pac J Allergy Immunol 2016;34(1): 59–64.

70. Jares EJ, Sanchez-Borges M, Cardona-Villa R, et al. Multinational experience with hypersensitivity drug reactions in Latin America. Ann Allergy Asthma Immunol 2014;113(3):282–9.

71. Dona I, Blanca-Lopez N, Cornejo-Garcia JA, et al. Characteristics of subjects experiencing hypersensitivity to non-steroidal anti-inflammatory drugs: patterns of response. Clin Exp Allergy 2011;41(1):86–95.

72. Mori F, Atanaskovic-Markovic M, Blanca-Lopez N, et al. A Multicenter Retrospective Study on Hypersensitivity Reactions to Nonsteroidal Anti-Inflammatory Drugs (NSAIDs) in Children: A Report from the European Network on Drug Allergy (ENDA) Group. J Allergy Clin Immunol Pract 2020;8(3): 1022–1031 e1021.

73. Arikoglu T, Aslan G, Batmaz SB, et al. Diagnostic evaluation and risk factors for drug allergies in children: from clinical history to skin and challenge tests. Int J Clin Pharm 2015;37(4):583–91.

74. Piccorossi A, Liccioli G, Barni S, et al. Epidemiology and drug allergy results in children investigated in allergy unit of a tertiary-care paediatric hospital setting. Ital J Pediatr 2020;46(1):5.

75. Arikoglu T, Aslan G, Yildirim DD, et al. Discrepancies in the diagnosis and classification of nonsteroidal anti-inflammatory drug hypersensitivity reactions in children. Allergol Int 2017;66(3):418–24.

76. Yilmaz Topal O, Kulhas Celik I, Turgay Yagmur I, et al. Results of NSAID provocation tests and difficulties in the classification of children with nonsteroidal anti-inflammatory drug hypersensitivity. Ann Allergy Asthma Immunol 2020;125(2): 202–7.

77. Hassani A, Ponvert C, Karila C, et al. Hypersensitivity to cyclooxygenase inhibitory drugs in children: a study of 164 cases. Eur J Dermatol 2008; 18(5):561–5.

78. Blanca-Lopez N, JT M, Dona I, et al. Value of the clinical history in the diagnosis of urticaria/angioedema induced by NSAIDs with cross-intolerance. Clin Exp Allergy 2013;43(1):85–91.

79. Sanchez-Borges M, Capriles-Hulett A. Atopy is a risk factor for non-steroidal anti-inflammatory drug sensitivity. Ann Allergy Asthma Immunol 2000;84(1): 101–6.

80. Yilmaz O, Ertoy Karagol IH, Bakirtas A, et al. Challenge-proven nonsteroidal anti-inflammatory drug hypersensitivity in children. Allergy 2013;68(12): 1555–61.

81. Cavkaytar O, Arik Yilmaz E, Karaatmaca B, et al. Different Phenotypes of Non-Steroidal Anti-Inflammatory Drug Hypersensitivity during Childhood. Int Arch Allergy Immunol 2015;167(3):211–21.

82. Cousin M, Chiriac A, Molinari N, et al. Phenotypical characterization of children with hypersensitivity reactions to NSAIDs. Pediatr Allergy Immunol 2016;27(7): 743–8.

83. Atanaskovic-Markovic M, Gaeta F, Gavrovic-Jankulovic M, et al. Diagnosing multiple drug hypersensitivity in children. Pediatr Allergy Immunol 2012;23(8): 785–91.

84. Tugcu GD, Cavkaytar O, Sekerel BE, et al. Actual drug allergy during childhood: Five years' experience at a tertiary referral centre. Allergol Immunopathol (Madr) 2015;43(6):571–8.

85. Topal E, Celiksoy MH, Catal F, et al. The value of the clinical history for the diagnosis of immediate nonsteroidal anti-inflammatory drug hypersensitivity and safe alternative drugs in children. Allergy Asthma Proc 2016;37(1):57–63.

86. Misirlioglu ED, Toyran M, Capanoglu M, et al. Negative predictive value of drug provocation tests in children. Pediatr Allergy Immunol 2014;25(7):685–90.

87. Topal OY, Ilknur KC, Irem YT, et al. Negative predictive value of provocation tests for nonsteroidal anti-inflammatory drugs in children. Allergy Asthma Proc 2020; 41(4):285–9.

88. Doña I, Blanca-López N, Jagemann LR, et al. Response to a selective COX-2 inhibitor in patients with urticaria/angioedema induced by nonsteroidal anti-inflammatory drugs. Allergy 2011;66(11):1428–33.

89. Corzo JL, Zambonino MA, Munoz C, et al. Tolerance to COX-2 inhibitors in children with hypersensitivity to nonsteroidal anti-inflammatory drugs. Br J Dermatol 2014;170(3):725–9.

90. Singalavanija S, Limpongsanurak W. Stevens-Johnson syndrome in Thai children: a 29-year study. J Med Assoc Thai 2011;94(Suppl 3):S85–90.

91. Li L, Zheng S, Chen Y. Stevens-Johnson syndrome and acute vanishing bile duct syndrome after the use of amoxicillin and naproxen in a child. J Int Med Res 2019;47(9):4537–43.

92. Dibek Misirlioglu E, Guvenir H, Bahceci S, et al. Severe Cutaneous Adverse Drug Reactions in Pediatric Patients: A Multicenter Study. J Allergy Clin Immunol Pract 2017;5(3):757–63.

93. Liccioli G, Mori F, Parronchi P, et al. Aetiopathogenesis of severe cutaneous adverse reactions (SCARs) in children: A 9-year experience in a tertiary care paediatric hospital setting. Clin Exp Allergy 2020;50(1):61–73.

94. Pena MA, Perez S, Zazo MC, et al. A Case of Toxic Epidermal Necrolysis Secondary to Acetaminophen in a Child. Curr Drug Saf 2016;11(1):99–101.

95. Cekic S, Canitez Y, Sapan N. Evaluation of the patients diagnosed with Stevens Johnson syndrome and toxic epidermal necrolysis: a single center experience. Turk Pediatri Ars 2016;51(3):152–8.

96. Kim GY, Anderson KR, Davis DMR, et al. Drug reaction with eosinophilia and systemic symptoms (DRESS) in the pediatric population: A systematic review of the literature. J Am Acad Dermatol 2020;83(5):1323–30.

97. Dilek N, Ozkol HU, Akbas A, et al. Cutaneous drug reactions in children: a multicentric study. Postepy Dermatol Alergol 2014;31(6):368–71.

98. Singvijarn P, Manuyakorn W, Mahasirimongkol S, et al. Association of HLA genotypes with Beta-lactam antibiotic hypersensitivity in children. Asian Pac J Allergy Immunol 2021;39(3):197–205.

99. Lin YF, Yang CH, Sindy H, et al. Severe cutaneous adverse reactions related to systemic antibiotics. Clin Infect Dis 2014;58(10):1377–85.

100. Ferrandiz-Pulido C, Garcia-Patos V. A review of causes of Stevens-Johnson syndrome and toxic epidermal necrolysis in children. Arch Dis Child 2013;98(12): 998–1003.

101. McPherson T, Exton LS, Biswas S, et al. British Association of Dermatologists' guidelines for the management of Stevens-Johnson syndrome/toxic epidermal necrolysis in children and young people, 2018. Br J Dermatol 2019;181(1): 37–54.

102. Copaescu A, Gibson A, Li Y, et al. An Updated Review of the Diagnostic Methods in Delayed Drug Hypersensitivity. Front Pharmacol 2021;(1928):11.
103. Bergmann MM, Caubet JC. Role of in vivo and in vitro Tests in the Diagnosis of Severe Cutaneous Adverse Reactions (SCAR) to Drug. Curr Pharm Des 2019; 25(36):3872–80.
104. Santiago F, Goncalo M, Vieira R, et al. Epicutaneous patch testing in drug hypersensitivity syndrome (DRESS). Contact Derm 2010;62(1):47–53.
105. Lehloenya RJ, Isaacs T, Nyika T, et al. Early high-dose intravenous corticosteroids rapidly arrest Stevens Johnson syndrome and drug reaction with eosinophilia and systemic symptoms recurrence on drug re-exposure. J Allergy Clin Immunol Pract 2021;9(1):582–584 e581.
106. Iammatteo M, Lezmi G, Confino-Cohen R, et al. Direct Challenges for the Evaluation of Beta-Lactam Allergy: Evidence and Conditions for Not Performing Skin Testing. J Allergy Clin Immunol Pract 2021;9(8):2947–56.
107. Ibáñez MD, Rodríguez del Río P, Lasa EM, et al. Prospective assessment of diagnostic tests for pediatric penicillin allergy: From clinical history to challenge tests. Ann Allergy Asthma Immunol 2018;121(2):235–44.e233.
108. Barni S, Mori F, Sarti L, et al. Utility of skin testing in children with a history of non-immediate reactions to amoxicillin. Clin Exp Allergy 2015;45(9):1472–4.
109. Kulhas Celik I, Turgay Yagmur I, Yilmaz Topal O, et al. Diagnostic value and safety of penicillin skin tests in children with immediate penicillin allergy. Allergy Asthma Proc 2020;41(6):442–8.

The Use of Electronic Health Records to Study Drug-Induced Hypersensitivity Reactions from 2000 to 2021

A Systematic Review

Fatima Bassir, MPH[a,b,1,*], Sheril Varghese, B.A.[a,1],
Liqin Wang, PhD[c], Yen Po Chin, MD, MBI[c], Li Zhou, MD, PhD[c]

KEYWORDS

- Drug hypersensitivity • Electronic health record • Allergy documentation
- Drug allergy label • Allergy epidemiology

KEY POINTS

- The widespread adoption of electronic health records has greatly enhanced the ability to study the epidemiology and management of a broad range of drug hypersensitivity reactions.
- There is a clear need for accurate drug allergy labeling, given that many patients are incorrectly labeled with a β-lactam allergy, undermining antimicrobial stewardship efforts.
- Although intended to promote safe drug prescribing practices, allergy alerting mechanisms lack specificity and clinical relevance, contributing to excessive override rates and alert fatigue.
- Accurate and complete clinical documentation in electronic health records is necessary to optimize the use of clinical decision support for drug hypersensitivity prevention.

Author Contributions: Please see author statement.
This research was supported with funding from the Agency for Healthcare Research and Quality (AHRQ) grant R01HS025375 and the National Institute of Allergy and Infectious Diseases (NIAID) of National Institute of Health (NIH) grant 1R01AI150295.
[a] Division of General Internal Medicine and Primary Care, Department of Medicine, Brigham and Women's Hospital, 399 Revolution Drive, Suite 1315, Somerville, MA 02145, USA; [b] Division of General Internal Medicine and Primary Care, Brigham and Women's Hospital, 399 Revolution Drive, Suite 1315, Somerville, MA 02145, USA; [c] Division of General Internal Medicine and Primary Care, Department of Medicine, Brigham and Women's Hospital, Harvard Medical School, 399 Revolution Drive, Suite 1315, Somerville, MA 02145, USA
[1] F. Bassir and S. Varghese have contributed equally to this work.
* Corresponding author. Division of General Internal Medicine and Primary Care, Brigham and Women's Hospital, 399 Revolution Drive, Suite 1315, Somerville, MA 02145.
E-mail address: fbassir@bwh.harvard.edu

Immunol Allergy Clin N Am 42 (2022) 453–497
https://doi.org/10.1016/j.iac.2022.01.004
0889-8561/22/© 2022 Elsevier Inc. All rights reserved.

INTRODUCTION

The severe morbidity and mortality caused by drug hypersensitivity reactions (DHRs) make them a serious public health concern.[1] For example, penicillin allergies are estimated to be responsible for approximately 75% of fatal anaphylactic cases in the United States, which cause 500 to 1000 deaths per year.[2] Although there has been increasing recognition of the importance of DHRs, their true incidence remains largely unknown.

With the rapid growth of information technology, the adoption and use of electronic health records (EHR) have greatly increased over the past several decades. The 2009 federal stimulus plan's Meaningful Use initiative significantly accelerated the EHR adoption process.[3] EHRs have since transformed the field of DHR research, significantly improving our ability to study epidemiology, prevention, case identification, and management of DHRs. With accumulated longitudinal data, EHRs have made it possible to identify large patient cohorts for clinical epidemiologic and pharmacogenetic studies and efficiently identify risk factors of DHRs.[4] The ability to identify large study cohorts would not have been possible without the centralized EHR and advanced computing techniques. Furthermore, the use of EHRs has paved the way for clinical decision support systems (CDSS), which have significantly enhanced safe drug prescribing practices and antimicrobial stewardship. Nevertheless, challenges still exist in using EHRs for clinical practice and research. We continue to see challenges and opportunities for improvements in drug allergy documentation, drug allergy delabeling, CDSS (eg, the counterproductive nature of overly frequent allergy alerts that contribute to clinician fatigue), and the epidemiology of DHRs.

Although prior efforts have been made to review the use of EHRs in specific areas of DHR research, there are no systematic reviews focused on the general utilization of EHR in this field. Our goal is to provide a comprehensive systematic review of the use of EHRs over the past 2 decades in DHR research across a broad spectrum of research topics.

MATERIALS AND METHODS
Data Sources and Searches

This review was conducted in compliance with the 2009 Preferred Reporting Items for Systemic Reviews and Meta-Analyses (PRISMA) statement.[5] We conducted systematic database searches to retrieve relevant articles from several databases, including PubMed, the Cumulative Index to Nursing and Allied Health Literature (CINAHL), Web of Science, ScienceDirect, and Ovid. Bias could not be evaluated according to the PRISMA guidelines because of the heterogeneity of study types included in the review. Through an iterative process, we refined our search queries and included our final search queries and articles retrieved in eTable 1 in the Supplement.

Inclusion and Exclusion Criteria

Inclusion criteria for this review required that all articles are (1) published between January 1, 2000, and June 30, 2021; (2) written in the English language; (3) included title, author(s), and abstract; and (4) mentioned EHR use and DHR in the abstract. Reviews and conference abstracts were excluded.

Study Selection

Search results from each query were exported, and duplicates were eliminated. The retrieved studies were screened by 3 independent reviewers (FB, SV, and YC) to assess whether they met the inclusion criteria. Via an iterative process, the reviewers identified major research topics across included studies. Then, 2 reviewers used the abstract to classify each study into one of the research topics. Any disagreements were adjudicated by a third reviewer (LW) via discussion until consensus was reached. Full-text reviews were conducted to extract relevant information from articles that were included in the review, including research topic(s), DHR discussed, and EHR database used if applicable.

RESULTS

We identified a total of 433 articles through our database search and included 140 articles in this systematic review (**Fig. 1**). Six main research topics were identified: (1) epidemiologic analysis of drug allergies (observational studies), (2) documentation of drug hypersensitivity (clinical documentation), (3) case management, (4) clinical decision support, (5) case identification, and (6) genetic studies. **Table 1** shows the definition and distribution of the articles to the 6 research topics.

Research Trends Over Time

Most of the articles (n = 129, 92.1%) were published in or after 2012 (**Fig. 2**), with the number of articles peaking in 2019 (n = 25, 17.9%). Articles discussing clinical

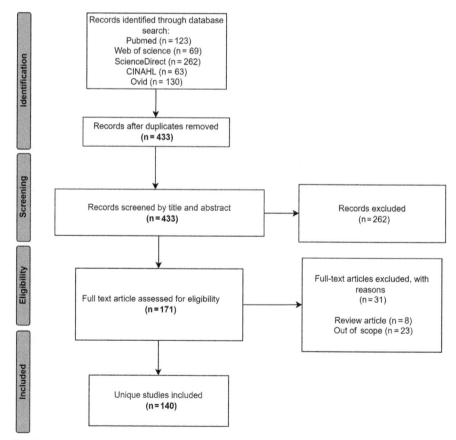

Fig. 1. Preferred Reporting Items for Systematic Reviews and Meta-Analyses (PRISMA) 2009 flow diagram. "Out of scope" were articles that were off topic, not written in English, or did not have an abstract.

Table 1
Overview of research topics for included articles (n = 140)

Research Topic	Description of Relevant Articles	n (%)
Observational Studies	Epidemiologic analysis of drug hypersensitivity, including incidence, prevalence, and risk factors of hypersensitivity reactions and drug-induced reactions using EHRs Excluded: articles primarily focusing on clinical treatment comparison	61 (43.6%)
Clinical Documentation	Documentation of drug hypersensitivity, such as evaluation of how well drug allergies were recorded or labeled in EHR	27 (19.3%)
Case Management	Review of allergy challenge testing and therefore delabeling in EHRs	22 (15.7%)
Clinical Decision Support	Overview of CDSS, including allergy alerts and clinician prescription order entry systems Excluded: If study did not focus on clinical utility or drug hypersensitivity	18 (12.9%)
Case Identification	Studies used EHR data to identify diverse patient cohorts or clinical cases with drug hypersensitivity	9 (6.4%)
Genetic Studies	Analysis of the relationship between genetic variation and drug hypersensitivity reactions	3 (2.1%)

documentation and observational studies were published throughout the review period. Dissimilarly, articles studying case management and genetic associations were published later in the study time window, starting from 2016 and 2019, respectively. The largest category of studies was observational studies (61 [43.6%]) followed by clinical documentation (27 [19.3%]), case management (22 [15.7%]), clinical decision support (CDS; 18 [12.9%]), case identification (9 [6.4%]), and genetic studies (3 [2.1%]).

RESEARCH TOPICS
Observational Studies

Observational studies, the largest category, included 61 epidemiologic studies (43.6%) of DHRs (**Table 2**). They were primarily designed as retrospective cohort analyses, using EHR data to identify patient cohorts, report the prevalence of adverse drug reactions (ADRs), and elucidate clinical associations with medication use. The main subcategory was dedicated to the discussion of the antibiotic drug class (n = 15, 24.6%), examining the prevalence of ADRs to β-lactams and secondary antibiotics.[6–13] Notably, the literature consistently reported that a significant proportion of ADRs (15.3%[14] -53.5%[15]) in hospitalized patients were attributed to antibiotics, specifically penicillin. The preponderance of research on penicillin allergies indicates the need for an accurate account of penicillin-related reactions, and improved care in the face of growing antimicrobial resistance.[9] Seven studies broadly examined the general incidence of DHRs in hospital systems, reporting rates as high as 35.5%[16]; however, the incidence rates among studies are not easily comparable as the study population and inclusion criteria varied. Common risk factors are sex,

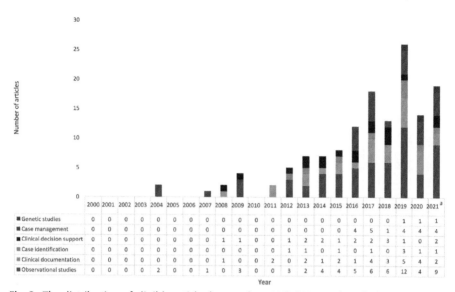

	2000	2001	2002	2003	2004	2005	2006	2007	2008	2009	2010	2011	2012	2013	2014	2015	2016	2017	2018	2019	2020	2021[a]
■ Genetic studies	0	0	0	0	0	0	0	0	0	0	0	0	0	0	0	0	0	0	0	1	1	1
■ Case management	0	0	0	0	0	0	0	0	0	0	0	0	0	0	0	0	0	4	5	1	4	4
■ Clinical decision support	0	0	0	0	0	0	0	0	1	1	0	0	1	2	2	1	2	2	3	1	0	2
■ Case identification	0	0	0	0	0	0	0	0	0	0	0	0	1	1	0	1	0	1	0	3	1	1
■ Clinical documentation	0	0	0	0	0	0	0	0	1	0	0	2	0	2	1	2	1	4	3	5	4	2
■ Observational studies	0	0	0	0	2	0	0	1	0	3	0	0	3	2	4	4	5	6	6	12	4	9

Year

Fig. 2. The distribution of eligible articles by year (n = 140). [a]2021 only includes articles published between January 1, 2021, and June 30th, 2021.

age, and having at least one documented allergy.[6,10,17] Females and older-aged patients in nearly all study populations exhibited higher rates of reported drug allergies.[12,14,15,18–20]

Observational articles applied different methods to extract information from select EHR sections. Nearly all antibiotic-focused studies[7–11,13,14,31,33,38–41] among other studies[18,26–28,30,34,36,49,57,59,61,62] (n = 25, 41.0%) explicitly referenced documented allergies and the problem list in EHRs. Several studies (n = 15, 24.6%) referenced using International Classification of Diseases, Ninth Revision (ICD-9) or International Classification of Diseases, Tenth Revision (ICD-10) codes for the purposes of identifying study cohorts or measuring the prevalence of specific comorbidities.[12,14,17,26,27,29,32,39,44,48,55,59,61,66] Six studies (9.8%) also used free-text comments and structured allergy entries with coded reactions to extract information.[26,28,36,43,57,59]

Clinical Documentation

Clinical documentation, a primary subject of this review, included a total of 27 articles (19.3%; **Table 3**). Seventeen studies assessed the accuracy of documentation and found that drug hypersensitivity records were incomplete and inconsistent with incorrectly labeled or categorized DHRs.[67–83] The documentation inaccuracies were mostly identified by retrospective chart reviews; however, 5 articles assessed documentation accuracy through patient interviews[72–74] and qualitative interviews with clinical staff.[76,77] There was significant heterogeneity in the delegation of drug hypersensitivity documentation among intake staff, pharmacists, physicians, registered nurses, nurse practitioners, physician assistants, and medical record technicians.

Five studies assessed approaches for improving drug allergy documentation, in particular, documentation completeness.[84–88] This was done by a pharmacist-driven protocol,[84] patient-facing medication reconciliation,[85] a novel standard format for recording drug allergies,[86] the use of CDS alerts based on antibiotic test dose results,[88] and an electronic version of a drug calendar.[87] Two articles discussed

Table 2
Summary of articles categorized as observational, organized by specific drug classes, general or specific adverse drug reactions, or both

Article	EHR Database/Data Source	Sample Size	Primary EHR Components[a]	Findings: Prevalence/Incidence, Risk Factors, Outcome, Other
Drug: Antibiotics (n = 15)				
Apter et al,[21] 2004	UK General Practice Research Database	3.4 million	D	57 of 3014 patients (0.15%) who had an allergic-like event after the first prescription experienced another event to the second prescription.
Albin et al,[7] 2014	Internal Medicine Associates Clinic of Mount Sinai Hospital/Epic EHR	1348	A, D	Documented reactions to penicillin allergy are rash (37%), hives (18.9%), and swelling (11.8%), and was most prevalent in African Americans, then Caucasians and Asians. Risk factors for penicillin allergy: sex (female)
May et al,[22] 2016	Mayo Clinic	927	A, D	IV penicillin did not increase risk of allergy in children (OR, 0.84).
Crotty et al,[10] 2017	NSLIJ Huntington Hospital, Huntington, NY	175	A, D	89% of 175 patients who received at least one dose of cefepime, ceftriaxone, cefoxitin, cephalexin, or meropenem had self-reported allergy to penicillin. 20% reported incidence of rash, whereas 63% said unknown reaction. 8 patients had an allergic reaction to penicillin, whereas 2 patients had an ADR to amoxicillin and piperacillin/tazobactam. Risk factor: history of self-reported allergy can increase risk of cross-sensitivity reactions, type of drug (cephalosporin)

Study	Source	N	Code	Findings
West et al.,[12] 2019	ResearchOne, UK	2.3 million	A, D	The prevalence of penicillin allergy was 5.9%. Risk factors: age (older), sex (female), and comorbidities
Liang et al,[13] 2020	Kaiser Permanente Southern California	6.1 million	A, B	More patients who received parenteral penicillin reported new allergic reactions (0.84%) than those who received oral penicillin (0.74%). 0.097% and 0.065% of parenteral and oral exposures, respectively, were confirmed anaphylaxis cases.
Lager et al,[6] 2009	University of Michigan Health System	211	A, D	Incidence of allergic-type reaction to carbapenem was 11% in patients with reported penicillin allergy, 5.2 times greater than those who did not report a penicillin allergy. Risk factor: documented penicillin allergy
Beltran et al,[8] 2015	Nationwide Children's Hospital Enterprise Data Warehouse (Epic EHR)	513	A, D	Cephalosporin resulted in one documented case of nonanaphylactic reaction when used as surgical prophylaxis. Clindamycin, the most common cephalosporin, produced an adverse rate of 1.5% in patients with penicillin allergy.
Macy et al,[23] 2015	Kaiser Permanente Southern California (Health Connect)	1.0 million	A, B, D	There were higher reports of allergy to cephalosporin among women (0.56%) than among men (0.43%). Anaphylaxis occurred in 5 oral exposures and 8 parenteral exposures. Clostridium difficile infection within 90 d (0.91%), nephropathy (0.15%), and all-cause death within 1 d (0.10%) were the most common serious ADR. No correlation with drug allergy history.

(continued on next page)

Table 2
(continued)

Article	EHR Database/Data Source	Sample Size	Primary EHR Components[a]	Findings: Prevalence/Incidence, Risk Factors, Outcome, Other
Blumenthal et al,[9] 2016	Partners HealthCare System—Mass General Brigham (Epic EHR)	96	A, D	ADR was observed in 21% of inpatient patients who received ceftaroline. No increased risk of ADR for patients with reported β-lactam allergy.
Alvarez-Arango et al,[24] 2021	Johns Hopkins Health System Corporation (JHHS) and Mass General Brigham (MGB) (Epic EHR)	4.5 million	A, D	0.3% of patients had documented vancomycin allergy with 42.1% reporting immediate phenotypes and 20.7% delayed reactions. 32% hypersensitivity reactions presented as rash and 16% as red man syndrome.
Butler et al,[11] 2018	Seattle Children's Hospital, University of Washington School of Medicine	17,496	B, D	1% of penicillin-allergic patients who received cefazolin experienced perioperative adverse drug reactions. Vancomycin associated with greater rates of ADR as prophylaxis.
Fosnot et al,[25] 2021	UCHealth System-Health Data Compass Data Warehouse project	690	A, D	Probable DHRs occurred in 0.9% of patients who received cefazolin, 1.4% of patients who received clindamycin, and 1.1% of patients who received vancomycin, not varying significantly.
Macy et al,[14] 2009	Kaiser Permanente	1127	A	15.3% of drug allergy reports reported at least one allergy to one antibiotic class. Risk factors: female, older age, and drug type (highest incidence w/sulfa class)
Salden et al,[17] 2015	Academic Health Care Center Terwijde at Leidsche Rijn Utrecht	8288	A	2.0% of sample had recorded allergy to β-lactams in the Dutch primary care system. Risk factors: age (very young), sex (female), and comorbidities (asthma, allergies, and skin disorders)

DRUG: Cancer therapy-related drugs (n = 7)

Lal et al,[26] 2009	University of Texas M. D.-Anderson Cancer Center	3746	D	Weekly paclitaxel infusions result in 1.5% rate of DHRs.
Kim et al,[27] 2012	Seoul National University Bundang Hospital	393	D	The prevalence rate of DHRs to oxaliplatin is 10.7%. Risk factors: higher dosage of oxaliplatin and lower dosage of dexamethasone
Jung et al,[28] 2014	Seoul National University Hospital	658	B, D	49.5% of patients who received rituximab experienced infusion-related reactions. Risk factors: certain types of lymphoma (CLL, intravascular B-cell lymphoma), high dosage, and rate of injection in first 30 min
Levin et al,[29] 2017	Partners HealthCare System—Mass General Brigham	67	A, D	51% of patients who experienced grade 1 reaction to rituximab can be safely rechallenged.
Welborn et al,[30] 2018	University of Texas MD Anderson Cancer Center	17	D	70.6% of patients with cutaneous ADE to tremelimumab experienced pruritis. Other reactions include eczematous dermatitis, morbilliform rash, vitiligo, xerosis, acneiform rash, and psoriasiform dermatitis.
Shazib et al,[31] 2020	Dana-Farber/Brigham and Women's Cancer Center	13	D	Of 13 patients, 4 had oral-only immune-related ADEs to programmed cell death-1 inhibitors. 10 had lichenoid lesions, 2 with erythema multiforme, 1 with graft vs host disease reactivation, and 8 with or without ulcerations.
Keiser et al,[32] 2021	University of Texas MD Anderson Cancer Center	64	B, D	91% of patients with cutaneous adverse events to immune checkpoint inhibitors were treated with topical steroids, oral antihistamines, or topical antihistamines, and 70% recovered from rash over 4 mo.

(continued on next page)

Table 2
(continued)

Article	EHR Database/Data Source	Sample Size	Primary EHR Components[a]	Findings: Prevalence/ Incidence, Risk Factors, Outcome, Other
DRUG: NSAIDs (n = 2)				
Blumenthal et al,[33] 2017	Partners HealthCare System (PHS)— Partners Enterprise Allergy Repository (PEAR)	62,719	A, B, C, D	1.7% had an ADR to prescription NSAIDs, 18.3% of which were hypersensitivity reactions. Risk factors: drug hypersensitivity reaction history, sex (female), autoimmune disease, and those who were prescribed the maximum standing NSAIDs dose
Li et al,[34] 2021	Partners HealthCare System	47,114	A, B, D	7.7% of patients with chronic back pain had active aspirin or NSAID adverse reaction.
DRUG: Opioids (n = 1)				
Inglis et al,[35] 2021	Royal Adelaide Hospital, Australia (Sunrise)	231,62 3	A, C, D	15.9% of ADR reports were due to opioids, with 64.7% reported as allergy and 35.3% as intolerance.
DRUG: Radiocontrast media (RCM)-related compounds (n = 4)				
Dillman et al,[36] 2007	University of Michigan Health System	78,353	D	The reaction frequency to IV gadolinium is 007%. 74% of reactions were mild, 19% were moderate, and 7% were severe. 50% had at least one risk factor to IV gadolinium reaction. Risk factors: allergic-like contrast reaction, a prior allergic reaction to a substance other than contrast media, or documented asthma

Power et al,[37] 2016	University Health Network, Toronto	19,074	D	The reaction rate to gadobutrol is 0.32% and the per-patient reaction basis was 0.43%. Risk factors: previous allergic-like reaction to gadolinium, previous reaction to any substance, history of asthma
Young et al,[38] 2019	NHS Tayside, Health Informatics Center, University of Dundee	22,897	D	0.01% of patients had DHRs to gadolinium-based contrast agents.
Lakshmanadoss et al,[39] 2012	Johns Hopkins Health System	234	D	71% of patients had a previous recorded allergy to iodinated contrast agents, 24% to iodine, and 5% to both. Most patients (77%) had skin rashes or unspecified reactions, whereas 8.5% had anaphylaxis.
DRUG: Statin (n = 1)				
Robison et al,[40] 2014	Intermountain HealthCare system (Murray, UT)	10,789	B, D	Patients with statin intolerance had a higher history of hypothyroidism (30.2%) compared with the control group (21.5%).
DRUG: Other (n = 3)				
Paisansinsup et al,[41] 2013	Park Nicollet Health Services EHR	1268	D	3.79% of patients prescribed allopurinol experienced an ADR. Risk factors: sex (female), older age, diabetes mellitus, diuretic use, and presence of tophi associated with possible ADR
Hall et al,[42] 2018	The Health Improvement Network, UK	70	C, D	Observed-to-expected ratio was 3.3 and 1.5 for convulsions and thrombocytopenia for those who received Optaflu, a trivalent seasonal influenza vaccine.

(continued on next page)

Table 2
(continued)

Article	EHR Database/Data Source	Sample Size	Primary EHR Components[a]	Findings: Prevalence/Incidence, Risk Factors, Outcome, Other
Laird et al,[43] 2020	UCHealth System	868	B, D	0.461% of patients who received fosaprepitant as prophylaxis for chemotherapy-related nausea had a systemic hypersensitivity reaction.
Adverse Drug Reaction (ADR): Broad/general overview (n = 6)				
Kidon and See,[44] 2004	KK Women's and Children's Hospital, Singapore	672	D	2.2% of pediatric patients had recorded ADR, 70% of which were due to antibiotics, specifically β-lactams. 18.5% were due to NSAIDs in Singapore. Risk factors: older age, male gender, and presence of asthma or other chronic disease
Macy et al,[15] 2014	Kaiser Permanente Southern California, Health Connect	105,614	B, D	The most common allergies in hospitalized patients were due to penicillin (16.7%), other nonantibiotics (12.7%), narcotics (11.7%), sulfonamides antibiotics (10.2%), and NSAIDs (7.1%), which altogether accounted for 58.4% of reported allergies. Risk factors: sex (female) and age (older)
Saager et al,[45] 2015	Cleveland Clinic Perioperative Health Documentation System	264	D	Overall incidence of intraoperative hypersensitivity reaction was 0.148%. 2 of 10,000 operations resulted in severe hypersensitivity reactions.

Study	Source	N	Rating	Findings
Zhou et al,[16] 2016	Partners HealthCare System/Partners' Enterprise-wide Allergy Repository (PEAR)	1.8 million	A, D	35.5% of patients reported at least one drug allergy with 1.95 allergies/patient. Risk factors: female sex, Caucasian race, antibiotic, statin, and ACE inhibitor use
Mendes et al,[46] 2019	Portuguese Catalog of Allergies and Other Adverse Reactions (CPARA)	380	D	0.4% of inpatients (380 patients) had DHRs over a 5-year period, 52.8% of which were associated with antibiotics, mainly β-lactam antibacterial use. 47.6% ADR were skin and subcutaneous tissue disorders and 41.3% were immune system disorders, specifically anaphylactic reactions (37.4%).
ADR: Anaphylaxis (n = 3)				
Wong et al,[20] 2019	Partners HealthCare System/Partners' Enterprise-wide Allergy Repository (PEAR)	2.7 million	A, C, D	13.8% of patient population had documented DHRs. 53.1% were associated with immediate reaction phenotypes. Risk factors: female sex, race/ethnicity, and drug type
Goh et al,[47] 2018	National University Hospital, KK Women's and Children's Hospital, and Tan Tock Seng Hospital, Singapore	426	B	45% of anaphylaxis cases were children in Singapore. Risk factors: food type and drug type
Dhopeshwarkar et al,[48] 2019	Partners HealthCare System/Partners' Enterprise-wide Allergy Repository (PEAR)	1.7 million	A, D	1.1% of patient population had at least one drug-induced anaphylaxis reaction. Risk factors: female sex, white race, and drug type

(continued on next page)

Table 2
(continued)

Article	EHR Database/Data Source	Sample Size	Primary EHR Components[a]	Findings: Prevalence/Incidence, Risk Factors, Outcome, Other
Rangkakulnuwat et al,[49] 2020	Chiang Mai University (CMU) Hospital, Chiang Mai, Thailand	433	B	Overall incidence of anaphylaxis in Asia was 3.9 cases of 100,000 visits, 84% of which were experienced in adults. Drug-induced anaphylaxis was more common in adults than children (19.8% vs 8.1%). NSAIDs (7.4%) and antimicrobials were the most common culprit drugs. 11.4% of cases had unknown cause. Risk factors: food, drug exposure, age, and sex
ADR: SCAR (n = 6)				
Ou-Yang et al,[50] 2013	Taiwan National Health Insurance Research Database	554	D	15.5% of outpatient and hospitalized patients in Taiwan were hospitalized twice due to SJS/TEN. Penicillin and cephalosporin (27%, 27%) were the main culprit agents for first hospitalization.
Micheletti et al,[51] 2018	18 US academic medical centers	377	D	89.7% of SJS/TEN cases were due to medication, mainly trimethoprim/sulfamethoxazole (26.3%) and β-lactams (12.4%).
Park et al,[52] 2019	Multicenter, Gangnam Severance Hospital, South Korea	745	D	Allopurinol was the causative drug in 14.2% of SCAR cases. Other culprit drugs are anticonvulsants (22.5%), β-lactams (21.1%), and NSAIDs (10.3%).

Study	Institution	N	ADR	Findings
De Bustros et al,[53] 2021	Loyola University Medical Center	163	D	Anticonvulsants (30%), trimethoprim-sulfamethoxazole (19%), β-lactams (11%), NSAIDs (8.4%), and allopurinol (8.4%) were identified the most probable culprit in SJS/TEN cases.
Zhang et al,[54] 2019	Penn State Hershey Medical Center	35	B, D	35 patients (5.9% of larger patient cohort) had documented SCAR, including 54.3% of DRESS, 22.8% of SJS, 17.1% of TEN, and 2.9% of AGEP, 2.9% of TEN, and SJS/TEN overlap.
Ma et al,[55] 2021	Chang Gung Memorial Hospital Linkou Branch, Taiwan	119	D	Of patients with SJS/TEN and overlap syndrome, 46.2% had severe ocular complications.
ADR: Other (n = 7)				
Macy et al,[18] 2012	Kaiser Permanente Southern California (Health Connect)	2.4 million	A	2.1% of health plan members had 3 or more allergies reported and can be diagnosed with multiple drug intolerance syndrome. Risk factors: female sex, age, drug type, and anxiety associated
Banerji et al,[56] 2017	Partners HealthCare System	135,000	A, C, D	Incidence of ACE inhibitor angioedema is 0.07% and 0.23% within the first month and first year of use, respectively.
Read et al,[57] 2017	Royal Brisbane and Women's Hospital, Gold Coast University Hospital, Australia	70	D	Only 9 cases of 70 reported erythema multiforme diagnoses in children met the criteria for erythema multiforme, with most being misdiagnosed.
Blumenthal et al,[58] 2018	Partners HealthCare System/Partners' Enterprise-wide Allergy Repository (PEAR)	746,888	A, B, C, D	The overall prevalence rate was multiple drug intolerance syndrome was 6.4% and 1.2% for multiple drug allergy syndrome. Risk factors for MDIS: female sex, older age, greater weight, prior hospitalizations, and multiple medical comorbidities

(continued on next page)

Table 2
(continued)

Article	EHR Database/Data Source	Sample Size	Primary EHR Components[a]	Findings: Prevalence/ Incidence, Risk Factors, Outcome, Other
Braswell et al,[59] 2019	University of Florida, the Medical College of Wisconsin, and Inform Diagnostics Research Institute	56	D	Of patients with lichenoid granulomatous dermatitis, most were diagnosed with drug eruption (39.3%, n = 22) and lichenoid keratosis (19.6%, n = 11).
Jimenez et al,[19] 2019	Cleveland Clinic	2.0 million	D	70.9% had no allergies; 27.4% had 1–4 allergies; 1.5% had 5–9 allergies; and 0.22% had >9 allergies in the patient population. Rates of mental health and somatic syndrome disorder increased with more allergies. Risk factors: female sex
Leigh et al,[60] 2019	University of Pennsylvania Health Systems	1218	A, B, D	Overall incidence of eosinophilic esophagitis is 0.034% in patient population. There may be a correlation with smoking.
BOTH Drug/ADR (n = 6)				
Silverman et al,[61] 2016	University of Pennsylvania Health Systems	220	A	12.4% of patients without chronic urticaria had a self-reported penicillin allergy. There was a 14.5% rate and 4.6% of chronic urticaria in patients with and without self-reported penicillin allergy, respectively.
Lin et al,[62] 2017	Penn State College of Medicine/Medical Center	138	D	In 78 pediatric reactions to vancomycin, 92% were consistent with red man syndrome. Of 60 children prescribed linezolid, 82% were unnecessarily avoiding vancomycin without prior reaction to vancomycin.

Coleman et al,[63] 2019	Yale-New Haven Hospital	98	D	Most rashes were associated with immune checkpoint inhibitors: pembrolizumab (35/103 rashes), nivolumab (33/103 rashes), and ipilimumab/nivolumab (17/103 rashes).
Jung et al,[64] 2019	Yonsei University Wonju College of Medicine, South Korea	1253	D	The prevalence of DRESS cases among patients prescribed antituberculosis drugs is 1.2%. Ethambutol (53.5%) and rifampin (26.7%) are the most common culprit drugs.
Fukasawa et al,[65] 2021	JMDC Claims Database, Japan	355	B, D	In Japan, the odds ratio of SJS/TEN for anticonvulsant, including carbamazepine (OR, 68.00) and lamotrigine (OR, 36.00) were significantly increased.
Sim et al,[66] 2021	Chonnam National University Hospital, South Korea	27	D	48% of 27 patients with drug fever or maculopapular exanthem had multiple drug hypersensitivity syndrome. The most common culprit agent was ethambutol and rifampin, followed by pyrazinamide and isoniazid.

Abbreviations: ADR, adverse drug reaction; DRESS, drug reaction with eosinophilia and systemic symptoms; IV, intravenous; NSAIDs, Non-steroidal anti-inflammatory drugs; OR, odds ratio; RCM, Radiocontrast media; SCAR, severe cutaneous adverse reactions.

[a] A, allergy list/problem list; B, ICD codes; C, free-text or structured data in the allergy list; D, other/unspecified.

Table 3
Summary of articles related to clinical documentation

Drugs of Interest Assessed	Study Design	Articles	Summary of Findings
Assessing Documentation Accuracy (n = 17)			
General	Retrospective review	Hsu et al,[67] 2011;Goldblatt et al,[68] 2017; Blumenthal et al,[71] 2017; Foremen et al,[69] 2020; Rukasin et al,[70] 2020	Drug allergy histories on smart cards are incomplete in many cases and have inconsistent formats.[67] Only 27% of SJS/TEN patients had all implicated drugs noted in the outpatient (primary care) record.[68] Allergies tend to accumulate over time with comparatively few allergy deletions.[71] Only 45.1% (n = 1671/ 3705) of reactions consistent with intolerance (eg, "nausea," "diarrhea") were correctly categorized as such.[69] EHR transitions pose a significant risk for EHR-related errors, which can be compounded by human error.[70]
	Cross-sectional	Reinhart et al,[75] 2008; Lyons et al,[73] 2015; Kiechle et al.,[72] 2018; Kabakov et al,[74] 2019	Allergy information was successfully entered in 84.6% of hospital admissions with a significantly lower rate (37.5%) among whose ethnicity groups, on average, have lower rates of English fluency.[75] Three studies[72–74] reported that discrepancies between medication allergies recorded in EHRs and those elicited in interviews are common.
	Qualitative interview	Fernando et al,[77] 2014; De Clercq et al,[76] 2020	Most drug reactions are likely to go unreported to and/or

(continued on next page)

Table 3 *(continued)*			
Drugs of Interest Assessed	**Study Design**	**Articles**	**Summary of Findings**
			unrecognized by health care professionals or are inaccurately recorded.[77] Family physicians and pharmacists perceive that few documented antibiotic allergies are in fact correct.[76]
β-Lactam	Retrospective review	Moskow et al,[78] 2016	Among all patients with a documented β-lactam allergy, 36.2% had an empty or missing allergy reaction description in their EHR.[78]
Penicillin	Retrospective review	Rimawi et al,[79] 2013; Inglis et al,[80] 2017	36% of the 55 patients with proven penicillin tolerance who revisited the hospital within a year had penicillin allergy redocumented.[79] Penicillin adverse drug reaction categorization was inconsistent. 10.1% of reports entered as allergy had reaction descriptions that were consistent with intolerance and 31.0% of the entered intolerances had descriptions consistent with allergy.[80]
	Prospective/ interventional	Staicu et al,[81] 2017	Severe or life-threatening penicillin allergies were underreported in nearly half of patients (43%).[81]
Contrast agents		Deng et al,[82] 2019; Ananthakrishnan et al,[83] 2021	Most 40,669 contrast allergen records were low quality (69.1%) rather than intermediate (19.4%) or high quality (11.5%).[82]

(continued on next page)

Table 3
(*continued*)

Drugs of Interest Assessed	Study Design	Articles	Summary of Findings
			Iodinated contrast media premedication prompts in the EHR are often erroneous because of inaccurate coding, incomplete data, and reaction misclassification.[83]
Improving drug allergy documentation (n = 10)			
General	Prospective/ interventional	Young et al,[87] 2011; Burrell et al,[84] 2013; Lesselroth et al.,[85] 2015; Masaharu et al,[86] 2018; Goss et al,[93] 2018; Soyer et al,[89] 2019; Wang et al,[90] 2020	Using an electronic version of a drug calendar considerably increased the ease and efficiency of completing dermatology consultations.[87] A pharmacy-driven initiative intended to improve the completeness of drug allergy/intolerance documentation was associated with modest success.[84] A patient-facing medication reconciliation and allergy review kiosk.[85] A novel standard format for recording allergy information resulted in increased allergy documentation and decreased adverse drug events.[86] A comprehensive value set to improve the consistency and accuracy of adverse reaction documentation in the allergy module was developed including 1106 concepts.[93] Structured intervention led to an increase in quality of coding and reduction in discrepancies coded by medical record technicians and pharmacovigilance teams.[89]

(*continued on next page*)

Table 3 *(continued)*			
Drugs of Interest Assessed	**Study Design**	**Articles**	**Summary of Findings**
	Retrospective review	Vethody et al,[91] 2021	A dynamic reaction picklist developed using EHR data and a statistical measure was superior to the static picklist and suggested proper reactions for allergy documentation.[90] Patients with multiple drug allergy labels can be safely delabeled to multiple drugs in 1 visit.[91]
β-Lactam	Prospective/ interventional	Wright et al,[88] 2019	Allergy documentation of antibiotic test dose results increased with use of CDS. The addition of electronic alerting increased allergy documentation to 66.7% from 51.3% in the prealert period. In addition to a greater likelihood of updating, updates were made significantly faster in the postalert period.[88]
Penicillin	Retrospective review	Lachover-Roth et al,[92] 2019	Penicillin allergy annulling via oral challenge test proved to be safe and effective.[92]

Abbreviations: SJS, Stevens-Johnson syndrome; TEN, toxic epidermal necrolysis.

improving the quality of drug allergy documentation,[89,90] and 3 articles focused on allergy testing and delabeling inappropriate allergies.[88,91,92] Quality improvement of drug allergy documentation was done through designing a dynamic reaction pick list,[90] a comprehensive value set for encoding reactions,[93] and a structured intervention for medical record technicians and pharmacovigilance teams.[89] Two articles addressed the safety of delabeling,[91,92] and another study focused on the likelihood and speed of updating allergies using CDS alerts based on antibiotic test dose results.[88]

Case Management

There were 22 articles (15.7%) discussing the management of DHRs using the EHR to identify and stratify patients who would benefit from the evaluation of drug allergies and

Table 4
Summary of articles related to case management

Focus/Intervention	Drug of Interest	Articles	Summary of Findings
Antimicrobial Stewardship (n = 19)			
Evaluation of documented β-lactam allergies	All β-lactam antibiotics	Abrams et al,[110] 2016	ICD-9 codes and billing codes were used to identify patients who had underdone assessment for suspected β-lactam antibiotic allergies for retrospective chart review. Following intradermal testing and oral challenge, 96% of patients with prior history of β-lactam allergy were advised they could safely reintroduce β-lactam antibiotics.
		Blumenthal et al,[99] 2019	This retrospective cohort study identified 1046 test doses challenges prompted by an electronic guideline for hospitalized patients with reported β-lactam allergies. The antimicrobial stewardship intervention was safe with only 3.8% of patients with β-lactam allergy histories had a hypersensitivity reaction. Cephalosporin allergy histories conferred a 3-fold risk.
		Kwon et al,[101] 2019	Allergies were updated for 474 patients (45%), with records specified (82%), deleted (16%), and added (8%). A retrospective review of patients with a history of β-lactam allergies in the EHR found that 15% (6/40) showed a positive cefazolin skin test result compared with only 1.36% (178/13,113) of cases with no such history.
		Shaw et al,[109] 2020	A retrospective review of 589 eligible patients with β-lactam allergies who underwent allergy service consult, found that changes in the allergy record were recommended for 62% of patients (n = 371); however, the allergy record was updated after the consult in only 74.9% of patients (n = 278).

Penicillins	Chen et al,[96] 2017	A specialized algorithm was used to flag and prioritize eligible inpatients in the EHR for penicillin skin tests and challenges resulting in the removal of penicillin allergy labels in 228 subjects (90.5%) and the use of β-lactams in 85 (38%) of patients who tested negative.
	Sundquist et al,[97] 2017	The EHR was screened to identify patients with a history of penicillin allergy and a total of 37 patients were recruited for penicillin skin testing and oral challenge. None of the patients had a positive skin test or oral challenge; however, 2 patients (5%) experienced reactions within 24 h.
	Kuder et al,[104] 2020	A retrospective review of pregnant women who underwent penicillin allergy evaluation via skin test found that 44 patients (95.6%) received negative results and 18 patients (39%) completed oral challenge and did not experience adverse reactions.
	Wolfson et al,[100] 2021	A retrospective study of the pregnant patients with penicillin allergies in the EHR found that of 220 patients skin tested, 209 (95%) had their penicillin allergy label safely removed and penicillin allergy testing was associated with significantly reduced broad-spectrum antibiotic use and increased first-line β-lactam antibiotic use.
General	Iammatteo et al,[102] 2017	A 5-y retrospective chart review of patients who underwent at least 1 single-blind placebo-controlled graded drug challenge was conducted. The reaction rate to drug and placebo was similar during β-lactam challenges (9.4% vs 8.2%; $P = .9$) and during nonsteroidal anti-inflammatory drug challenges (14% vs 7%, $P = .5$), respectively.

(continued on next page)

Table 4
(continued)

Focus/Intervention	Drug of Interest	Articles	Summary of Findings
Evaluation of allergy for treatment optimization	All β-lactam antibiotics	Sigona et al,[107] 2016	A pharmacist-driven β-lactam allergy interview was effective in switching 65% of eligible patients to β-lactam therapy and identifying discrepancies between confirmed allergies and those documented in the EHR in 87%. Medical providers accepted 87.5% of pharmacists' antimicrobial recommendations.
	Penicillins	McDanel et al,[103] 2017	β-Lactam allergy screening using an electronic best practice advisory and Drug Allergy Clinic referral in orthopedic surgery patients resulted in higher cefazolin use in patients evaluated in the clinic vs those not evaluated (90% vs 77%) and lower use of non-β-lactam antibiotics (16% vs 27%).
		Blumenthal et al,[106] 2017	Both application with clinical decision support and penicillin skin test increased the use of penicillin and cephalosporin antibiotics among inpatients reporting penicillin allergy by nearly 2-fold and 6-fold, respectively.
		Ramsey and Staicu,[108] 2018	Inpatients with penicillin allergies receiving moxifloxacin, intravenous vancomycin, aztreonam, daptomycin, or linezolid were identified through an EHR report and a penicillin allergy history algorithm was used to determine eligibility for penicillin skin testing. Forty-seven patients (94%) were skin-test negative and were subsequently transitioned to β-lactam antibiotic and no patients experienced immediate adverse reaction.
		Englert and Weeks,[94] 2019	Patients with documented penicillin allergy (type I, immunoglobulin E [IgE]-mediated) who were prescribed alternate antibiotics enrolled in a pharmacist-driven PST service to facilitate

	Kuruvilla et al,[105] 2020	delabeling of inaccurate penicillin allergies in the EHR. Of 22 patients, all were negative, and 68.2% (15) were successfully transitioned to β-lactam antibiotics reducing the use of fluoroquinolones and vancomycin. Using an institutional algorithm for antibiotic selection in penicillin-allergic surgical patients (n = 2296), treatment with cephalosporin increased from 22% at baseline to 80% after algorithm implementation without severe adverse reactions.
Other antibiotics	Lin et al,[98] 2020	Patients with antibiotic allergy labels which interfered with the preferred antibiotic treatment were identified through physician recommendation in the EHR and 42 patients received oral challenges. In 40 of these patients (95%), no allergic reaction was observed, and the preferred antibiotic treatment was given. Two patients (5%) developed a nonsevere skin reaction after a drug challenge and continued an alternative antibiotic regimen
Improvement of desensitization	All β-lactam antibiotics	Pandya et al,[111] 2021	A clinician survey found that the creation of standardized electronic β-lactam antibiotic desensitization order sets results in increased overall efficiency.
Assessment of alternate antibiotic use		Mancini et al,[112] 2021	Of 2276 inpatients receiving antibiotics for pneumonia at 95 US hospitals, 450 (20%) had a documented penicillin and/or cephalosporin allergy. Inpatients with this documented allergy and pneumonia were less likely to receive recommended β-lactams and more likely to receive carbapenems and fluoroquinolones.

(continued on next page)

Table 4
(continued)

Focus/Intervention	Drug of Interest	Articles	Summary of Findings
Referral for allergy delabeling	Penicillins	Wang et al,[95] 2021	Using an attending physician educational session and Best Practice Advisory in the EHR, referrals to the allergy clinic increased for penicillin-class drug allergies from 1.9% to 13.7% after the educational session with a further increase to 27.8% after the Best Practice Advisory.
Nonantibiotic drug desensitization and rechallenge (n = 3)			
Assess outcomes of drug desensitization	General	Murray et al,[115] 2016	A retrospective review of EHR of patients undergoing drug desensitization found that of 69 patients, desensitization was completed with no cutaneous reaction in 85% of patients. Reported histories of urticaria and labored breathing during prior exposure were significant in identifying patients who might have a reaction during desensitization.
Risk stratification and evaluation of taxane re-exposure	Taxane	Picard et al,[114] 2016	EHR of patients who had been treated for taxane-related DHRs was retrospectively reviewed to identify patients for re-exposure to taxanes. Of 138 patients desensitized, 29 (21%) had an immediate and 20 (14%) had delayed DHRs with the procedure. Of 49 patients challenged, 2 (4%) had mild immediate and 1 (2%) had delayed DHRs with the procedure.
Assessing safety of chemotherapy drug rechallenge protocol	Chemotherapy drugs	Wu,[113] 2019	Patients who attempted rechallenge with paclitaxel, docetaxel, carboplatin, and oxaliplatin were identified through retrospective chart review. The first rechallenge cycle was completed successfully in 43/46 patients (93.5%) and 42/46 patients (91.3%) were hypersensitivity reaction-free throughout the treatment course under the rechallenge protocol.

to increase the efficiency and safety of desensitization (**Table 4**). Predominantly, research focused on antimicrobial stewardship including 15 studies on delabeling inappropriate antibiotic allergy labels and optimizing treatment,[94–110] one evaluating the safety and efficiency of antibiotic desensitization,[111] and one assessing antibiotic use in patients with antibiotic allergy documentation.[112] Delabeling and treatment optimization efforts were accomplished through retrospective review of antibiotic evaluation history,[99] a computerized guideline application with decision support,[106] patient interview,[107] and the stratification of patients in the EHR with antibiotic allergy labels as candidates for penicillin skin testing (PST),[94,95,108] oral challenges,[98,102] or both.[96,97,103,110] Other studies focused on the management of DHRs induced by cancer treatments including one study which retrospectively assessed chemotherapy drug rechallenges[113] and one which stratified patients with taxane-related DHRs for skin testing.[114] Finally, one study retrospectively reviewed patients undergoing desensitization and found that it was safe for patients with no alternatives for therapy but noted that urticaria and labored breathing were risk factors for having a reaction during desensitization.[115]

CDS

Eighteen studies (12.9%) reviewed the use of automated CDS in EHRs, including drug allergy alerting mechanisms and override rates (**Table 5**). Eleven of these studies measured the prevalence of allergy alerts, specifically, drug allergy and drug-drug interaction alerts, the most common types of CDS alerts.[116] Medication-related alerts made up nearly three-quarters of all inpatient alert[116] with most drug-allergy alerts triggered by narcotics.[117,118] These studies also evaluated how frequently clinicians overrode drug alerts, reporting override rates as high as 93%.[119] Of these overrides, approximately 80% of these allergy alert overrides were deemed appropriate. Even so, Wong and colleagues, 2018 determined that inappropriately overridden allergy alerts are 6 times more likely to trigger ADRs compared with those that are appropriately overridden.[120]

Seven studies explored tools that can be used to evaluate[121] and modify CDS by adding or eliminating certain alerts.[122–126] Two studies evaluated clinician behavior after reducing allergy alerts for β-lactam antibiotics, a commonly documented patient allergy.[125,126] Interestingly, both studies noted that the reduction[126] and even the elimination of allergy alerts[125] did not lead to a significant increase in DHRs. Three other studies created CDS alerts, including premedication alerts for when patients were prescribed radiocontrast media[122,123] and drug-gene interaction alerts to prevent future DHRs,[124] thereby promoting tailored alerts for specific drug interactions. Altogether, these studies intended to improve CDSS while reducing ADRs and medication errors in clinical settings.

Case Identification

Among 9 articles (6.4%) allocated to the case identification category, 3 focused on identifying DHRs using unstructured data,[134–136] 2 using structured data,[137,138] and 4 using a combination of both (**Table 6**).[139–142] Studies using unstructured data used text processing techniques like natural language processing (NLP) and free-text searches. Wolfson and colleagues used free-text searches of drug reaction with eosinophilia and systemic symptoms (DRESS) syndrome-related keywords to identify a large DRESS syndrome cohort (n = 69) from a database consisting of 3.1 million patients.[134] Similarly, Epstein and colleagues developed an algorithm that uses RxNorm[143] and NLP to identify drug allergies with accuracy, precision, recall, and F-measure of above 97%.[136] Case identification research using structured data

Table 5
Summary of articles related to clinical decision support systems (n = 18)

Focus/Intervention	Allergens	Alert Type	Articles	Clinical Setting	Summary of Findings
Descriptive Study Design (n = 11)					
Measure of allergy alerts and overrides	Food, drug, environment	Food/drug allergy and intolerance alerts	González-Gregori et al,[116] 2012	Inpatient	Alerts were mainly caused by drugs (74.4%), followed by foods (12.6%) and materials (4.8%).
	Drug	Drug allergy alerts, drug-drug interaction alerts	Lin et al,[127] 2008	Inpatient	Clinicians indicated alerts were overly frequent, with low specificity and high sensitivity. 93% of drug alerts were overridden. More drug-drug alerts were overridden (87%–95.1%) compared with drug allergy alerts (81%–90.9%).
			Weingart et al,[128] 2009	Inpatient; Outpatient	Alerts containing immune-mediated (72.8%) and life-threatening reactions (74.1%) were overridden. Narcotics triggered most drug alerts (48%).
			Carspecken et al,[129] 2013	Inpatient; Pediatric hospital	
			Bryant et al,[119] 2014	Inpatient	
			Topaz et al,[117] 2016	Inpatient	
			Wong et al,[120] 2018	Inpatient, Outpatient	46.0% and 68.8% of definite anaphylaxis drug-allergy interaction alerts were overridden in inpatient and outpatient settings, respectively. 83.9% of inpatient overrides and 100% of outpatient overrides were appropriate.
		Drug-allergy, drug-drug interaction, geriatric and renal alerts	Wong et al.,[130] 2017	Inpatient; Intensive Care Unit	Between commercial and internally developed EHR, physicians experienced more alerts and overrode more alerts with the commercial EHR. (commercial: n = 5535; legacy: n = 1030).

Create Clinical Decision Support	Drug	Alert type	Author, year	Setting	Findings
		Opioid allergy alerts	Wong et al.,[131] 2018	Inpatient; Intensive Care Unit	81.6% of alert overrides were appropriate in the intensive care unit. However, inappropriate overrides were 6 times more likely to result in an ADE compared with appropriate overridden alerts.
			Ariosto, D,[118] 2014	Inpatient	At least 89% of opioid allergy alerts that make up almost a third of visible alerts were overridden. Physicians are more likely to override opioid alerts than advanced practice nurses.
			Genco et al.,[132] 2016	Inpatient; Emergency department	34.6% of visible alerts are opioid alerts. Of these alerts, 96.3% were overridden.
Interventional Study Design (n = 7)					
Create Clinical Decision Support	Radiocontrast media agents	Premedication alerts	Bae et al,[122] 2013	Inpatient	There was a significant increase in premedication rates; however, only Bae et al noticed a significant reduction in breakthrough reactions.
	Drug	Drug-gene interaction alerts	Benson et al,[123] 2017 Dolin et al,[124] 2018	NA	With the use of clinical decision support and pharmacogenetic sequencing data, genomics-EHR integration can lead to drug-gene interaction alerts.
	NA	NA	Garabedian et al.,[133] 2019	Outpatient	Redesigning CPOE structure to allow physicians to enter the indication, or reason for medication first, before prescribing will improve usability and user satisfaction while minimizing medication error.

(continued on next page)

Table 5
(continued)

Focus/Intervention	Allergens	Alert Type	Articles	Clinical Setting	Summary of Findings
Modified Alerting Rules	β-Lactam antibiotics	β-Lactam alerts	Macy et al.,[125] 2021	Inpatient, Outpatient	Elimination of cephalosporin alerts increased cephalosporin use, decreased second line of antibiotic treatment without significantly increasing anaphylaxis
			Buffone et al,[126] 2021	Inpatient	7.7% of patients were alerted for a β-lactam prescription, whereas 92.3% of patients were no longer alerted under the adjusted rules when prescribed a β-lactam antibiotic with a different side chain. They did not report any incidence of anaphylaxis.
Evaluation Tool for Clinical Decision Support		Therapeutic Duplication, Drug-Dose (single and daily), Drug-Allergy, Drug-Route, Drug–Drug, Drug-Diagnosis, Drug-Age, Drug-Labs, Drug-Renal, Monitoring, Nuisance Orders	Cho et al.,[121] 2015	NA	Using the Leapfrog CPOE evaluation tool, errors were captured in Therapeutic Duplication and Drug-Drug Interaction alerts, mainly.

Abbreviation: CPOE, computerized provider order entry.

Table 6
Summary of articles related to case identification

Article	Search Method	Reaction Analyzed	Sample Size	Summary of Findings
Unstructured data (n = 3)				
Epstein et al,[136] 2013	RxNorm and NLP	Adverse drug events	N/A	A high-performing algorithm was used to identify medication allergies with a specificity of 90.3% and 85% in the training and testing data, respectively. Accuracy, precision, recall, and F-measure for medication allergy matches were all above 98% in the training data set and above 97% in the testing data set for all allergy entries
Wolfson et al,[134] 2019	Free-text keyword search of allergy module	DRESS syndrome	69	Of 538 hypersensitivity reactions identified, 69 patients (2.18 in 100,000 patients) had DRESS syndrome.
DeLozier et al,[135] 2021	Text processing system	SJS/TEN and torsades de pointes	138	The automated recruitment system resulted in the capture of 138 true cases of drug-induced rare events, improving recall from 43% to 93%
Structured data (n = 2)				
Davis et al,[137] 2015	ICD-9 codes	SJS/TEN	475–875	Patients with the ICD-9 codes introduced after 2008 were more likely to be confirmed as cases (OR, 3.32; 95% CI 0.82, 13.47) than those identified in earlier years. The likelihood of case status increased with length of hospitalization. Applying the probability of case status to the 56 591 potential cases, we estimated 475–875 to be valid SJS/TEN cases.
Saff et al.,[138] 2019	ICD-9 codes and E codes	Allergic drug reactions	409	Specific ICD-9 codes can identify patients with allergic drug reactions, with antibiotics accounting for almost half of true reactions. Most patients with codes 693.0, 995.1, 708, and 995.0 had allergic drug reactions, with 693.0 as the highest yield code. An aggregate of multiple specific codes consistently identifies a cohort of patients with confirmed allergic drug reactions.

(continued on next page)

Table 6
(continued)

Article	Search Method	Reaction Analyzed	Sample Size	Summary of Findings
Combination of structured and unstructured data (n = 4)				
Kim et al,[142] 2012	Procedure codes and International Classification for Nursing Practice terms	Contrast-media-induced hypersensitivity reactions	266	An EHR-based electronic search method was highly efficient and reduced the charts that needed to be reviewed by 96% (28/759)
Cahill et al,[140] 2017	ICD-9 codes and an informatics algorithm	AERD	593	An informatics algorithm can successfully identify both known and previously undiagnosed cases of AERD with a high positive predictive value. Involvement of an allergist/immunologist significantly increases the likelihood of an AERD diagnosis.
Fukasawa et al,[141] 2019	ICD-10 codes and informatics algorithms using clinical course and medical encounters	SJS/TEN	N/A	One algorithm, consisting of a combination of clinical course for SJS/TEN, medical encounters for mucocutaneous lesions from SJS/TEN, and items to exclude paraneoplastic pemphigus, but not ICD-10 codes, showed a sensitivity of 76.9%, specificity of 99.0%, positive predictive value of 40.5%, negative predictive value of 99.8%, and diagnostic odd ratio of 330.00.
Banerji et al,[139] 2020	ICD-9 codes and NLP	Allergic drug reactions	335	Among the 335 confirmed positive cases, NLP identified 259 true cases, resulting in a recall/sensitivity of 77% (range, 26% to 100%). Among the 390 negative cases, NLP achieved a specificity of 89% (range, 69% to 100%).

Abbreviations: AERD, aspirin-exacerbated respiratory disease; DRESS, drug reaction with eosinophilia and systemic symptoms; NLP, natural language processing; SJS, Stevens-Johnson syndrome; TEN, toxic epidermal necrolysis.

used ICD-9 codes and E codes.[137,138] Davis and colleagues and Saff and colleagues used ICD-9 codes to identify inpatient ADRs and Stevens-Johnson syndrome (SJS)/toxic epidermal necrolysis (TEN) cases, respectively, from large patient populations.[137,138]

Most of the studies reviewed (n = 4, 44.4%) used a combination of structured and unstructured data for case identification. Banerji and colleagues have used ICD-9 codes to identify DHRs followed by a rule-based NLP algorithm to search free-text clinical notes and discharge summaries.[139] They found that the use of ICD-9 codes alone resulted in a positive predictive value (PPV) of 46% (range, 18% to 79%) compared with a PPV of 86% (range, 69% to 100%) with the combination of ICD-9 codes and NLP. Alternatively, Kim and colleagues developed an EHR-based surveillance system using signals from standardized search terms within the international classification of nursing terms, and order codes for procedures that used contrast media, antihistamine, and epinephrine with a sensitivity of 66.7%, a specificity of 99.6%, and a negative predictive value of 99.7%.[142]

GENETIC STUDIES

The genetic studies included 3 articles (2.1%) focused on investigating the contribution of genetic variation to DHRs. Zheng and colleagues conducted genome-wide association studies (GWAS) for ADRs in 14 common drug/drug groups for 81,739 patients.[144] They identified 7 genetic loci significantly associated with ADRs, which were consistent with additional expression quantitative trait loci and phenome-wide association analyses. They applied an approach that included a combination of prospective identification of cases and identification of cases in the Vanderbilt University Medical Center (VUMC) BioVu repository that links the EHR to DNA. Konvinse and colleagues reported a strong association between the HLA-A*32:01 and vancomycin-induced DRESS syndrome in a population of predominantly European ancestry.[145] In their study, 19 (82.6%) of 23 vancomycin-associated DRESS syndrome cases had HLA-A*32:01 compared with 0 (0%) of 46 vancomycin-tolerant comparators matched by sex, race, and age using their BioVU deidentified EHR database. Lastly, Krebs and colleagues uncovered an association between HLA-*55:01 and self-reported penicillin allergy by extracting EHR data from over 1.1 million individuals, which was also replicated in 23andMe and VUMC BioVu.[146]

DISCUSSION

We examined the use of EHRs in drug hypersensitivity literature by systematically reviewing articles in this field from 5 scientific databases from 2000 to 2021. We found that relevant studies fall into 6 study categories: observational studies, allergy documentation, case management, CDS, case identification, and genetic studies. We discuss the major findings in each study category, identify gaps and challenges that the field is currently facing, and outline the future directions.

Observational Studies

Overall, EHR-dependent analyses promote the use of extensive clinical data to build an epidemiologic profile for DHRs and culprit drugs. With access to millions of medical records, reviewing EHRs conveniently increases sample size as demonstrated by Macy and colleagues,[18] Wong and colleagues,[20] and Alvarez-Arango et al.[24] Furthermore, the retrospective use of EHRs allows for rare conditions, such as DRESS syndrome, to be studied in greater detail, which would otherwise be difficult for conditions that already have a low prevalence and incidence rate.[51,54] In a similar vein, EHRs are used to study periodic trends, measuring the prevalence of DHRs throughout many years.[13,46,54] Nonetheless, the retrospective design is considered a limitation as it is difficult to establish a clear temporal association compared with prospective cohort studies.

Furthermore, it was not consistently communicated what sections of EHRs were analyzed or how they analyzed EHRs. This heterogeneity is a limitation that cannot be always identified. Of the studies that defined their search methods, several studies used ICD codes to identify patients with the ADR or comorbidity of interest while a few others developed algorithms[34,65] and searched key terms in EHRs.[22,54,59] The problem list and allergy module were frequently used to measure the prevalence of allergies. Only 10% of studies highlighted the use of automated processes, like NLP, to extract information from free-text entries.[16,20,24,30,33] Thirteen percent of the studies used a combination of the problem list, ICD codes, and the allergy module. With the profound growth of EHR literature, observational EHR studies should clarify how medical information was extracted for the data extraction to be considered transparent, replicable, and reliable. In addition, the fact that allergy information has been documented in different places and often unreliably in the EHR highlights that allergy documentation needs to be systematically improved with reconciliation mechanisms in place, which is also discussed below.

Clinical Documentation

There was a consensus among the articles reviewed that there is a high rate of incomplete and inaccurate drug hypersensitivity documentation. This is especially concerning in cases that involve severe morbidity and high mortality rates including SJS/TEN and DRESS cases. Goldblatt and colleagues found that in 26 cases of SJS/TEN, only 27% of patients had all implicated drug notes in the outpatient primary record.[68] Similarly, Rukasin and colleagues reported that 5% of 511 patients had inaccurate descriptions for confirmed severe reactions like SJS/TEN, DRESS, or anaphylaxis, yet these errors were not identified and corrected for patients with new encounters after a system-wide EHR transition.[70]

Sources of inaccurate documentation include lack of training and misconceptions among clinical staff responsible for documentation. Foreman and colleagues found that only 45.1% of reactions consistent with intolerance (eg, "nausea," "diarrhea") were correctly categorized as such.[69] Likewise, Inglis and colleagues observed that of 5023 ADRs to penicillins, 95% were labeled as allergy rather than intolerance (n = 250, 5.0%), which is consistent with the known overdiagnosis of penicillin allergy in the hospital and other populations. Errors also stem from the failure to delete inaccurate allergies and redocument deleted allergies. Blumenthal and colleagues found that allergies tend to accumulate over time with relatively few allergy deletions, and Topaz and colleagues reported that over 50% of drug allergy alerts were triggered for previously tolerated medications, which undermines the purpose of CDS alerts.[117]

Successful approaches to improving DHRs documentation include creating standard formats for allergy recording[86] and implementing interventions to improve training and communication between medical record technicians and pharmacovigilance teams.[89] Concerted efforts should be made to educate clinicians documenting DHRs to improve the accuracy and completeness of records. Delabeling inappropriate allergies of multiple drugs in a single visit and delabeling after a negative oral challenge test were safe and effective methods to correct allergy documentation.[91,92] Furthermore, the involvement of patients in updating drug allergy records including allowing patients to review and update their allergy records could reduce allergy record errors.

Case Management

Most patients with β-lactam allergy documentation do not have "true" β-lactam allergies.[110] This leads to the overuse of antibiotics with potential lower efficacy, such as fluoroquinolones and vancomycin, harming individual and public health.[95] Hence, a priority of antimicrobial stewardship is to delabel inaccurate antibiotic allergies to optimize future treatments. The EHR is an essential tool for identifying and stratifying patients who would benefit from the evaluation of antibiotics allergies through skin tests, oral challenges, or patient interviews. In addition, misconceptions about cross-reactivity or shared hypersensitivity between β-lactams also contribute to the use of less optimal antibiotic alternatives. This presents an opportunity for the use of CDS applications to determine appropriate antibiotic alternatives[106] and evaluate the safety for drug rechallenges[113] and desensitization.[114]

Clinical Decision Support

Though the Medicare and Medicaid EHR Incentive Programs encouraged the installation of CPOE systems to promote EHR usage, it has become increasingly evident that the high prevalence of allergy alerts and override rates jeopardizes patient safety and increases alert fatigue.[119] EHR literature centered on CDS critically evaluates the effectiveness of current CDS alerts and calls for only essential allergy alerting mechanisms in response to the frequency of alert overrides. It is important to recognize that approximately 80% of these overrides are considered appropriate, suggesting that many alerts are not clinically relevant or useful; the fact that both Macy and colleagues, 2021 and Buffone and colleagues, 2021 have demonstrated that the reduction of β-lactam alerts does not result in serious ADR reflects that our current alert rules need to be modified.[125,126] Still, there should be a greater concern for the 20% of alerts that are overridden but are in fact clinically relevant. Owing to alert fatigue, clinicians may not be sensitized to the alerts that highlight allergens that can trigger severe DHRs. More research must actively explore and modify CDS to minimize the overwhelming number of alert overrides and improve clinical workflow.

Case Identification

Optimizing methods for the identification of DHRs in the EHR is important for studying the epidemiology of these reactions and for participant recruitment for prospective clinical studies including those assessing genetic risk factors. This includes real-time monitoring of EHR surveillance and the retrospective review of structured and unstructured EHR data which is especially essential for rare reactions like SJS/TEN that carry high mortality risk. The use of such optimized identification methods greatly reduced the amount of time and cost-intensive manual chart reviews. Kim and colleagues reported a reduction in the number of charts that needed to be manually reviewed by 96% using their electronic search strategy for contrast media hypersensitivity reactions.[142] Furthermore, using a combination of case identification methods with structured data like ICD-9 and ICD-10 codes and unstructured data with text can greatly increase PPV compared with the use of structured data alone.[139] Future studies could leverage advanced computational and informatics technologies (eg, NLP and machine learning) and diverse data sources for more efficient and accurate case identification and phenotyping.

Genetic Studies

Understanding genetic associations could facilitate the adoption of preventative, predictive, and diagnostic strategies to improve drug safety. Such studies have been limited by small sample sizes; however, Zheng and colleagues have used "drug allergy" labels from EHRs to obtain a large sample size from their DNA Biobank for GWAS.[144] Their high-throughput framework can be replicated to accelerate the discovery of drug response genetic association and improve precision medicine. Similarly, the discovery of HLA associations holds substantial promise for the prevention of severe cutaneous adverse drug reactions like DRESS syndrome, which to date have shown strong associations with HLA class I alleles.

Limitations

This review has several limitations. Although we repeatedly refined our search query to broadly capture relevant articles, it is possible we did not include relevant studies in our systematic review because we only extracted literature from 5 databases. We also excluded research letters, literature without abstracts, non-English studies, which may contribute to selection bias and limit generalizability. It is also worth noting that due to the heterogeneity of the studies included, we were not able to evaluate bias consistently. In addition, the research categories were subjectively defined after the initial screening, and each article was placed in one category based on the predominant research theme. Hence, there may be important themes that are not studied extensively in this review and articles that fall into multiple categories.

SUMMARY

EHRs present a rich source of clinical information that has been increasingly used to study drug hypersensitivity across diverse research topics. By leveraging large EHR databases, studies have been able to elucidate the epidemiology and genetic associations of DHRs. A growing number of studies has innovatively applied advanced informatics methods, including NLP, to analyze unstructured allergy data for case identification. Nonetheless, poor standardization and quality of allergy documentation jeopardize patient safety and pose a significant challenge to case identification.

In addition, the overuse of CDS alerts counters their utility while also contributing to clinician fatigue. Improvement of clinical documentation, more selective use of CDS alerts, and strategies to harmonize data from different sources are critical future avenues for drug hypersensitivity research.

CLINICS CARE POINTS

- Emphasis should be placed on the completeness and accuracy of drug hypersensitivity reaction documentation to prevent future reactions.
- Drug allergy records need to be regularly updated to avoid unnecessary reliance on suboptimal substitutes.
- Evaluation of drug allergies through skin tests, oral challenges, and patient interviews are safe and effective methods for delabeling inappropriate drug allergies.
- To minimize alert fatigue which compromises patient safety, it is critical for hospital systems to increase the specificity of allergy alerts.

DISCLOSURE

F. Bassir, S. Varghese, L. Wang, and Y.P. Chin report no disclosures. L. Zhou receives research funding from IBM Watson Health.

SUPPLEMENTARY DATA

Supplementary data related to this article can be found online at https://doi.org/10.1016/j.iac.2022.01.004.

REFERENCES

1. Rawlins MD, Thompson JW. Pathogenesis of adverse drug reactions. In: Davies DM, editor. Textbook of adverse drug reactions. Oxford (UK): Oxford University Press; 1977.
2. Ruby Pawankar M, Canonica GW, Holgate ST, Lockey RF. White book on allergy 2011- 2012. Executive summary. Milwaukee, WI: World Allergy Organization; 2011.
3. Evans RS. Electronic health records: then, now, and in the future. Yearb Med Inform 2016;25(S 01):S48–61.
4. Chiriac AM, Macy E. Large health system databases and drug hypersensitivity. J Allergy Clin Immunol Pract 2019;7(7):2125–31.
5. Moher D, Liberati A, Tetzlaff J, et al. Preferred reporting items for systematic reviews and meta-analyses: the PRISMA statement. PLoS Med 2009;6(7): e1000097.
6. Lager S, White B, Baumann M, et al. Incidence of cross- sensitivity with carbapenems in documented penicillin-allergic patients. J Pharm Technology 2009; 25(3):159–63.
7. Albin S, Agarwal S. Prevalence and characteristics of reported penicillin allergy in an urban outpatient adult population. Allergy Asthma Proc 2014;35(6): 489–94.
8. Beltran RJ, Kako H, Chovanec T, et al. Penicillin allergy and surgical prophylaxis: Cephalosporin cross-reactivity risk in a pediatric tertiary care center. J Pediatr Surg 2015;50(5):856–9.
9. Blumenthal KG, Kuhlen JL, Weil AA, et al. Adverse drug reactions associated with ceftaroline use: a 2-center retrospective cohort. J Allergy Clin Immunol Pract 2016;4(4):740–6.
10. Crotty DJ, Chen XJC, Scipione MR, et al. Allergic reactions in hospitalized patients with a self-reported penicillin allergy who receive a cephalosporin or meropenem. J Pharm Pract 2017;30(1):42–8.
11. Butler DF, Lee BR, Suppes S, et al. Variability of surgical prophylaxis in penicillin-allergic children. Infect Control Hosp Epidemiol 2018;39(12):1480–3.
12. West RM, Smith CJ, Pavitt SH, et al. Warning: allergic to penicillin': association between penicillin allergy status in 2.3 million NHS general practice electronic health records, antibiotic prescribing and health outcomes. J Antimicrob Chemother 2019;74(7):2075–82.
13. Liang EH, Chen LH, Macy E. Adverse reactions associated with penicillins, carbapenems, monobactams, and clindamycin: a retrospective population-based Study. J Allergy Clin Immunol Pract 2020;8(4):1302–13.e2.
14. Macy E, Poon K-YT. Self-reported Antibiotic Allergy Incidence and Prevalence: Age and Sex Effects. Am J Med 2009;122(8):778.e1-e7.
15. Macy E, Contreras R. Health care use and serious infection prevalence associated with penicillin "allergy" in hospitalized patients: a cohort study. J Allergy Clin Immunol 2014;133(3):790–6.
16. Zhou L, Dhopeshwarkar N, Blumenthal KG, et al. Drug allergies documented in electronic health records of a large healthcare system. Allergy 2016;71(9): 1305–13.

17. Salden OA, Rockmann H, Verheij TJ, et al. Diagnosis of allergy against beta-lactams in primary care: prevalence and diagnostic criteria. Fam Pract 2015; 32(3):257–62.

18. Macy E, Ho NJ. Multiple drug intolerance syndrome: prevalence, clinical characteristics, and management. Ann Allergy Asthma Immunol 2012;108(2):88–93.

19. Jimenez XF, Shirvani N, Hogue O, et al. Polyallergy (multiple chemical sensitivity) is associated with excessive healthcare utilization, greater psychotropic use, and greater mental health/functional somatic syndrome disorder diagnoses: a large cohort retrospective study. Psychosomatics 2019;60(3):298–310.

20. Wong A, Seger DL, Lai KH, et al. Drug hypersensitivity reactions documented in electronic health records within a large health system. J Allergy Clin Immunol Pract 2019;7(4):1253–60.e3.

21. Apter AJ, Kinman JL, Bilker WB, et al. Represcription of penicillin after allergic-like events. J Allergy Clin Immunol 2004;113(4):764–70.

22. May SM, Hartz MF, Joshi AY, et al. Intrapartum antibiotic exposure for group B Streptococcus treatment did not increase penicillin allergy in children. Ann Allergy Asthma Immunol 2016;116(2):134–8.

23. Macy E, Contreras R. Adverse reactions associated with oral and parenteral use of cephalosporins: A retrospective population-based analysis. J Allergy Clin Immunol 2015;135(3):745–52.e5.

24. Alvarez-Arango S, Yerneni S, Tang O, et al. Vancomycin Hypersensitivity Reactions Documented in Electronic Health Records. J Allergy Clin Immunol Pract 2021;9(2):906–12.

25. Fosnot S, Currier K, Pendell J, et al. Comparison of immediate hypersensitivity reactions to preoperative antibiotics in patients labeled as penicillin allergic. Surgery 2021;170(3):777–82.

26. Lal LS, Gerber DL, Lau J, et al. Retrospective evaluation of weekly paclitaxel hypersensitivity reactions reported utilizing an electronic medical record system at a tertiary cancer center. Support Care Cancer 2009;17(10):1311–5.

27. Kim M, Kang S, Lee S, et al. hypersensitivity reactions to oxaliplatin: clinical features and risk factors in Koreans. Asian Pac J Cancer Prev 2012;13(4):1209–15.

28. Jung JW, Kang HR, Lee SH, et al. The incidence and risk factors of infusion-related reactions to rituximab for treating B cell malignancies in a single tertiary hospital. Oncology 2014;86(3):127–34.

29. Levin AS, Otani IM, Lax T, et al. Reactions to Rituximab in an Outpatient Infusion Center: A 5-Year Review. J Allerg Clin Immunol Pract 2017;5(1):107–13.e1.

30. Welborn M, Kubicki SL, Garg N, et al. Retrospective chart review of cutaneous adverse events associated with tremelimumab in 17 patients. Am J Clin Dermatol 2018;19(6):899–905.

31. Shazib MA, Woo SB, Sroussi H, et al. Oral immune-related adverse events associated with PD-1 inhibitor therapy: A case series. Oral Dis 2020;26(2):325–33.

32. Keiser MF, Patel AB, Altan M. Cutaneous toxicities in lung cancer patients on immune checkpoint inhibitor therapy. Clin Lung Cancer 2021;22(3):195–200.e1.

33. Blumenthal KG, Lai KH, Huang M, et al. Adverse and hypersensitivity reactions to prescription nonsteroidal anti-inflammatory agents in a large health care system. J Allergy Clin Immunol Pract 2017;5(3):737–43.e3.

34. Li L, Chang Y, Song S, et al. Impact of reported NSAID "allergies" on opioid use disorder in back pain. J Allergy Clin Immunol 2021;147(4):1413–9.

35. Inglis JM, Caughey GE, Smith W, et al. Documentation of adverse drug reactions to opioids in an electronic health record. Intern Med J 2021;51(9):1490–6.

36. Dillman JR, Ellis JH, Cohan RH, et al. Frequency and severity of acute allergic-like reactions to gadolinium-containing i.v. contrast media in children and adults. AJR Am J Roentgenol 2007;189(6):1533–8.

37. Power S, Talbot N, Kucharczyk W, et al. Allergic-like reactions to the MR imaging contrast agent gadobutrol: a prospective study of 32 991 consecutive injections. Radiology 2016;281(1):72–7.

38. Young LK, Matthew SZ, Houston JG. Absence of potential gadolinium toxicity symptoms following 22,897 gadoteric acid (Dotarem®) examinations, including 3,209 performed on renally insufficient individuals. Eur Radiol 2019;29(4): 1922–30.

39. Lakshmanadoss U, Lindsley J, Glick D, et al. Incidence of amiodarone hypersensitivity in patients with previous allergy to iodine or iodinated contrast agents. Pharmacotherapy 2012;32(7):618–22.

40. Robison CD, Bair TL, Horne BD, et al. Hypothyroidism as a risk factor for statin intolerance. J Clin Lipidol 2014;8(4):401–7.

41. Paisansinsup T, Breitenstein MK, Schousboe JT. Association between adverse reactions to allopurinol and exposures to high maintenance doses: implications for management of patients using allopurinol. JRC: J Clin Rheumatol 2013;19(4): 180–6.

42. Hall GC, Davies PTG, Karim MY, et al. Observational safety study of specific outcomes after trivalent cell culture seasonal influenza vaccination (Optaflu(®)) among adults in THIN database of electronic UK primary healthcare records. Pharmacoepidemiol Drug Saf 2018;27(1):52–8.

43. Laird CM, Glode AE, Schwarz K, et al. Evaluation of fosaprepitant- associated hypersensitivity reactions at a National Cancer Center. J Oncol Pharm Pract 2020;26(6):1369–73.

44. Kidon MI, See Y. Adverse drug reactions in Singaporean children. Singapore Med J 2004;45(12):574–7.

45. Saager L, Turan A, Egan C, et al. Incidence of intraoperative hypersensitivity reactions: a registry analysis: a registry analysis. Anesthesiology 2015;122(3): 551–9.

46. Mendes D, Alves C, Loureiro M, et al. Drug-induced hypersensitivity: A 5-year retrospective study in a hospital electronic health records database. J Clin Pharm Ther 2019;44(1):54–61.

47. Goh SH, Soh JY, Loh W, et al. Cause and Clinical Presentation of Anaphylaxis in Singapore: From Infancy to Old Age. Int Arch Allergy Immunol 2018; 175(1–2):91–8.

48. Dhopeshwarkar N, Sheikh A, Doan R, et al. Drug-Induced Anaphylaxis Documented in Electronic Health Records. J Allergy Clin Immunol Pract 2019;7(1): 103–11.

49. Rangkakulnuwat P, Sutham K, Lao-Araya M. Anaphylaxis: ten-year retrospective study from a tertiary-care hospital in Asia. Asian Pac J Allergy Immunol 2020; 38(1):31–9.

50. Ou-Yang C, Agustianty S, Wang H-C. Developing a data mining approach to investigate association between physician prescription and patient outcome – A study on re- hospitalization in Stevens–Johnson Syndrome. Comput Methods Programs Biomed 2013;112(1):84–91.

51. Micheletti RG, Chiesa-Fuxench Z, Noe MH, et al. Stevens-Johnson syndrome/toxic epidermal necrolysis: a multicenter retrospective study of 377 adult patients from the United States. J Invest Dermatol 2018;138(11):2315–21.

52. Park HJ, Yun J, Kang DY, et al. Unique clinical characteristics and prognosis of allopurinol-induced severe cutaneous adverse reactions. J Allergy Clin Immunol Pract 2019;7(8):2739–49.e2733.

53. de Bustros P, Baldea A, Sanford A, et al. Review of culprit drugs associated with patients admitted to the burn unit with the diagnosis of Stevens- Johnson syndrome and toxic epidermal necrolysis syndrome. Burns 2021;S0305-4179(21) 00220-5.

54. Zhang C, Van DN, Hieu C, et al. Drug-induced severe cutaneous adverse reactions: Determine the cause and prevention. Ann Allergy Asthma Immunol 2019; 123(5):483–7.

55. Ma DH, Tsai TY, Pan LY, et al. Clinical Aspects of Stevens-Johnson syndrome/ toxic epidermal necrolysis with severe ocular complications in Taiwan. Front Med 2021;8:661891.

56. Banerji A, Blumenthal KG, Lai KH, et al. Epidemiology of ACE inhibitor angioedema utilizing a large electronic health Record. J Allergy Clin Immunol Pract 2017;5(3):744–9.

57. Read J, Keijzers GB. Pediatric Erythema Multiforme in the Emergency Department: More Than "Just a Rash. Pediatr Emerg Care 2017;33(5):320–4.

58. Blumenthal KG, Li Y, Acker WW, et al. Multiple drug intolerance syndrome and multiple drug allergy syndrome: Epidemiology and associations with anxiety and depression. Allergy 2018;73(10):2012–23.

59. Braswell DS, Hakeem A, Walker A, et al. Lichenoid granulomatous dermatitis revisited: A retrospective case series. J Am Acad Dermatol 2019;81(5):1157–64.

60. Leigh LY, Spergel JM. An in-depth characterization of a large cohort of adult patients with eosinophilic esophagitis. Ann Allergy Asthma Immunol 2019;122(1): 65–72.e61.

61. Silverman S, Localio R, Apter AJ. Association between chronic urticaria and self- reported penicillin allergy. Ann Allergy Asthma Immunol 2016;116(4): 317–20.

62. Lin SK, Mulieri KM, Ishmael FT. Characterization of Vancomycin Reactions and Linezolid Utilization in the Pediatric Population. J Allergy Clin Immunol Pract 2017;5(3):750–6.

63. Coleman E, Ko C, Dai F, et al. Inflammatory eruptions associated with immune checkpoint inhibitor therapy: a single-institution retrospective analysis with stratification of reactions by toxicity and implications for management. J Am Acad Dermatol 2019;80(4):990–7.

64. Jung H, Park S, Shin B, et al. Prevalence and clinical features of drug reactions with eosinophilia and systemic symptoms syndrome caused by antituberculosis drugs: a retrospective cohort study. ALLERGY Asthma Immunol Res 2019;11(1): 90–103.

65. Fukasawa T, Takahashi H, Takahashi K, et al. Risk of Stevens-Johnson syndrome and toxic epidermal necrolysis associated with anticonvulsants in a Japanese population: Matched case–control and cohort studies. Allergol Int 2021;70(3): 335–42.

66. Sim DW, You HS, Yu JE, et al. High occurrence of simultaneous multiple-drug hypersensitivity syndrome induced by first-line anti-tuberculosis drugs. World Allergy Organ J 2021;14(7):100562.

67. Hsu M-H, Yen J-C, Chiu W-T, et al. Using health smart cards to check drug allergy history: the perspective from Taiwan's experiences. J Med Syst 2011; 35(4):555–8.

68. Goldblatt C, Khumra S, Booth J, et al. Poor reporting and documentation in drug-associated Stevens-Johnson syndrome and toxic epidermal necrolysis - lessons for medication safety. Br J Clin Pharmacol 2017;83(2):224–6.

69. Foreman C, Smith WB, Caughey GE, et al. Categorization of adverse drug reactions in electronic health records. Pharmacol Res Perspect 2020;8(2):04.

70. Rukasin CRF, Henderlight S, Bosen T, et al. Implications of electronic health record transition on drug allergy labels. J Allergy Clin Immunol Pract 2020;8(2):764–6.

71. Blumenthal KG, Acker WW, Li Y, et al. Allergy entry and deletion in the electronic health record. Ann Allergy Asthma Immunol 2017;118(3):380–1.

72. Kiechle ES, McKenna CM, Carter H, et al. Medication allergy and adverse drug reaction documentation discrepancies in an Urban, Academic Emergency Department. J Med Toxicol 2018;14(4):272–7.

73. Lyons N, Rankin S, Sarangarm P, et al. Disparity in patients' self-reported and charted medication allergy information. [Comparative Study, Journal Article, Research Support, Non-U.S. Gov't]. Southampt Med J 2015;108(6):332–6.

74. Kabakov A, Rhodes NJ, Wenzel R. Discrepancies between patient self-reported and electronic health record documentation of medication allergies and adverse reactions in the acute care setting: room for improvement. J Pharm Technology 2019;35(4):139–45.

75. Reinhart K, Corbo T, Ewen E, et al. The impact of ethnicity and gender on agreement of severe allergy history between inpatient and outpatient electronic medical records. Pharm Pract (Granada) 2008;6(4):197–200.

76. De Clercq K, Cals JWL, de Bont EGPM. Inappropriate antibiotic allergy documentation in health records: a Qualitative Study on Family Physicians' and Pharmacists' Experiences. Ann Fam Med 2020;18(4):326–33.

77. Fernando B, Morrison Z, Kalra D, et al. Approaches to recording drug allergies in electronic health records: qualitative study. PLoS One 2014;9(4):e93047.

78. Moskow JM, Cook N, Champion-Lippmann C, et al. Identifying opportunities in EHR to improve the quality of antibiotic allergy data. J Am Med Inform Assoc 2016;23(e1).

79. Rimawi RH, Shah KB, Cook PP. Risk of redocumenting penicillin allergy in a cohort of patients with negative penicillin skin tests. J Hosp Med 2013;8(11):615–8.

80. Inglis JM, Caughey GE, Smith W, et al. Documentation of penicillin adverse drug reactions in electronic health records: inconsistent use of allergy and intolerance labels. Intern Med J 2017;47(11):1292–7.

81. Staicu ML, Plakosh M, Ramsey A. Prospective evaluation of electronic medical record penicillin allergy documentation at a tertiary community teaching hospital. Ann Allergy Asthma Immunol 2017;119(1):94–5.

82. Deng F, Li MD, Wong A, et al. Quality of documentation of contrast agent allergies in electronic health records. J Am Coll Radiol 2019;16(8):1027–35.

83. Ananthakrishnan L, Parrott DT, Mielke N, et al. Fidelity of electronic documentation for reactions prompting premedication to iodinated contrast media. J Am Coll Radiol 2021;18(7):982–9.

84. Burrell C, Tsourounis C, Quan D, et al. Impact of a pharmacist- driven protocol to improve drug allergy documentation at a University Hospital. Hosp Pharm 2013;48(4):302–7.

85. Lesselroth B, Adams K, Tallett S, et al. Usability evaluation of a medication reconciliation and allergy review (MRAR) Kiosk: a methodological approach for analyzing user interactions. Stud Health Technol Inform 2015;218:61–7.

86. Masaharu N, Ryusuke I. Implementation and effect of a novel electronic medical record format for patient allergy information..."building continents of knowledge in oceans of data: The Future of Co-Created eHealth," EFMI, Medical Informatics Europe (MIE), April 24-26th, 2018, Gothenburg, Sweden. Stud Health Technol Inform 2018;247:51–5.

87. Young AL, Marji J, Grossman ME. Drug hypersensitivity in the age of electronic medical records. J Drugs Dermatol 2011;10(12):1430–1.

88. Wright A, Rubins D, Shenoy ES, et al. Clinical decision support improved allergy documentation of antibiotic test dose results. J Allergy Clin Immunol Pract 2019; 7(8):2919–21.

89. Soyer J, Necsoiu D, Desjardins I, et al. Identification of discrepancies between adverse drug reactions coded by medical records technicians and those reported by the pharmacovigilance team in pediatrics: An intervention to improve identification, reporting, and coding. Arch de Pédiatrie. 2019;26(7):400–6.

90. Wang L, Blackley SV, Blumenthal KG, et al. A dynamic reaction picklist for improving allergy reaction documentation in the electronic health record. J Am Med Inform Assoc 2020;27(6):917–23.

91. Vethody C, Yu R, Keck JM, et al. Safety, efficacy, and effectiveness of delabeling in patients with multiple drug allergy labels. J Allergy Clin Immunol Pract 2021; 9(2):922–8.

92. Lachover-Roth I, Sharon S, Rosman Y, et al. Long-term follow-up after penicillin allergy delabeling in ambulatory patients. J Allergy Clin Immunol Pract 2019; 7(1):231–5.

93. Goss FR, Lai KH, Topaz M, et al. A value set for documenting adverse reactions in electronic health records. J Am Med Inform Assoc 2018;25(6):661–9.

94. Englert E, Weeks A. Pharmacist-driven penicillin skin testing service for adults prescribed nonpreferred antibiotics in a community hospital. Am J Health Syst Pharm 2019;76(24):2060–9.

95. Wang H, Kozman M, Pierce H, et al. A quality improvement initiative to improve primary care referral rates for penicillin allergy delabeling. Ann Allergy Asthma Immunol 2022;28(1):33–8.

96. Chen JR, Tarver SA, Alvarez KS, et al. A proactive approach to penicillin allergy testing in hospitalized patients. J Allergy Clin Immunol Pract 2017;5(3):686–93.

97. Sundquist BK, Bowen BJ, Otabor U, et al. Proactive penicillin allergy testing in primary care patients labeled as allergic: outcomes and barriers. Postgrad Med 2017;129(8):915–20.

98. Lin L, Nagtegaal JE, Buijtels PCAM, et al. Antimicrobial stewardship intervention: optimizing antibiotic treatment in hospitalized patients with reported antibiotic allergy. J Hosp Infect 2020;104(2):137–43.

99. Blumenthal KG, Li Y, Hsu JT, et al. Outcomes from an inpatient beta-lactam allergy guideline across a large US health system. [Journal Article, Research Support, N.I.H., Extramural, Research Support, Non-U.S. Gov't]. Infect Control Hosp Epidemiol 2019;40(5):528–35.

100. Wolfson AR, Mancini CM, Banerji A, et al. Penicillin allergy assessment in pregnancy: safety and impact on antibiotic use. J Allergy Clin Immunol Pract 2021; 9(3):1338–46.

101. Kwon JW, Kim YJ, Yang MS, et al. Results of intradermal skin testing with cefazolin according to a history of hypersensitivity to antibiotics. J Korean Med Sci 2019;34(50):30.

102. Iammatteo M, Ferastraoaru D, Koransky R, et al. Identifying allergic drug reactions through placebo-controlled graded challenges. The Journal of Allergy and Clinical Immunology Practice 2017;5(3):711–7.e2.

103. McDanel DL, Azar AE, Dowden AM, et al. Screening for beta-lactam allergy in joint arthroplasty patients to improve surgical prophylaxis practice. Proceedings of the 26th Annual Meeting of AAHKS, November 10 – 13, 2016: Dallas, Texas. 2017;32(9, Supplement):S101-S108.

104. Kuder MM, Lennox MG, Li M, et al. Skin testing and oral amoxicillin challenge in the outpatient allergy and clinical immunology clinic in pregnant women with penicillin allergy. Ann Allergy Asthma Immunol 2020;125(6):646–51.

105. Kuruvilla M, Sexton M, Wiley Z, et al. A streamlined approach to optimize perioperative antibiotic prophylaxis in the setting of penicillin allergy labels. J Allergy Clin Immunol Pract 2020;8(4):1316–22.

106. Blumenthal KG, Wickner PG, Hurwitz S, et al. Tackling inpatient penicillin allergies: Assessing tools for antimicrobial stewardship. J Allergy Clin Immunol 2017;140(1):154–61.e156.

107. Sigona NS, Steele JM, Miller CD. Impact of a pharmacist-driven beta-lactam allergy interview on inpatient antimicrobial therapy: a pilot project. J Am Pharm Assoc 2016;56(6):665–9.

108. Ramsey A, Staicu ML. Use of a penicillin allergy screening algorithm and penicillin skin testing for transitioning hospitalized patients to first-line antibiotic therapy. J Allergy Clin Immunol Pract 2018;6(4):1349–55.

109. Shaw BG, Masic I, Gorgi N, et al. Appropriateness of beta-lactam allergy record updates after an allergy service consult. J Pharm Pract 2020;33(3):243–6.

110. Abrams EM, Wakeman A, Gerstner TV, et al. Prevalence of beta-lactam allergy: a retrospective chart review of drug allergy assessment in a predominantly pediatric population. Allergy Asthma And Clin Immunol 2016;12:59.

111. Pandya A, Gregory E, Cherian S, et al. Implementation of EMR-based standardized antibiotic desensitization protocols and its impact on providers. Allergy And Asthma Proceedings 2021;42(2):160–6.

112. Mancini CM, Wimmer M, Schulz LT, et al. Association of penicillin or cephalosporin allergy documentation and antibiotic use in hospitalized patients with pneumonia. J Allergy Clin Immunol Pract 2021;9(8):3060–8.e3061.

113. Wu H-L. Retrospective evaluation of a rechallenge protocol in patients experiencing hypersensitivity reactions with prior chemotherapy in a tertiary hospital. J Oncol Pharm Pract 2019;25(6):1388–95.

114. Picard M, Pur L, Caiado J, et al. Risk stratification and skin testing to guide reexposure in taxane-induced hypersensitivity reactions. J Allergy Clin Immunol 2016;137(4):1154–64.e2.

115. Murray TS, Rice TW, Wheeler AP, et al. Medication desensitization: characterization of outcomes and risk factors for reactions. Ann Pharmacother 2016;50(3):203–8.

116. González-Gregori R, Dolores Hernández Fernandez De Rojas M, López-Salgueiro R, et al. Allergy alerts in electronic health records for hospitalized patients. Ann Allergy Asthma Immunol 2012;109(2):137–40.

117. Topaz M, Seger DL, Slight SP, et al. Rising drug allergy alert overrides in electronic health records: an observational retrospective study of a decade of experience. J Am Med Inform Assoc 2016;23(3):601–8.

118. Ariosto D. Factors Contributing to CPOE Opiate Allergy Alert Overrides. AMIA Annu Symp Proc 2014;2014:256–65.

119. Bryant AD, Fletcher GS, Payne TH. Drug interaction alert override rates in the Meaningful Use era: no evidence of progress. Appl Clin Inform 2014;5(3): 802–13.

120. Wong A, Seger D, Slight S, et al. Evaluation of 'definite' anaphylaxis drug allergy alert overrides in inpatient and outpatient settings. Drug Saf 2018;41(3): 297–302.

121. Cho I, Lee J, Choi S, et al. Acceptability and feasibility of the Leapfrog computerized physician order entry evaluation tool for hospitals outside the United States. Int J Med Inform 2015;84(9):694–701.

122. Bae YJ, Hwang YW, Yoon SY, et al. The Effectiveness of automatic recommending system for premedication in reducing recurrent radiocontrast media hypersensitivity reactions. PLoS One 2013;8(6):e66014.

123. Benson JC, McKinney AM, Hines P, et al. Use of Clinical Decision Support to Increase Premedication Regimen Homogeneity. J Am Coll Radiol 2017;14(4): 509–16.

124. Dolin RH, Boxwala A, Shalaby J. A Pharmacogenomics clinical decision support service based on FHIR and CDS Hooks. Methods Inf Med 2018;57(S 02): e115–23.

125. Macy E, McCormick TA, Adams JL, et al. Association between removal of a warning against cephalosporin use in patients with penicillin allergy and antibiotic prescribing. JAMA Netw Open 2021;4(4):e218367.

126. Buffone B, Lin Y-C, Grant J. β-lactam exposure outcome among patients with a documented allergy to penicillins post-implementation of a new electronic medical record system and alerting rules. JAMMI: J Assoc Med Microbiol Infect Dis Can 2021;6(2):104–13.

127. Lin C, Payne TH, Nichol WP, et al. Evaluating clinical decision support systems: monitoring CPOE order check override rates in the Department of Veterans Affairs' Computerized Patient Record System. J Am Med Inform Assoc 2008;15(5): 620–6.

128. Weingart SN, Massagli M, Cyrulik A, et al. Assessing the value of electronic prescribing in ambulatory care: A focus group study. Int J Med Inform 2009;78(9): 571–8.

129. Carspecken CW, Sharek PJ, Longhurst C, et al. A clinical case of electronic health record drug alert fatigue: consequences for patient outcome. Pediatrics 2013;131(6):e1970–3.

130. Wong A, Wright A, Seger DL, et al. Comparison of Overridden Medication-related Clinical Decision Support in the Intensive Care Unit between a Commercial System and a Legacy System. Appl Clin Inform 2017;8(3):866–79.

131. Wong A, Amato MG, Seger DL, et al. Prospective evaluation of medication-related clinical decision support over-rides in the intensive care unit. BMJ Qual Saf 2018;27(9):718–24.

132. Genco EK, Forster JE, Flaten H, et al. Clinically inconsequential alerts: the characteristics of opioid drug alerts and their utility in preventing adverse drug events in the Emergency Department. Ann Emerg Med 2016;67(2):240–8.e3.

133. Garabedian PM, Wright A, Newbury I, et al. Comparison of a prototype for indications- based prescribing with 2 commercial prescribing systems. JAMA Netw Open 2019;2(3):e191514.

134. Wolfson AR, Zhou L, Li Y, et al. Drug reaction with eosinophilia and systemic symptoms (DRESS) syndrome identified in the electronic health record allergy module. J Allergy Clin Immunol Pract 2019;7(2):633–40.

135. DeLozier S, Speltz P, Brito J, et al. Real-time clinical note monitoring to detect conditions for rapid follow-up: A case study of clinical trial enrollment in drug-induced torsades de pointes and Stevens-Johnson syndrome. J Am Med Inform Assoc 2021;28(1):126–31.

136. Epstein RH, St Jacques P, Stockin M, et al. Automated identification of drug and food allergies entered using non-standard terminology. J Am Med Inform Assoc 2013;20(5):962–8.

137. Davis RL, Gallagher MA, Asgari MM, et al. Identification of Stevens-Johnson syndrome and toxic epidermal necrolysis in electronic health record databases. Pharmacoepidemiol Drug Saf 2015;24(7):684–92.

138. Saff RR, Li Y, Santhanakrishnan N, et al. Identification of inpatient allergic drug reactions using ICD-9-CM Codes. J Allergy Clin Immunol Pract 2019;7(1):259–64.e251.

139. Banerji A, Lai KH, Li Y, et al. Natural language processing combined with ICD-9-CM codes as a novel method to study the epidemiology of allergic drug reactions. J Allergy Clin Immunol Pract 2020;8(3):1032–8.e1031.

140. Cahill KN, Johns CB, Cui J, et al. Automated identification of an aspirin-exacerbated respiratory disease cohort. J Allergy Clin Immunol 2017;139(3):819–25.e816.

141. Fukasawa T, Takahashi H, Kameyama N, et al. Development of an electronic medical record-based algorithm to identify patients with Stevens-Johnson syndrome and toxic epidermal necrolysis in Japan. PLoS One 2019;14(8):e0221130.

142. Kim M-H, Park C-H, Kim D-I, et al. Surveillance of contrast-media-induced hypersensitivity reactions using signals from an electronic medical recording system. Ann Allergy Asthma Immunol 2012;108(3):167–71.

143. Nelson SJ, Zeng K, Kilbourne J, et al. Normalized names for clinical drugs: RxNorm at 6 years. J Am Med Inform Assoc 2011;18(4):441–8.

144. Zheng NS, Stone CA, Jiang L, et al. High-throughput framework for genetic analyses of adverse drug reactions using electronic health records. PLoS Genet 2021;17(6):e1009593.

145. Konvinse KC, Trubiano JA, Pavlos R, et al. HLA-A*32:01 is strongly associated with vancomycin-induced drug reaction with eosinophilia and systemic symptoms. J Allergy Clin Immunol 2019;144(1):183–92.

146. Krebs K, Bovijn J, Zheng N, et al. Genome-wide Study Identifies Association between HLA-B*55:01 and self-reported penicillin allergy. Am J Hum Genet 2020;107(4):612–21.

Moving?

Make sure your subscription moves with you!

To notify us of your new address, find your **Clinics Account Number** (located on your mailing label above your name), and contact customer service at:

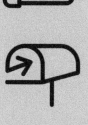

Email: journalscustomerservice-usa@elsevier.com

800-654-2452 (subscribers in the U.S. & Canada)
314-447-8871 (subscribers outside of the U.S. & Canada)

Fax number: 314-447-8029

Elsevier Health Sciences Division
Subscription Customer Service
3251 Riverport Lane
Maryland Heights, MO 63043

*To ensure uninterrupted delivery of your subscription, please notify us at least 4 weeks in advance of move.

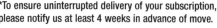

Printed and bound by CPI Group (UK) Ltd, Croydon, CR0 4YY

03/10/2024

01040474-0012